Essentials of
Physical Pharmacy

Second Edition

Essentials of Physical Pharmacy

Second Edition

Derle Deeliprao V.

(Ph.D.)

MVP's College of Pharmacy, Nasik,
Director,4
All India council for Technical Education,
New Delhi. 110 001

Sai Hanuman Sagar Boddu

(Ph.D.)

School of Pharmacy
University of Missouri-Kansas City
5211 Health Sciences Building
2464 Charlotte Street
Kansas City, MO 64108-2718

Pharma Med PRESS
An Imprint of Pharma Book Syndicate

PharmaMed Press
An imprint of Pharma Book Syndicate

A unit of BSP Books Pvt., Ltd.

4-4-309/316, Giriraj Lane,
Sultan Bazar, Hyderabad - 500 095.

Published by

PharmaMed Press

An imprint of Pharma Book Syndicate

A unit of BSP Books Pvt. Ltd.

4-4-309/316, Giriraj Lane, Sultan Bazar, Hyderabad - 500 095.

Phone: 040-23445605, 23445688; Fax: 91+40-23445611

e-mail: info@pharmamedpress.com

ISBN : 978-93-52300-52-5 (HB)

Dedicated to

Our Parents

Preface to Second Edition

Pharmacy profession is pursued equally by students from biological and mathematical background. Like other fields, students entering the pharmacy profession need to understand certain basic principles in the field of pharmacy. The subject of Physical Pharmacy deals with the application of fundamental physicochemical principles in order to overcome the problems related to the development and characterization of various dosage forms. Most of the pharmacy professionals entering the pharmaceutical industries often lack these fundamentals in physical pharmacy. This book is designed to acts a quick reference on various topics of physical pharmacy.

This book is derived from the first edition of our textbook "Essentials of Physical Pharmacy", published by Pharma Book Syndicate, in the year 2006. Our first edition consisted of fifteen chapters and was a huge success. This gave us the momentum to elaborate the book with inclusion of more chapters. Our teaching experience in pharmaceutics and physical pharmacy over many years, guided us in designing the chapters and their contents.

It is my pleasure to acknowledge the tireless efforts of many scientists who contributed for the development of subject. We thanks to M/S. PharmaMed Press who are responsible for the publication of the book. We hope that the contents in this book will help graduate students in all pharmacy colleges throughout the country. Finally, we would like to thank all our readers who inspired us and made us to come out with the second edition of ***"Essentials of Physical Pharmacy"***.

- Authors

Preface to First Edition

Physical Pharmacy is one of the important subjects for a pharmacy student. The purpose of introducing this subject in the first or second year graduate curriculum is to make the students thoroughly acquainted with the fundamental concepts, which helps them in successive years. However, the purpose is not served due to complexities in understanding the subject from the other textbooks existing in the market.

This book ***Essentials of Physical Pharmacy*** is mainly designed to remove the phobia from the minds of students towards physical pharmacy. The author's experience in the subject has shown them that it is often difficult for the students to understand an oversimplified presentation than the one that is rigorous enough to engender some insight into the relevance of material. This was the primary objective in designing the contents of the book.

The unique feature of this book is the presentation of fundamental concepts in a lucid, disentangled and self-explanatory form. This book consists of 15 chapters. Each chapter includes discussion of important experiments and investigations followed by a set of problems. This approach helps the students to evaluate themselves. In order to avoid imposing the students to memorize isolated definitions, a glossary is included.

It is my pleasure to acknowledge the tireless efforts of many scientists who contributed for the development of subject. I would specially place on record the help rendered by Mr. Sagar S.H. Boddu while writing this book. I also thank M/s. Pharma Book Syndicate who are responsible for the publication of the book.

- Author

Greek Alphabets

Alpha	Α	α
Beta	Β	β
Delta	Δ	δ
Gamma	Γ	γ
Epsilon	Ε	ε
Eta	Η	η
Theta	Θ	θ
Iota	Ι	ι
Kappa	Κ	κ
Lambda	Λ	λ
Mu	Μ	μ
Nu	Ν	ν
Pi	Π	π
Sigma	Σ	σ
Tau	Τ	τ
Psi	Ψ	ψ
Omega	Ω	ω
Zeta	Ζ	ζ
Rho	Ρ	ρ
Chi	Χ	χ
Phi	Φ	ϕ
Upsilon	ϒ	υ
Omicron	Ο	ο
Xi	Ξ	ξ

Contents

CHAPTER 1

States of Matter

Generally matter can be categorized into gases, liquids and solids. A gaseous state is characterized by its nature to occupy the complete available space and changes in volume with respect to the temperature and pressure. Liquids on the otherhand take the shape of the container in which it is placed. Solids differ markedly from gases and liquids as they have definite shape and the changes in volume with the variation in temperature and pressure is very small. Solids have fixed spatial intermolecular relationships.

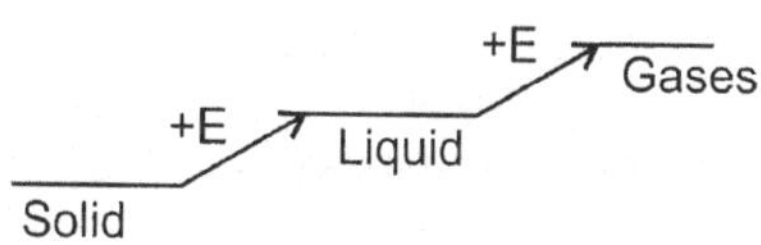

Apart from the above mentioned categories some molecules exhibit a fourth phase termed as mesophase (Greek, meso, middle) which falls between liquid and crystalline states. This phase is also termed as liquid crystalline state. Each of these states is also known as phase. Generally, as the temperature rises, matter moves to a more active state. Things only move from one phase to another by physical means. If energy is added (like increasing temperature or increasing pressure) or if energy is taken away (like freezing or decreasing pressure) one can observe a physical change. Recently, a fourth state of matter known as plasma has been introduced. Plasma state consists of a highly ionized gas that usually occurs at high temperature. Ionic attractions and repulsions that exist between the molecules give these compositions distinct properties.

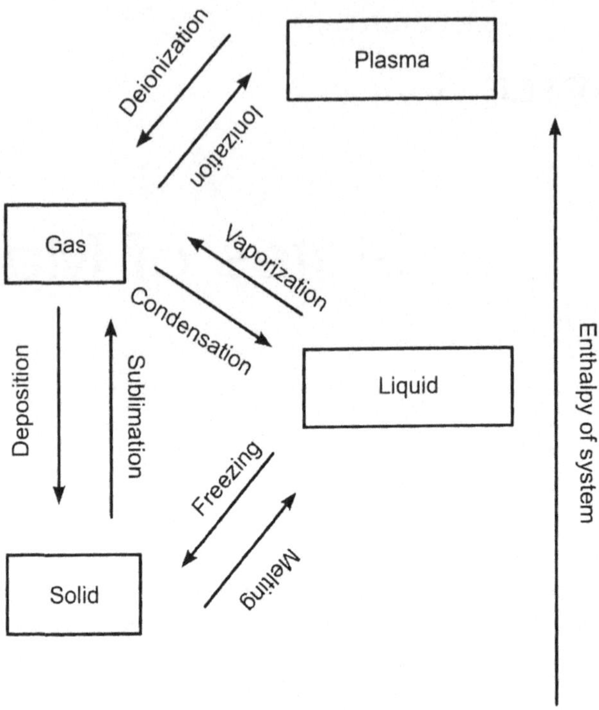

Summary of properties of the states of matter

Solids	Liquids	Gases
very high intermolecular forces	weak intermolecular forces	negligible intermolecular forces
vibration of the consisting molecules about fixed (equilibrium) positions	molecules can slide past one another but they cannot break	random (or) free motion
small interparticle distances	small empty spaces	large empty spaces
high density	medium density	low density
no (or) less compressibility	medium compressible	high compressibility
definite shape	takes shape of container	no shape
definite volume	definite volume	no definite volume

Binding Forces Between Molecules

A knowledge of binding forces existing between the molecules helps in better understanding about the states of matter, viz., gases, liquids and solids. From pharmaceutical point of view these forces play a very important role in studying the interfacial phenomena, stabilization of emulsions, flocculation of suspensions, flow properties of powders/granules etc.

(a) Repulsive and Attractive Forces

Whenever two molecules are brought together, the like charges present on them account for the repulsive forces between the molecules which prevents them from interpenetration. Similarly the opposite charges will account for attractive forces. The repulsive force increases exponentially with decrease in distance between the molecules. At a particular distance an equilibrium is established between the two forces and at this point the repulsive force becomes equal to attractive force. At this position the potential energy of system is minimum.

Van der Waals Forces : It is a combination of Keesom forces, Debye's forces and London attractions.

(i) ***Dipole-Dipole (or) Keesom Forces :*** These are the weak attractive forces which operates when large number of dipolar molecules are brought together.

$$\overset{\delta+}{H} \text{---} \overset{\delta-}{Cl} \text{ - - - - } \overset{\delta+}{H} \text{---} \overset{\delta-}{Cl}$$

(ii) ***Dipole-Induced dipole (or) Debye Forces :*** Induced dipoles are formed when a nonpolar molecule is kept close to permanent dipole. These interactions are also called Debye's interactions.

(iii) ***Induced dipole-Induced dipole (or) London attractions :*** These attractions come into play when nonpolar molecules induce polarity into other molecules.

(b) Ion-Dipole and Ion-Induced Dipole Forces

These forces account for the solubility of ionic crystalline substances in water. These forces act between polar (or) nonpolar molecules and ions

$$I_2 + K^+ I^- \rightarrow K^+ I_3^-$$

The above reaction accounts for the solubility of iodine in potassium iodide solution. In dipolar molecules cations have attraction towards oxygen atoms of water molecules and anions have attraction towards hydrogen atoms. These forces play a very important role in solubilizing dipolar molecules.

Hydrogen Bond

This type of bond exists between the molecules containing hydrogen atom and a strongly electronegative atoms like nitrogen, oxygen, fluorine, bromine etc. The small hydrogen atom has positive charge which accounts for the bond formation. Some examples of the molecules that form hydrogen bonds are given below :

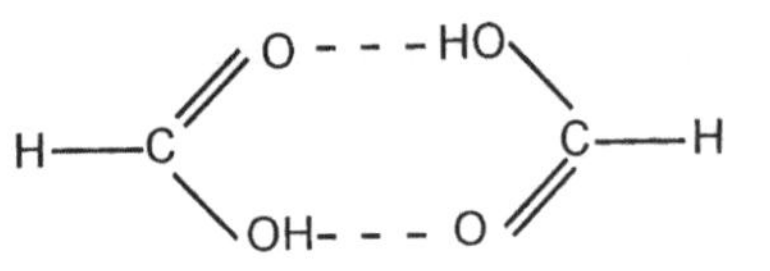

Dimers of formic acid

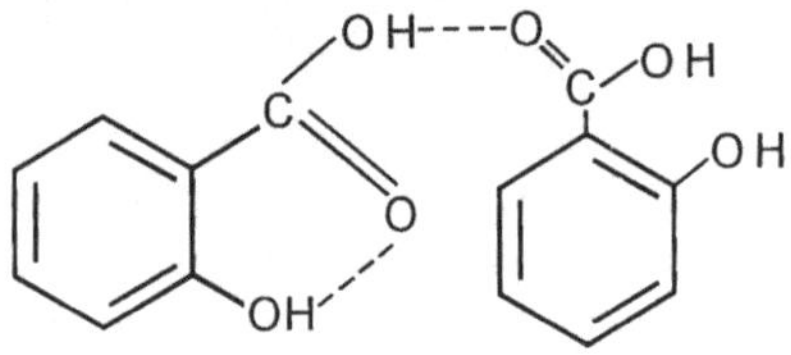

Inter and Intra molecular bonding of salicylic acid.

Relative approximate strength of bonds

Bond type	Relative strength
Ionic bonds	1000
Hydrogen bonds	100
Dipole-dipole	10
London (*Van der Waals*) Forces	1

A sample of gas is always defined by the parameters like pressure, volume, temperature and number of moles.

Pressure : It is the force exerted by gas molecules on unit area of container walls

Units = atmosphere or mm Hg or pascals

1 atm = 760 mm Hg = 1.013×10^5 pa.

Volume : It is always taken as the volume of the container.

Units = mL or Litres or Cubic centimeters

Temperature : It is generally measured in kelvins or absolute degree.

$$\text{Kelvin} = (\text{K}) = {}^{o}\text{C} + 273$$

1. ***Boyle's Law***

Robert Boyle in the year 1660 found that any gas at constant temperature and mass has volume that is inversely proportional to pressure.

Mathematically,

$$V \alpha\ 1/P \text{ or } PV = K = \text{constant.}$$

or $$P_1V_1 = P_2V_2. \qquad [T, n \text{ are constants}]$$

2. ***Charle's Law***

Charle's in the year 1787 found that at constant pressure, the volume of fixed mass of gas is directly proportional to its absolute temperature.

Mathematically, $V \alpha\ T$ or $V/T = K$ [P is constant]

or $$\frac{V_1}{T_1} = \frac{V_2}{T_2}$$

3. ***Combined Gas Law***

According to this volume of a given sample of gas is directly proportional to absolute temperature and inversely proportional to pressure.

Mathematically,

$$V \alpha \frac{T}{P} \text{ or } \frac{PV}{T} = K \qquad [n \text{ is constant}]$$

or $$\frac{P_1\ V_1}{T_1} = \frac{P_2\ V_2}{T_2}$$

4. ***Gay Lussac's Law***

Joseph Gay Lussac observed that at constant volume, the pressure exerted by a fixed mass of gas is directly proportional to the absolute temperature.

Mathematically,

$$P\ \alpha\ T \text{ (or) } P = K\ T \qquad [V, n \text{ are constants}]$$

or $$\frac{P_1}{T_1} = \frac{P_2}{T_2}$$

5. *Avagadro's Law*

According to Avagadro, keeping the temperature and pressure constant, the volume of gas is directly proportional to amount of gas in moles.

Mathematically,

$$V \alpha n \text{ or } \frac{V_1}{n_1} = \frac{V_2}{n_2} \quad \text{[P, T are constants]}$$

6. Graham's law states that the rate at which gas molecules diffuse is inversely proportional to the square root of its density. Combining Graham's law with Avogadro's law we obtain the following equation.

$$\frac{Rate_1}{Rate_2} = \sqrt{\frac{M_2}{M_1}}$$

where:

$Rate_1$: rate of diffusion of the first gas

$Rate_2$: rate of diffusion for the second gas.

M_1 : molar mass of first gas

M_2 : molar mass of second gas

7. Dalton's law of partial pressures states that the pressure of a mixture of gases simply is the sum of the partial pressures of the individual components. Dalton's Law is as follows:

$$P_{total} = P_1 + P_2 + P_3 + ... + P_n,$$

where:

P_{Total} : total pressure of the gas

P_n : partial pressure of individual components.

8. Henry's law states that at constant temperature, the amount of a given gas dissolved in a given type and volume of liquid is directly proportional to the partial pressure of that gas in equilibrium with that liquid.

$$p = k_H C$$

Ideal-gas equation

According to the combined gas law's, the equation as discussed earlier.

$$\frac{P_1 V_1}{T_1} = \frac{P_2 V_2}{T_2}$$

or $$\frac{PV}{T} = \text{Constant}$$

So we can write it as $$\frac{PV}{T} = R$$

Considering R as a constant and number of moles of a gas is equal to 1. For n moles of gas the equation can be written as

$$PV = nRT. \quad \text{(Ideal - gas equation)}$$

R is called as Molar gas constant = 8.314×10^7 erg/Mol.deg. or 1.987 cal/Mol.deg. or 0.08205 lit.atm/Mol.deg.

Molecular Weight Determination

Using the ideal - gas equation we can find the approximate molecular weight value of any gas. The number of moles are replaced by g/M (where g is number of grams of gas sample and M is molecular weight of gas). So the equation can be written as

$$P\,V = \frac{g}{M}\,RT \text{ or } M = gRT/PV.$$

Van der Waals Equation for Real Gases

Real gases do not follow the ideal - gas equation. They are composed of finite volume of particles that tend to attract one another. So ideal gas equation is slightly modified in consideration to real gases.

Modified Equation

$$\left(P + \frac{a}{V^2}\right)(V - b) = RT \quad \text{[for 1 mole of gas]}$$

for n moles of gas

$$\left(P + \frac{an^2}{V^2}\right)(V - nb) = nRT$$

Where a/V^2 accounts for pressure correction and b corresponds to volume correction.

(i) Pressure Correction

Lets consider a molecule X randomly from a gas sample. It has got forces that act equally from all sides and so the net force acting is zero. Now consider another molecule Y from the gas sample which is about to hit the wall of container. This experiences a net inward pull and hence strikes the wall with a reduced velocity. Hence final pressure is

$$P = P_{ideal} - P_a$$

where, P_a the pressure correction factor is directly proportional to concentration of X type of molecules and concentration of Y type molecules.

In other words, the force exerted on a single molecule of Y is proportional to number of molecules in the bulk of gas, and consequently to its density (ρ). Further number of molecules striking the wall of any instant is also directly proportional to ρ. So P_a is proportional to ρ^2.

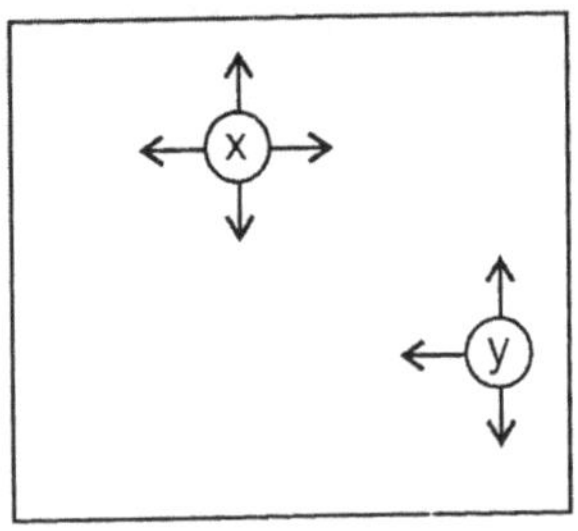

But $$\rho \propto \frac{n}{V}$$

So $$P_a \propto \frac{n}{V} \times \frac{n}{V}$$

or $$P_a = \frac{a\,n^2}{V^2}$$

where a = Proportionality constant

(ii) Volume Correction

According to ideal gas law the volume of gas is equal to volume of container. But ideal gas law did not take into consideration the volume occupied by the gas molecules. The volume correction term or the excluded volume (nb) must be substracted from V.

The final volume for a real gas is considered to be

$$V - nb$$

Generally excluded volume is four times the actual volume of molecules.

So, finally the Van der Waal's equation is

$$\left(P + \frac{an^2}{V^2}\right)(V - nb) = nRT.$$

$$\text{Units of} \quad a = \frac{\text{atm. liter}^2}{\text{Mol}^2}.$$

$$b = \text{Liter. Mol}^{-1}$$

Critical Phenomenon

Andres, in 1869 studied the liquefaction of gases by varying pressure and temperature. Any gas can be converted into liquid either by increasing pressure or decreasing temperature. Andres established that all gas molecules below critical temperature (T_c) can be liquified by increasing pressure. Critical temperature can also be defined as the temperature above which gas can not be in liquid state.

Critical Pressure (P_c) : It is the minimum pressure required to liquefy the gas at its critical temperature.

Critical Volume (V_c) : It is the volume occupied by a mole of gas at critical temperature and critical pressure.

Critical Phenomena : At critical temperature and critical pressure, any gas behaves similar to its liquid and is said to be in critical state. This phenomena is called Critical Phenomena.

Liquefaction of Gases

An discussed earlier any gas can be liquefied by increasing pressure or by decreasing temperature. The temperature above which liquefaction of gas does not take place is known as critical temperature. When a gas is cooled, it loses some of its kinetic energy in the form of heat and velocity of the molecules decreases. If pressure is applied to the gas the molecules are brought within the sphere of Van der Waals interaction forces and thus pass in to liquid state.

Methods of Liquefaction of Gas

Generally three techniques are used in liquefaction of gases :

1. ***Faraday's Method***

   This method is used to liquefy gases whose critical temperature is above (or) just below atmospheric temperature.

Faraday succeeded in liquifying a number of gases such as SO_2, CO_2, NO and Cl_2 by this method. The apparatus used consists of V - shaped tube, with one of its arm engaged in heating the reactants. The other arm is dipped in ice-mixture as shown in Fig. 1.1. It involves cooling of gases by using freezing mixture.

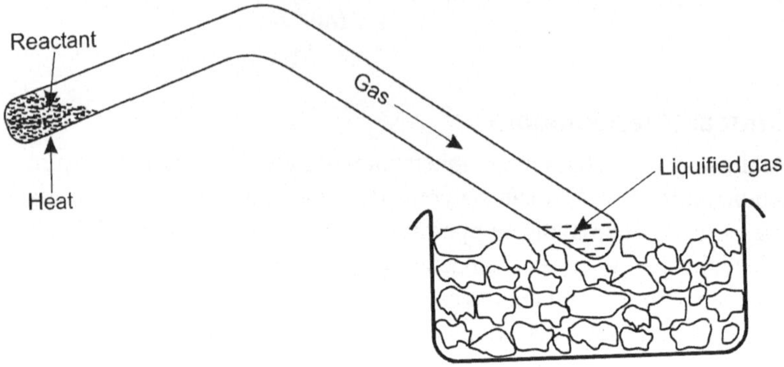

Fig. 1.1 Faraday's method for liquefaction of gas.

2. ***Linde's Method***

According to this method the gas is compressed to 200 atm, which is then allowed to pass through a pipe cooled by liquid ammonia as shown in Fig. 1.2.

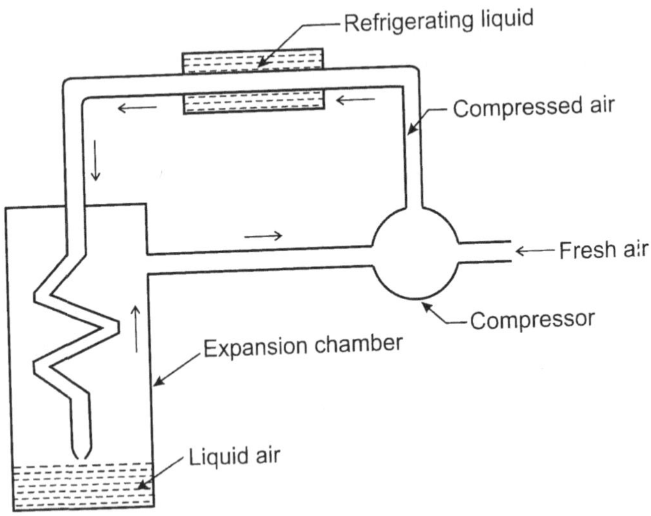

Fig. 1.2 Linde's Method for liquefaction of air.

The other end of the pipe has a narrow opening. The free expansion of gas through the narrow opening results in considerable drop of temperature and thereby liquefaction of gas. The main principle involved in this is Joule-Thomson effect, i.e, compressed gas is allowed to expand into region of low vapour pressure, which results in intense cooling of gas. The molecules in a compressed gas are very close and have appreciable forces of attraction. When the gas is allowed to expand through the area of low vapour pressure considerable amount of energy is utilized by the gas in overcoming the forces of attraction. This results in cooling of gas molecules and there by liquefaction of gas.

3. ***Claude's Method***

This method is quite similar to Linde's Method except for the cylinder and piston attachment. The compressed gas (200 atm) is allowed to pass through refrigerating liquid, which then enters the expansion chamber. Here, the gas is allowed to expand freely through narrow opening which results in cooling of gas. A part of gas also enters cylinder and pushes the piston in outward direction as shown in Fig. 1.3.

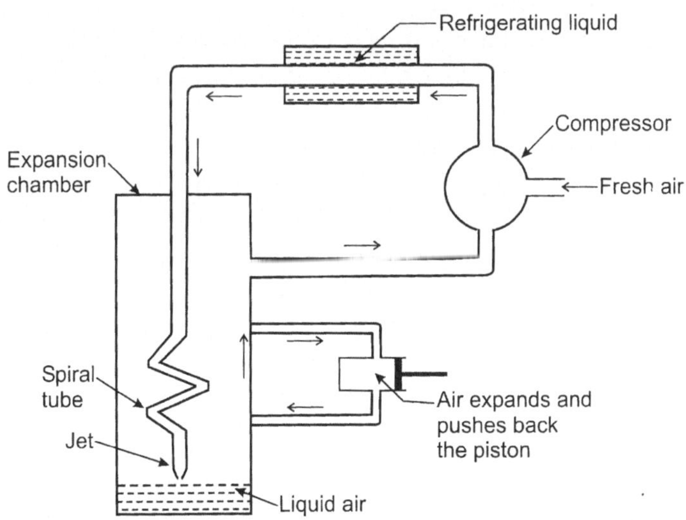

Fig. 1.3 Claude's method for liquefaction of air.

Thus a part of energy is utilized by the gas in doing mechanical work. This gas them enters the expansion chamber and cools the incoming gas.

Applications of Liquefaction to Aerosols

Aerosols is a broad term which encompasses body sprays, deodorants, perfumes and certain pharmaceutical drugs that are packaged in pressurised systems. It can defined as a system that depends on the power of compressed or liquified gas to expel the contents from the container. Various drugs which are suitable for this type of packing include local anesthetics, ergotamines, steroids, antiseptics etc. In aerosol systems the drug product is either dissolved or suspended in propellant (gas which is liquified under pressure).

By pressing the valve excess pressure is created inside the container, that expels the contents. As soon as the contents are exposed to atmospheric pressure, they are get evaporated and forms a fine spray. The pressure inside an aerosol container varies from 1-6 atm, that can be achieved by varying the proportions of propellants. Various propellants used in the manufacture of aerosols include Hydrocarbons (Propane, Butane etc.), Chlorofluorocarbon, Nitrogen, Nitrous Oxide etc.

The advantages of aerosol include :

1. Direct delivery of medicament to the affected area, such as spray, stream or stable foam.
2. Removal of contents without contamination.
3. Stability of the drug substance can be enhanced as they do not come in contact with moisture and oxygen.
4. Mechanical application can be avoided.

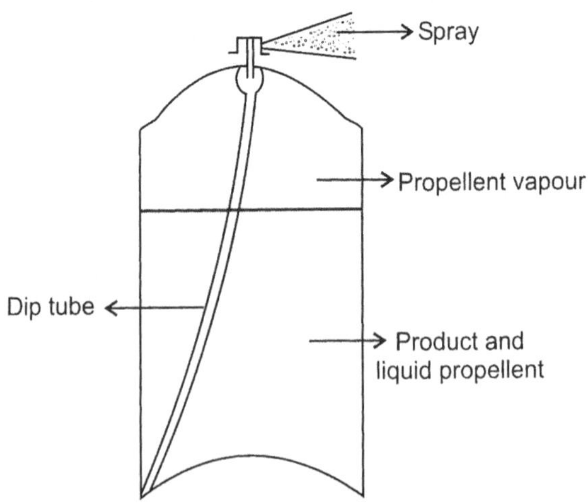

Fig. 1.4 Diagram of aerosol container.

Problems

1. Calculate the volume of gas at 0 °C and at 760 mm Hg. The gas occupies the volume of 30 ml at a temperature of 20 °C and pressure of 740 mm of Hg.

   Solution : Date given

   Volume occupied by gas = 30 ml = V_1

   Temperature = 20 °C = 273 + 20 = 293 °K

   Pressure = 740 mm Hg = P_1

   Equation for Volume

$$\frac{P_1 V_1}{T_1} = \frac{P_2 V_2}{T_2}$$

$$\frac{740 \times 30}{(273 + 20)} = \frac{760 \times V_2}{273}$$

$$V_2 = 27.2 \text{ ml}$$

2. Calculate the molecular weight of given liquid if 0.32 gm of liquid in vapour state occupies 300 ml at a pressure of 1 atm and temperature of 100 °C.

   Solution : Data given

   Weight of gas = 0.32 gm

   Temperature = 273 + 100 = 373 °K.

   Pressure = 1 atm

   Volume = 0.25 liters

   Equation for molecular weight

$$M = \frac{0.32 \times 0.082 \times 373}{1 \times 0.25} = 39.15 \text{ g/mole}$$

3. Calculate the root mean square velocity of given gas at 25 °C, having molecular weight 32.

   Temperature = 25 °C = 298 °K

   Molecular weight = 32

Equation for root mean square velocity = $\mu = \sqrt{\frac{3RT}{M}}$

$$= \sqrt{\frac{3 \times 8.314 \times 10^{7} \times 298}{32}}$$

$$= 4.82 \times 10^{4} \text{ cm/sec.}$$

CHAPTER 2

Physical Properties of Drug Molecules

The development of a formulation for any drug molecule is a tedious process. It needs to understand the various physical properties of drug molecules for developing a successful formulation.

These properties may be of three types :

(a) ***Additive Properties :*** These involve the simple addition of the properties of individual molecules.

For example if we consider the molecular weight of Methane (CH_4).

It involves the addition of individual molecular weight of each atom i.e., $4 \times$ mol.wt of H $+ 1 \times$ mol.wt of C.

(b) ***Constitutive Properties :*** These properties depends on the structural arrangement of atoms within the molecule.

E.g., : Spectrophotometry of compounds, optical rotation etc.

(c) ***Additive-Constitutive Properties :*** Some properties of the compounds depend both on number of individual atoms and the nature of attachment.

Ex : The Molar refraction of two compounds $H_3C - O - CH_3$ and C_2H_5OH having same molecular weight differs due to the variation in the nature of C – O linkage in two compounds.

Colligative properties depends mainly on the number of particles in a solution.

E.g., : Depression in freezing point.
Elevation in boiling point.
Vapour pressure lowering.
Osmotic pressure.

This topic deals with some of the important physical properties of the drug molecules.

Dielectric Constant : It is denoted by ε (epsilon). It is defined as the property of a substance to weaken the force of attraction between the two parallel conducting plates, such as the plate of electric condenser; when dipped in the solvent under study. It has no units as it is always compared with the vaccum.

Mathematically,

$$\varepsilon = C_m/C_o.$$

where, C_m = Capacitance of medium under study.

C_o = Capacitance, when the space in filled with vaccum.

Note : The value of C_o is equal to one.

Substance	Dielectric Constant
Water	80
Toulene	2.38
Benzene	2.27
Acetone	20.7

The Dielectric Constant can be determined by Oscillometry.

Molar Polarisation : To understand molar polarization we need to know about polarizability.

Polarizability is the ease with which the molecule can be polarised by an external force. It is denoted by α.

Mathematically,

$$m = \alpha F.$$

where, m = electrical moment of the induced dipole.

F = field intensity acting on a single molecule.

Concept

It can be shown from electrostatics that

$$\frac{\epsilon - 1}{\epsilon + 2} = \frac{4}{3}\pi n\alpha \qquad .....(2.1)$$

where, n is the number of molecules per unit volume.

If ρ is the density of medium between the charged plates, and M is its molecular weight, then number of molecules n in unit volume is Ne/M, where N is Avogadro's number. Eq. (2.1) is known as Clausius-Mossotti equation.

Substitution in above Eq. (2.1) we get

$$\left(\frac{\epsilon - 1}{\epsilon + 2}\right)\frac{M}{\rho} = \frac{4}{3}\pi N\alpha \qquad .....(2.2)$$

The LHS of Eq. (2.2) is denoted by P and is called molar polarization of the material; thus,

$$P = \left(\frac{\epsilon - 1}{\epsilon + 2}\right)\frac{M}{\rho} \qquad .....(2.3)$$

Since the applied field produces an induced charge in the molecule by relative displacement, or distortion, of electrons and nuclei, P is often called as "induced" or "distortion" polarization.

Permanent Dipole Moment

In the case of polar compounds we know that the positive and the negative charges are separated by a finite distance and hence the molecule will possess a permanent dipole moment. It is denoted by μ. The unit of μ is the debye, named after the scientist P. Debye.

$$1 \text{ debye} = 10^{-18} \text{ esu cm.}$$

This is derived by the multiplication of charge of the electron (10^{-10} esu) with the averge distance between charged centers on a molecule (10^{-8} cm).

Determination of Dipole Moment

(a) ***Vapour Temperature Method***

In this dielectric constant of a substance and its density of vapour are determined at series of temperatures. If the substance decomposes on heating then observations can be made under reduced pressures.

The total polarization is then calculated by using the Eq. (2.3).

But according to Debye $P = a + \frac{b}{T}$

where $a = \frac{4}{3}\pi N\alpha, \quad b = \frac{4}{3}\pi N\left(\frac{\mu^2}{3K}\right),$

$k = 1.38 \times 10^{-16}$ ergs per degree, N = Avogadro's number.

By plotting the values of P on Y-axis and $\frac{1}{T}$ on X-axis we obtain a straight line with slope equal to b. The dipole moment is calculated by equation, $\mu = 0.0128\sqrt{b} \times 10^{-18}$.

The other methods involved in the determination of dipole moment include Refraction Method and Dilute Solution Method which are not frequently used.

Significance of Dipole Moment

1. For drug-receptor binding.
2. In knowing the crystalline arrangement of substances composed of molecules with permanent dipole moments.
3. It also helps in determining the biological activity of certain compounds.

   E.g., : DDT (Insecticidal activity)

Refractive Index and Molar Refraction

The Refractive Index of a substance is the ratio of sine of the incident angle to the sine of refracted angle.

Mathematically,

$$n = \frac{Sin\, i}{Sin\, r}$$

or

$$= \frac{\text{Velocity of light in vaccum}}{\text{Velocity of light in medium}}$$

The refractive index is greater than 1 for substance denser than air.

It depends on the wavelength and temperature. The refractive index can be determined by Abb's Refractometer as seen in Fig. 2.2 and its ray diagram in Fig. 2.3.

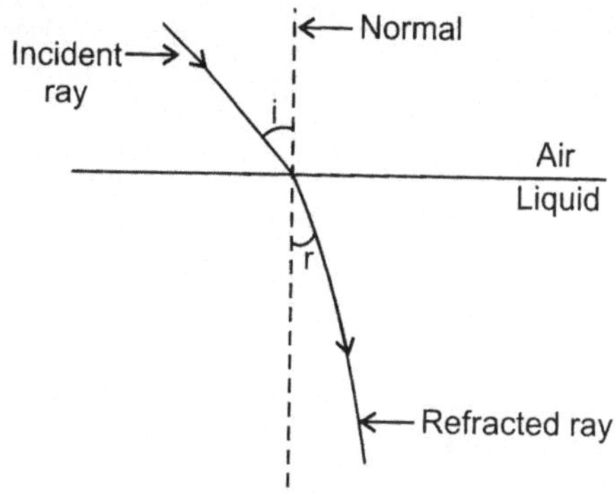

Fig. 2.1 Refraction of light.

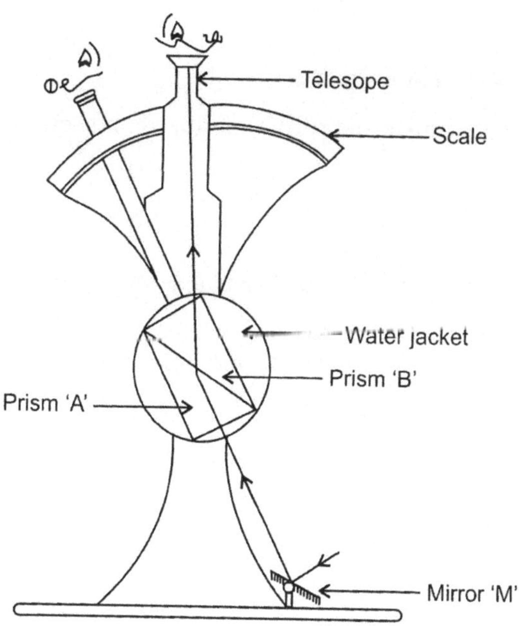

Fig. 2.2 Refraction of light.

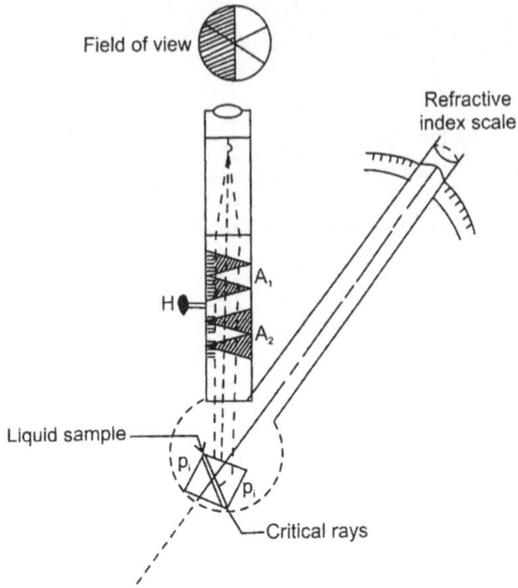

Fig. 2.3 Ray diagram of refractometer.

Molar Refraction : It is denoted by R_m.

It is partly additive and partly constitutive. It is given by the equation

$$R_m = \frac{n^2 - 1}{n^2 + 2}\left(\frac{M}{\rho}\right).$$

where, M is molecular weight and ρ is the density of compound.

Refractive index helps in identification, measuring the purity, and to determine the concentration of one substance dissolved in another.

Optical Rotation

An emerging beam of light has oscillations in a single plane is said to be plane polarised.

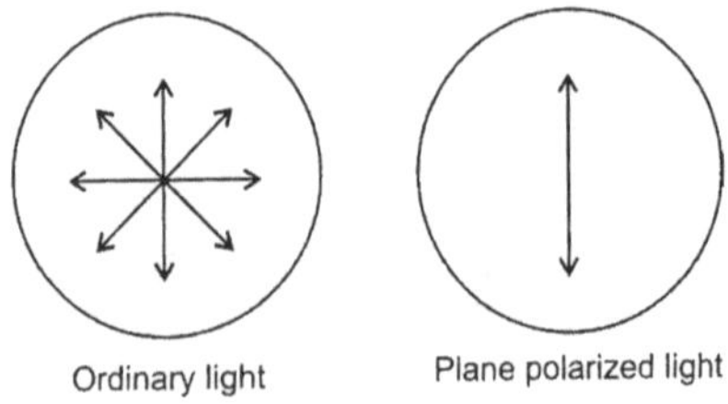

When this ordinary light is passed through Nicol prism a plane polarized light is emitted. Organic compounds having asymmetric carbon center have the tendency to rotate the plane polarized light. This property of the compounds is called optical activity. Based on the direction of rotation the compounds can be either dextrorotatory (rotation in clock wise direction) or levorotatory (rotation in anticlock wise direction).

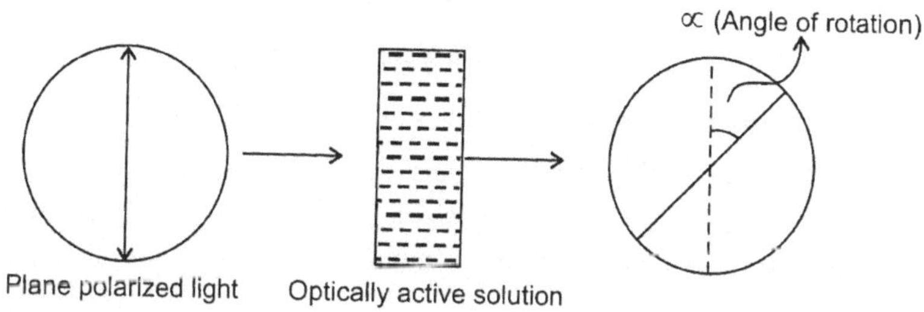

Fig. 2.4 Rotation of plane polarised light by optically active solution.

. Polarimeter is used in measurement of optical activity.

The Laurents polarimeter is widely used for measurement of optical activity as shown in Fig. 2.5.

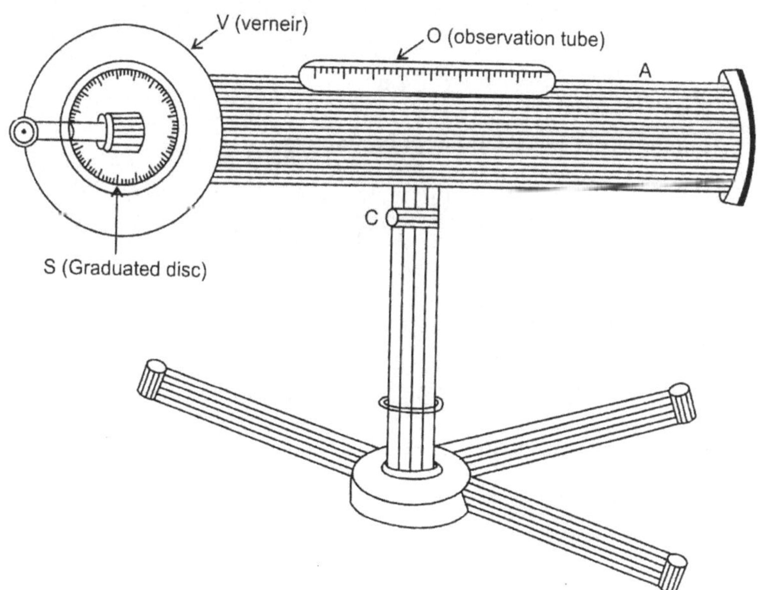

Fig. 2.5 Laurents polarimeter.

Specific Rotation

It is usually defined at particular temperature (t) and wave length (λ), generally the D-line of sodium. The rotation depends on the number of optically active molecules encountered.

Mathematically,

$$\text{Specification Rotation} = [\alpha]_\lambda^t = \frac{\alpha}{l \times c}$$

c = number of grams of optically active substance in Vml of solvent.

l = length of sample solution in decimeters. (1dm : 10 cm)

α = angle of rotation.

So, specific rotation can be defined as the observed angle of rotation at a concentration of 1 gm/ml and path length of 1 dm.

Problems

1. Compute the induced molar polarizability of chloroform. Given : Molecular weight of chloroform is 119 g/mol and density 1.43 g/cm^3. The dielectric constant is 4.8.

   Solution : Data given

   Molecular weight = M = 119 g/mol.

   Density = ρ = 1.43 g/cm³.

   Dielectric constant = ε = 4.8.

   Equation for induced molar polarizability

   $$P_i = \frac{(\epsilon - 1)}{(\epsilon + 2)} \times \frac{M}{\rho} = \frac{(4.8 - 1)}{(4.8 + 2)} \times \frac{119}{1.43}$$

   $$= 46.5 \text{ cm}^3/\text{mole}.$$

2. Compute the molar refraction of acetic acid. The density of acetic acid is 1.046 g/cc. The index of refraction, η, for sodium light is 1.3715 and molecular weight of acetic acid is 60.05 g/mole.

   Solution : Data given

   Density of acetic acid = 1.046 g/cc.

   Index of refraction = 1.3715

   Molecular weight = 60.05 g/mole

Equation for molar refraction

$$R_m = \left(\frac{\eta^2 - 1}{\eta^2 + 2}\right) \frac{M}{\rho}$$

$$= \left(\frac{(1.3715)^2 - 1}{(1.3715)^2 + 2}\right) \times \frac{60.05}{1.046}$$

$$= 13.03 \text{ cc/mole.}$$

3. Calculate the molar refraction of given sample having refractive index 1.3200, density is 0.6972 g/cc and molecular weight is 70.08.

 Solution : Data given

The refractive index	=	1.3200
Density	=	0.6972
Molecular weight	=	70.08

 Equation for molar refraction

$$R_M = \frac{\eta^2 - 1}{\eta^2 + 2} \cdot \frac{M}{\rho}$$

$$= \frac{(1.32)^2 - 1}{(1.32)^2 + 2} \times \frac{70.08}{0.6972}$$

$$= \frac{1.7424 - 1}{1.7424 + 2} \times 100.51$$

$$= \frac{0.7424}{3.7424} \times 100.51$$

$$= 19.93 \text{ CC}$$

4. A liquid having density 0.7910 g/cm^3 at 20° C. Calculate surface tension. [Molecular weight of liquid is 58.08 and parachor 62].

 Solution : Data given

 Density of liquid = 0.7910 g/cm^3

 Molecular weight = 58.08

 Parachor of liquid = 162

Equation for parachor

$$[P] = \left[\frac{M}{D}\right] y^{1/4}$$

$$162 = \frac{58.08}{0.7910} \cdot y^{1/4}$$

$$y = 23.7 \text{ dyne/cm}$$

5. A solution of sample has rotation of + 1.72° in a 20 cm polarimeter tube. Calculate the specific rotation. [Concentration used was 6 g/100ml].

Solution : Data given.

Rotation of given sample = + 1.72°

Length of tube = 20 cm = 2 dm

Equation for specific rotation,

$$[\alpha]_\lambda^t = \frac{\alpha}{l \times c} = \frac{1.72^\circ}{2 \times 0.06}$$

$$= + 14.3^\circ$$

If the molecular weight of given sample is 141.2, what is molar rotation of sample ?

Equation for molar rotation is

$$[M] = [\alpha]_\lambda^t \times M$$

$$= + 14.3 \times 141.2$$

$$= + 2019.6^\circ$$

CHAPTER 3

Phase Rule

The phase rule was first proposed by J. Willard Gibbs in 1876. It is a simple equation relating degrees of freedom (F), number of components (C), number of phases (P) in a system at equilibrium. The least number of independent variables or degrees of freedom (i.e. pressure, temperature, concentration, density) can be correlated with number of components and phases for any system at equilibrium in the following way.

$$F = C - P + 2$$

Degrees of Freedom

These are the minimum number of intensive variables required for defining a system completely. This is invariant if F = 0, univariant if F = 1 and, bivariant if F = 2.

Components

These are the least number of chemically distinct species that are present in a system. For example a system of ethyl alcohol and water has two components. Here chemically distinct species indicates the variation in chemical formula. The number of components present in a system containing water and its vapour is two as both are described by chemical formula H_2O.

Phases

It is a portion of a system that is distinctly separated from other portions by boundaries.

For a system of ice and water the number of phases are 2 (solid and liquid).

Condensed Systems : To reduce the complexity in the phase diagram we often consider pressure 1 atm and thus we neglect the vapour phase. These systems are called as condensed systems. For these systems we consider $F^1 = C - P + 1$. This is also called as *Reduced Phase Rule.* F^1 gives the remaining degrees of freedom.

Systems Containing Single Component

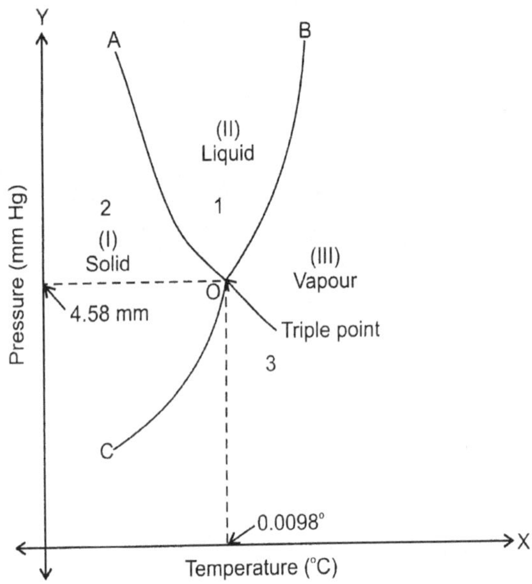

Fig. 3.1 Phase diagram of one - component system.

In the Fig. 3.1, O is the triple point where the three phases solid, liquid and vapour co-exist.

The number of degrees of freedom at triple point is

$$F = 1 - 3 + 2$$

$$= 0 \text{ (invariant system)}$$

This implies that point o can only lie at the point of intersection of the lines bounding the three phase regions.

Now if we consider points 1, 2, 3 in Fig. 3.1 the number of degrees of freedom are

$$F = 1 - 1 + 2$$
$$= 2 \text{ (bivariant system)}$$

This implies that it requires 2 variables to define the system. (i.e. pressure and temperature)

Systems Containing Two Components

For a two component system the phase rule can be written as

$$F = 4 - P$$

A two component system can be classified on the basis of miscibility as follows

(a) ***Completly Miscible Systems***

e.g., Ethyl alcohol and water

The number of degrees of freedom is given by

$$F = 4 - 1 = 3.$$

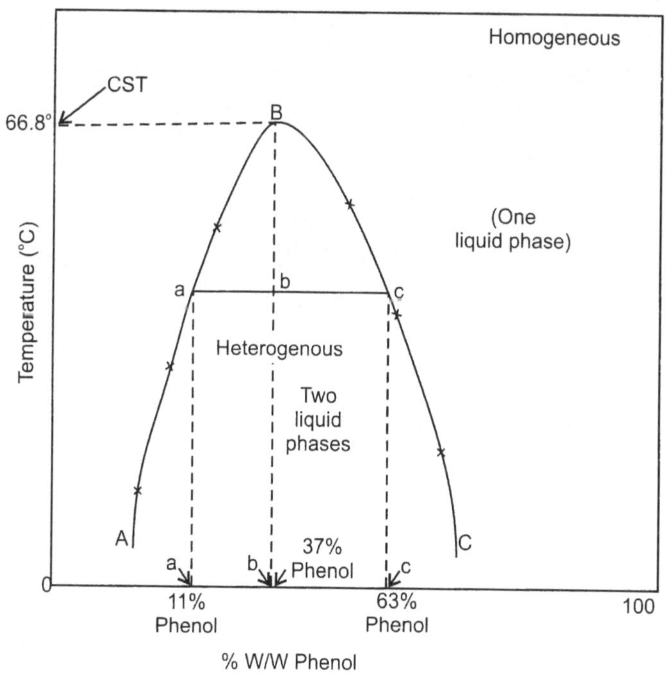

Fig. 3.2 Temperature-composition curve of phenol and water.

(b) *Partially Miscible Systems*

Under partially miscible systems phenol and water system is explicitly defined. The miscibility of phenol in water depends on concentration and temperature of the system.

By plotting the values of temperature on y-axis and percent w/w values of phenol on x-axis we obtain an inverted U - shaped curve as shown in Fig. 3.2. This curve implies that the temperature at which the miscibility appears between the 2 component increases with increase in %w/w value of phenol till certain point and then decreases gradually.

The maximum temperature at which the two-phase region exists is termed as upper consolute temperature or critical solution temperature (CST). This value is 66.8 °C for phenol-water system. The area under curve denotes system of two liquid phases and the region out side the curve denotes one liquid phase.

Interesting facts can be observed upon considering the line ac. This line is also called as tie line. Any point on the tie line represents a system which will separate into phases of constant composition at equilibrium. These phases are also known as conjugate phases.

Consider point b on the tie line. At this point

$$\frac{\text{Weight of phase A}}{\text{Weight of phase B}} = \frac{\text{length cb}}{\text{length ab}} = \frac{63-37}{37-11}$$

$$= \frac{26}{26} = 1.$$

i.e., at point b, the %w/w of phenol in the system is 37%.

which implies equal weights of phase A and phase B are present in the system.

Applying phase rule for the phenol and water system for the region outside the curve.

$$F = C - P + 2$$
$$= 2 - 1 + 2$$
$$= 3$$

Considering the system as condensed system the pressure can be neglected and value of F becomes equal to 2. So, the temperature and concentration of one component is required to define the system.

Applications

From formulation point of view these phase diagrams help in deciding concentration of each component that should taken so as to achieve a single liquid phase. A number of solutions containing different concentration of phenol are official in many pharmacopoeias. But phenol gets solidified at low ambient temperature which may lead to disturbances in the accuracy of dose. Mulley, experimentally concluded that the system of phenol and water exists in a single liquid phase up to 3.5 °C at 76% w/w of phenol concentration. But liquefied phenol, USP which contains approximately 90% w/w of phenol starts solidifying at about 17 °C. This makes the usage of liquid preparations impossible below 20 °C or room temperature.

Other examples of two component systems include Carbon disulfide - methyl alcohol, Water - aniline, Methyl alcohol - cyclohexane.

Some systems like triethylamine–water show lower consolute temperature up on varying temperature and concentration of triethylamine in the system. This is illustrated in Fig. 3.3.

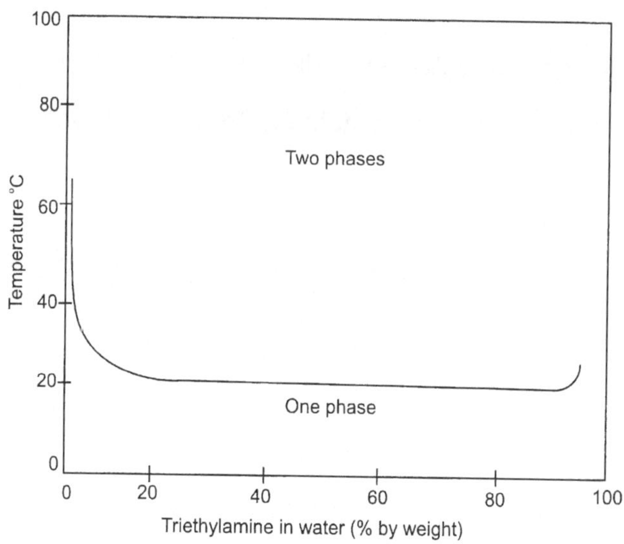

Fig. 3.3 Phase diagram of Triethylamine/water system.

Below lower consolute temperature the two components tend to miscibilize in all ratios. Certain systems tend to show both upper consolute temperature and lower consolute temperature.

Nicotine - water system is a popular example of this catagory. Fig. 3.4 depicts the phase diagram of Nicotine-water system.

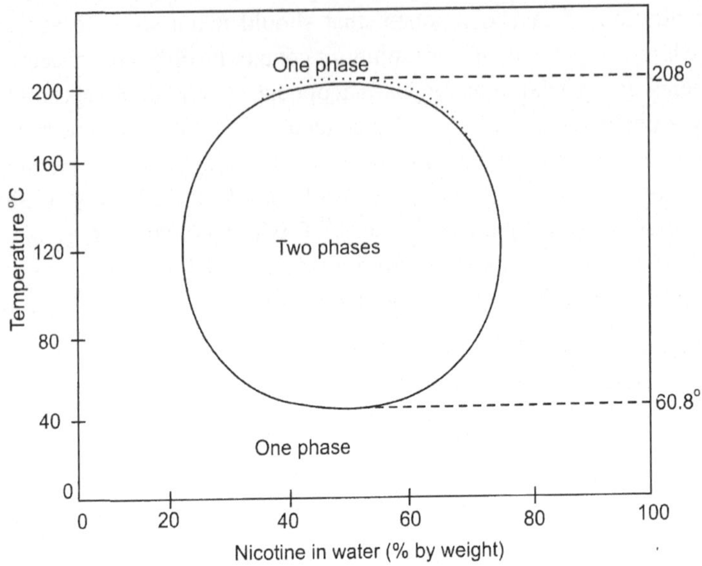

Fig. 3.4 Phase diagram of Nicotine / water system.

Two Component Systems Containing Solid and Liquid Phases

These systems are also called as Eutectic Mixtures. These systems contain two phases i.e., solid and liquid.

The two components are miscible as liquids but remain immiscible as solids.

We take into consideration the reduced phase rule to define these systems.

So $$F^1 = C - P + 1$$

A simple phase diagram is shown below in Fig 3.5.

AE - curve denotes the freezing of A. Point A denotes melting point of A. BE - Curve denotes freezing of B and point B denotes melting point of B.

Region above AEB denotes single phase system. Consider a point X as we come down along X, component A starts solidifying. Point E is called as Eutectic point. At this point solid A, solid B and liquid phase of A and B co-exist or exist in equilibrium. This temperature is denoted by T_{EP} or

Eutectic temperature. At this point F (number of degrees of freedom) becomes equal to zero, or invariant system.

At point E,

$$F = 2 - 3 + 1$$
$$= 0$$

At point X,

$$F = 2 - 1 + 1$$
$$= 2 \text{ (bivariant)}$$

At any point of curve AE or curve BE,

$$F = 2 - 2 + 1$$
$$= 1 \text{ (univariant)}$$

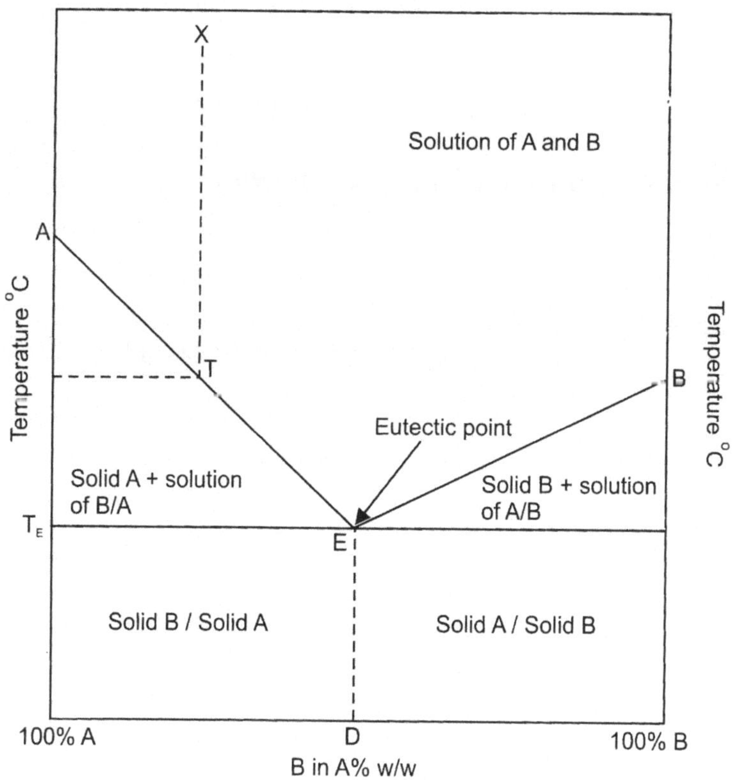

Fig. 3.5 Phase diagram of a system showing eutectic point.

Some examples of the system which fall into this category include Salol - Thymol, Salol - Camphor. Pure salol and pure thymol are completely misicible as liquids but immiscible as solids. The same holds true for mixtures of salol and camphor.

The eutectic point of salol-thymol system belong to the catagory of solid dispersions. As the name suggests solid dispersions are intimate crystalline compounds of one component dispersed in the other component.

The other category of solid dispersions include solid solution in which solid solute is dissolved in a solid solvent to give a mixed crystal. Solid dispersion is a technique used for increasing dissolution of poorly soluble drugs which improves bioavailability. Many compounds like PEG'S, sucrose etc are used in preparation of solid dispersions. The mechanisms by which solid dispersions improve the solubility include :

(a) Increasing wettability

(b) Reducing aggregation or agglomeration.

Systems Containing Three Components

With the increase in number of components in a system it becomes difficult to represent graphically using phase diagram. In a three component system the degrees of freedom are

$$F = 3 - 1 + 2 \quad \text{[for single phase]}$$
$$= 4$$

This accounts for temperature, pressure and concentration of any two components.

In case of condensed systems we get F = 3. For the sake of convenience we can maintain constant temperature, so that the value of 'F' equals to 2. Generally the phase diagrams for three component systems are represented by using a triangle whose vertices represents various components present in a system as shown in Fig. 3.6.

(a) Area inside the triangle represents all the possible combinations of A, B, C to give a three component system.

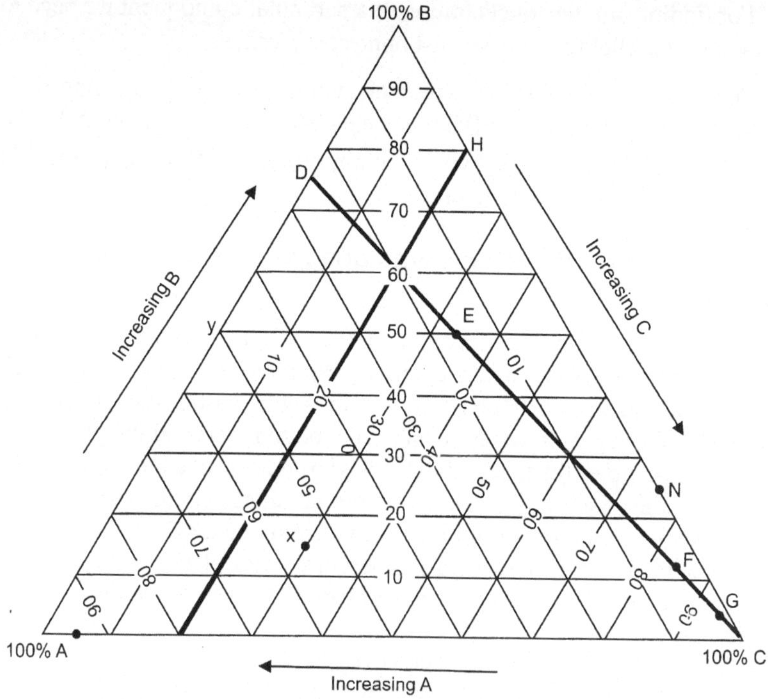

Fig. 3.6 Phase diagram for a three component system.

(b) At vertex A concentration of component A is 100% w/w. At vertex B concentration of component B is 100% w/w and at vertex C concentration of component C is 100% w/w.

(c) Up on going from A to B along the line AB the concentration of component B increases from 0 to 100% w/w. In the similar way the concentration of component C increases along the line BC and concentration of component A increases along a line CA.

(d) At any point inside the triangle the concentration of 3 components will be added up to 100% [concentration of A + concentration of B + concentration of C].

For example consider point P.

Concentration of component A = 40% w/w

Concentration of component B = 50% w/w

Concentration of component C = 10% w/w

Total concentration = 100% w/w

For finding out the concentration of a particular component we need to draw lines parallel to the base, just opposite to vextex.

For example we can determine concentration of A by drawing lines parallel to line BC. The line BC represents 0% w/w of component A. The line B′C′ represents 25% w/w of component A. Similarly line EH represents 20% w/w of component C.

Three component systems with one pair of partially miscible liquids

For system consisting of water and benzene we get a two phase system as the two components are miscible only to a slight extent. One phase is rich in benzene and the other phase is rich in water. As density of water is higher the phase rich in water occupies the bottom part and the phase rich in benzene occupies the top position. But with addition of a third component that has partial miscibility results in the formation of a single phase system. Earlier we discussed the miscibility of two-component system like phenol - water system with increasing temperature. The phase diagram for a three component system with one pair of partially miscible liquids is shown in Fig 3.7.

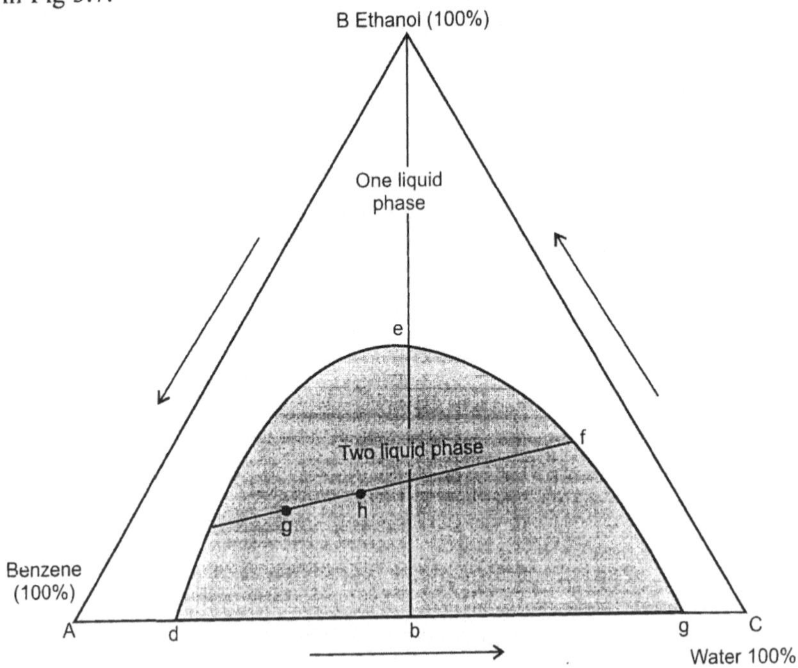

Fig. 3.7 Phase diagram for benzene/water/ethanol system.

The three components in the above phase diagram can be supposed to be benzene, water and ethanol. The shaded curve *defg* represents a two phase system of benzene and water. The region above the curve *defg* represents a single phase system. This curve *defg* is also termed as binodal curve which demarcates two phase region from single phase region.

In general, the area of the binodal decreases as the temperature is raised and miscibility is promoted.

Problems

1. The concentration of iodine between water and CCl_4 is determined as under :

   - Concentration of I_2 in water = 0.000421 0.00605 0.00966
   - Concentration of I_2 in CCl_4 = 0.003735 0.005368 0.08571

   Find out that these results the distribution law.

   Solution : Data given

   The concentration of I_2 in water and CCl_4 are given.

   Equation for distribution law.

   1. $$\frac{CI_2 - H_2O}{CI_2 - CCI_4} = \frac{0.000421}{0.003735} = 0.1127$$

   2. $$\frac{CI_2 - H_2O}{CI_2 - CCI_4} = \frac{0.000605}{0.005368} = 0.1127$$

   3. $$\frac{CI_2 - H_2O}{CI_2 - CCI_4} = \frac{0.00966}{0.08577} = 0.1126.$$

   Since these ratios are constant, distribution law is followed or obeyed.

2. In a distribution experiment the result of the distribution of benzoic acid between water and benzene are as under :

   - Concentration of benzoic acid in water
     0.0360 0.06235 0.09657 0.1237
   - Concentration of benzoic acid in benzene
     0.005735 0.009944 0.01538 0.01970

   Show that distribution law is obeyed.

Solution : Data given

Concentrations of benzoic acid in water and benzene are given

The distribution,

$$K = \frac{\text{Concentration of Benzoic acid} - H_2O}{\text{Concentration of Benzoic acid} - \text{Benzene}}$$

$$\frac{0.0360}{0.005735} = 6.277 \quad .....(i)$$

$$\frac{0.06235}{0.009944} = 6.270 \quad .....(ii)$$

$$\frac{0.09657}{0.01538} = 6.278 \quad .....(iii)$$

$$\frac{0.1237}{0.01970} = 6.279 \quad .....(iv)$$

All these values are constant thus obey the distribution law.

3. Results obtanied in some experiments on the distribution of succinic acid between water and ether are found as under

- Concentration of Succinic acid in H_2O
  0.127 0.345 0.587 0.757
- Concentration of succinic acid in ether :
  0.0275 0.0746 0.1271 0.1638

Solution : Data given

The concentrations of succinic acid in water and ether are given.

$$K = \frac{\text{Concentration of Succinic acid} - H_2O}{\text{Concentration of Succinic acid} - \text{ether}}$$

$$K = \frac{0.127}{0.0275} = 4.618 \quad .....(i)$$

$$K = \frac{0.345}{0.0746} = 4.624 \quad .....(ii)$$

$$K = \frac{0.587}{0.1271} = 4.618 \quad .....(iii)$$

$$K = \frac{0.757}{0.1638} = 4.621 \quad .....(iv)$$

All these values are constant. The distribution law is thus obeyed.

4. Acetic acid was shaken with CCl_4 and water. The following data was obtained.

$C_1\,(H_2O)$	:	6.02	8.37	11.45
$C_2\,(CCl_4)$	:	0.345	0.675	1.284

Assuming that acetic acid has single molecules in water show that it has double molecules in CCl_4.

$$K = \frac{C_1}{\sqrt{C_2}} = \frac{6.02}{\sqrt{0.345}} = 10.250 \quad .....(i)$$

$$K = \frac{8.37}{\sqrt{0.675}} = 10.188 \quad .....(ii)$$

$$K = \frac{11.45}{\sqrt{1.284}} = 10.105 \quad .....(iii)$$

These constant values for K indicates that acetic acid exists as double molecules in CCl_4.

CHAPTER 4

Thermodynamics

Thermodynamics (from the Greek thermos meaning heat and dynamis meaning power). The term thermodynamics was coined by Lord Kelvin in 1849. Historically, thermodynamics developed out of the need to increase the efficiency of early steam engines. Roughly, heat means "energy in transit" and dynamics relates to "movement", thus, in essence thermodynamics studies the movement of energy and how energy instills movement. *Energy can be defined as the capacity of a body to do work.* Energy is available in various forms like potential energy (due to the position), kinetic energy (due to motion), heat energy, chemical energy, electrical energy.

Units of Energy = ergs (C.G.S)

Joules (S.I. System)

1 Joule = 10^7 ergs.

Thermodynamics is a branch of science which deals with the heat changes accompanying a particular process.

An important concept in thermodynamics is the "System". A system is the region of universe under study. A system is separated from the remainder of universe by a boundary which may be imaginary or not, but which by convention delimits a finite volume. The possible exchange of work, heat, or matter between the system and surroundings take place across this boundary. Various types of systems are – or :

(a) Isolated System – matter and energy may not cross the boundary
(b) Adiabatic System – heat and matter may not cross the boundary
(c) Closed System – matter may not cross the boundary
(d) Open System – heat, work and matter may cross the boundary.

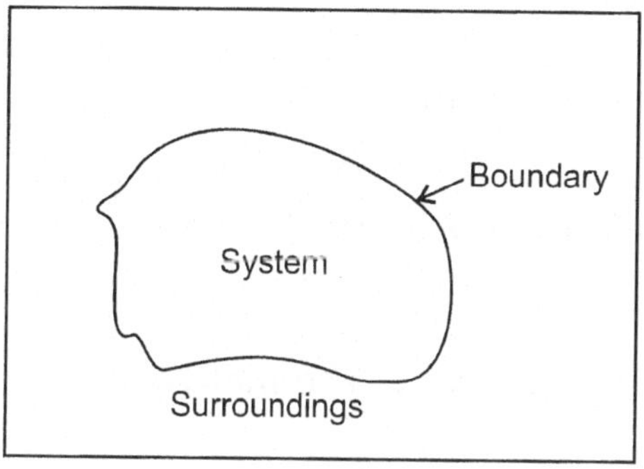

Law of Conservation of Energy or First law of Thermodynamics :

This can be stated in various forms

"*Energy can neither be created nor destroyed and may be converted from one form to another*".

"When a quantity of one kind energy disappeares an exactly equivalent amount of other form must be produced".

Mathematically it can be expressed as,

$$\Delta E = Q - W \qquad .....(4.1)$$

In differential form

$$dE = dQ - dW \qquad .....(4.2)$$

or $$\Delta E = Q - P\Delta V$$

where,

$\Delta E \;=\; E_B - E_A$ = change in the internal energy

Q = heat (It is denoted by +Q when heat is input and – Q when heat is output).

W = Work done (It is denoted by +W when work is input and –W when work is output).

Since in thermodynamics it is difficult to find absolute value of energy, it is always expressed as the difference in the final and initial states of system.

i.e., $$\Delta E = E_2 - E_1$$

When the process is adiabatic (i.e., neither heat is absorbed nor given out), then eq. (4.1) can be written as

$$\Delta E = -W \quad (Q = 0)$$

and when work done is zero then,

$$\Delta E = Q$$

Applications of First Law of Thermodynamics

Reversible and irreversible Process

A reversible process may be defined as one which can be performed in forward and reverse directions, so that all changes occuring in any part of the direct process are exactly reversed in the corresponding part of the reverse process, and only infinitesimal changes are produced.

A simple illustration of reversible process can be made by considering hypothetical case of water at its boiling point in a cylinder placed in a constant temperature bath. The cylinder is closed by means of a frictionless piston as shown in Fig. 4.1.

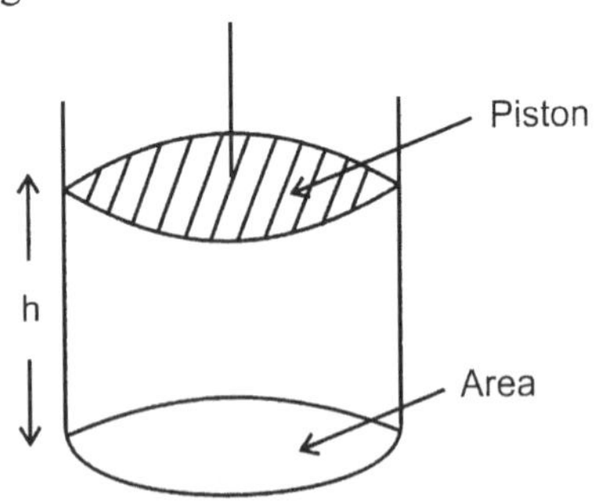

Fig. 4.1 Cylinder with weightless and frictionless piston.

If the external pressure is increased infinitesimally then small amount of vapour will condense, but this process will take place at such a slow rate that the system will not change and pressure above liquid remains unaltered. Although condensation is occuring, the system at every instant is in equilibrium. Similarly, if the external pressure is reduced slightly than the vapour pressure, the liquid will evaporate at an extremely slow rate, maintaining the system in equilibrium. The change may be regarded as a series of equilibrium states. Since, this process is always in a state of virtual thermodynamic equilibrium, being reversed by an infinitesimal change of pressure, it is said to be reversible. The work done by a system in an isothermal process is maximum when it is done reversibly.

A process is called irreversible if it cannot be reversed and if it is reversed, it cannot do so without leaving the surroundings permanently changed.

Reversible Isothermal Expansion of Gas at Constant Pressure

In this process the pressure remains constant throughout, since it is always equal to the equilibrium vapour pressure P of the liquid at the experimental temperature. Let ΔV be the change in volume. The work done by the system against opposing pressure is

$$W = P \times \Delta V \qquad \text{.....(4.3)}$$

or

$$P(V_2 - V_1)$$

Isothermal Work of Expansion against a Variable Pressure

As we have mentioned earlier the external pressure is only infinitesimally less than the pressure of an ideal gas in an isothermal expansion. So the external pressure can be replaced by gas equation P = nRT/V.

Substituting this in Eq. (4.3) we will get,

$$\int dw = nRT \int_{V_1}^{V_2} \frac{1}{V}\, dV.$$

$$W_{max} = nRT\, [lnV]_{1/1}^{V_2}$$

$$= nRT \left[ln \frac{V_2}{V_1}\right]$$

or

$$= 2.303\, nRT \left[\log \frac{V_2}{V_1}\right] \qquad \text{.....(4.4)}$$

According to Boyle's law, $P_1 V_1 = P_2 V_2$.

Replacing this in Eq. (4.4) gives

$$W_{max} = 2.303 \text{ nRT} \log \frac{P_1}{P_2}.$$

Heat Content : Consider a system at constant pressure or (enthalpy). By replacing ΔE by $E_B - E_A$. The Eq. (4.1) can be written as

$$(E_B - E_A) = Q_p - P(V_B - V_A)$$

$$\Rightarrow Q_p = (E_B + PV_B) - (E_A + PV_A)$$

By replacing E + PV with symbol H, we can write,

$$Q_P = H_B - H_A = \Delta H \quad .....(4.5)$$

The symbol H is used to represent heat content of a system at constant pressure.

Substituting ΔH for Q_P we get

$$\Delta H = \Delta E + P \Delta V \quad .....(4.6)$$

Heat Capacity

The heat capacity of a system is defined as quantity of heat required to raise the temperature of one mole of a substance by 1 degree. It is denoted by C. It is also known as molar heat capacity since we consider 1 mole of a pure substance.

$$C = \frac{q}{dT} \quad .....(4.7)$$

The heat capacity varies with temperature, it is defined for infinitesimally small value dT at constant volume. Eq. (4.7) may be represented as

$$C_V = \frac{q_v}{dT} \quad .....(4.8)$$

but at constant volume, d E = q_v (from first law) so Eq. (4.8) becomes

$$C_V = \left(\frac{\partial E}{\partial T}\right)_v \quad .....(4.9)$$

At constant pressure, the heat capacity is

$$C_p = \frac{q_P}{dT} \quad .....(4.10)$$

But $q_P = dH$ from Eq. (4.5), so

$$C_p = \left(\frac{\partial H}{\partial T}\right)_P \qquad .....(4.11)$$

Difference in Heat Capacities

By subtracting Eq. (4.9) from Eq. (4.11)

$$C_P - C_V = \left(\frac{\partial H}{\partial T}\right)_P - \left(\frac{\partial E}{\partial T}\right)_V$$

But H = E + PV.

$$C_P - C_V = \left(\frac{\partial E}{\partial T}\right)_P + P\left(\frac{\partial V}{\partial T}\right)_P - \left(\frac{\partial E}{\partial T}\right)_V \qquad .....(4.12)$$

Here dE is completely differential

$$\partial E = \left(\frac{\partial E}{\partial V}\right)_T^{dv} + \left(\frac{\partial E}{\partial T}\right)_T^{dT}$$

Upon dividing by ∂T and at constant pressure

$$\left(\frac{\partial E}{\partial T}\right)_P = \left(\frac{\partial E}{\partial V}\right)_T \left(\frac{\partial V}{\partial T}\right)_P + \left(\frac{\partial E}{\partial T}\right)_V \qquad .....(4.13)$$

Addition of Eq. (4.12) and Eq. (4.13) gives

$$C_P - C_V = \left[P + \left(\frac{\partial E}{\partial V}\right)_T\right]\left(\frac{\partial V}{\partial T}\right)_P \qquad .....(4.14)$$

The Eq. (4.14) represents general form of equation for difference in heat capacities of ideal gas.

Thermochemistry

Heat changes in chemical Reactions

The aspect of physical chemistry which deals with the heat changes accompanying a chemical reaction is known as thermochemistry. To a great extent it is based on first law of thermodynamics. A chemical reaction may be either exothermic (heat evolved) or endothermic (heat absorbed).

Generally the reaction proceeds under constant pressure or constant volume. One of these must be specified so as to conclude whether the reaction is exothermic or endothermic.

In practice the reactions proceed under atmospheric conditions so pressure is considered to be constant and heat changes (Q_P) is equal to ΔH. This quantity is often referred to as *heat of reaction*. If the reaction proceeds at constant volume then Q_V is equal to ΔE.

The heat changes accompanying a reaction involving solid carbon and gaseous oxygen to yield carbon dioxide gas as given below

$$C \text{ (solid)} + O_2 \text{ (gas)} \rightarrow CO_2 \text{ (gas)}$$

$$\Delta H = -94.05 \text{ kcal}$$

The above reaction proceeds with evolution of heat which implies that reactants contain 94.05 kcal in excess compared to the product.

Heat of Formation

It is the increase in heat content ΔH when 1 mole of substance is formed from its constituents. From the above mentioned example the heat of formation of CO_2 (gas) is – 94.05 Kcal.

Heats of formation per mole in Kcal at 25 °C.

1. NO : 27.5
2. N_2O : 17.0
3. H I : 6.0
4. NH_3 : 11.0
5. CO : 26.4

Heat of Combustion

It is defined as the change in heat content accompanying when of 1 mole of a compound undergoes combustion process.

Heats of combustion per mole in kcal at 25 °C.

Substance	$-\Delta H$
1. Ethane	368.5
2. Toluene	936
3. Ethanol	327
4. Methanol	171

Heat of Hydrogenation

It is defined as the increase in heat content when 1 mole of unsaturated hydrocarbon is converted in to corresponding saturated compound by gaseous hydrogen.

E.g. : $C_6 H_6 (s) + 3 H_2 (g) \rightarrow C_6 H_{12} (g)$

$\Delta H = -49.80$ Kcal

Thermochemical Laws

The quantity of heat required to decompose a compound into its elements is equal to the heat evolved when compound is formed from its element.

G. H. Hess in the year 1840 proposed second law. According to this law the heat changes in a chemical reaction is the same whether it takes place in one or several stages.

E.g. :

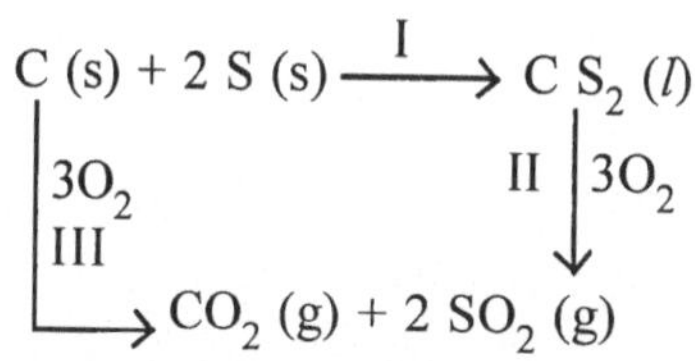

If ΔH_I, ΔH_{II} and ΔH_{III} are the heat content changes in the respective processes marked I, II and III, then from Hess's Law

$$\Delta H_I + \Delta H_{II} = \Delta H_{III}$$

Second Law of Thermodynamics

There is no body in the universe that can convert the entire energy into work. According to second law, "*It is impossible to construct a machine functioning in cycles that can convert heat completely into the equivalent amount of work without producing changes elsewhere*".

This practical impossibility of converting entire energy into work led to the coining of term "efficiency". *The amount of energy utilized for doing useful work is called free energy.*

The Efficiency of a Heat Engine

It is the fraction of the heat Q at the source converted into work W.

The efficicency of the engine : efficiency $= \frac{W}{Q}$.

Imagine a hypothetical steam engine operating reversibly between an upper temperature T_2 and a lower temperature T_1. It absorbs heat Q_2 from source. It converts the quantity W into work and returns heat Q_1 to the cold reservior or sink. The efficiency of such an engine can be given by the expression (Carnot, 1824).

$$\frac{W}{Q_2} = \frac{Q_2 - Q_1}{Q_2} \qquad .....(4.15)$$

Lord Kelvin used the ratio of two heat quntities Q_2 and Q_1 of the Carnot cycle to establish the Kelvin temperature scale.

$$\frac{Q_2}{Q_1} = \frac{T_2}{T_1} \qquad .....(4.16)$$

By combining Eq. (4.15) and Eq. (4.16) we can write,

$$\text{Efficiency} = \frac{Q_2 - Q_1}{Q_2} = \frac{T_2 - T_1}{T_2}$$

Entropy

From Eq. (4.15) and (4.16) we can obtain

$$\frac{W}{Q_2} = \frac{T_2 - T_1}{T_2}$$

or

$$W = Q_2 - T_1 \frac{Q_2}{T_2} \qquad .....(4.17)$$

The term $\frac{Q_2}{T_2}$ is denoted as entropy change of reversible process at T_2

and $\frac{Q_2}{T_1}$ is the entropy change of T_1.

From Eq. (4.16) we obtain

$$\frac{Q_2}{T_2} + \frac{Q_1}{T_1} = 0 \qquad .....(4.18)$$

or

$$\sum \frac{q}{T} = 0$$

Eq. (4.18) implies that the total entropy change in a reversible cycle is zero. But if we consider an irreversible cycle then,

$$\sum \frac{q}{T} > 0$$

Entropy and Probability

R.Clausius suggested second law of thermodynamics in terms of entropy. According to him the total amount of entropy in nature is always increasing. Consider molecules of gas in a cylinder. The probability that all the gas molecules will be equally spaced and move in an ordered manner relative to each other is very small. This is due to irregular collisions of the gas molecules between themselves and with walls of container. This state has got more probability to occur than the ordered state in the Fig. 4.2.

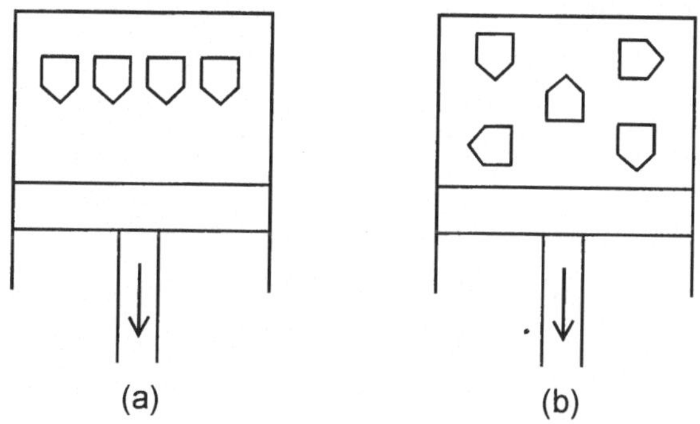

Fig. 4.2 Cyclinders containing gas molecules showing (a) low entropy; or orderliness, and (b) high entropy, or disorderliness.

Boltzmann Equation

$$S = k \ln W$$

where,

k = Boltzmann Constant = 1.38066×10^{-16} erg. deg^{-1}. $molecule^{-1}$.

W = Probability of system or number of configuration that system can assume.

Third Law of Thermodynamics

According to this law the probability of entropy of a pure crystalline substance is zero at absolute zero because the crystal arrangement must show the greatest orderliness at this temperature.

This is not applicable for supercooled liquids.

$$\Delta S = \int_0^T \frac{C_P}{T} dT$$

$$= 2.303 \int_0^T C_P \, d \log T. \qquad .....(4.19)$$

From T = 0° where S = O to T where S = S.

Using this law one can calculate the absolute entropies of pure crystalline substance.

Eq. (4.19) can be calculated by plotting values of C_p against log T and determining the area under the curve by the use of planimeter.

Free Energy Functions and Applications

Helmholtz Free Energy

It is also known as total work function.

Mathematically,

$$A = E - TS$$

for small change

$$dA = dE - TdS - SdT. \quad .....(4.20)$$

But

$$dS = \frac{dQ_{rev}}{T}$$

According to first law of thermodynamics

$$dQ = dE + PdV$$

$$\Rightarrow dS = \frac{dE + PdV}{T} \quad .....(4.21)$$

Substituting (4.21) into (4.20)

$$dA = -PdV - SdT$$

or

$$dA = -dW.$$

So the change in Helmholtz free energy (A) denotes the total work that can be obtained

Gibb's Free Energy

It is denoted by G.

Mathematically,

$$\Delta G = E + PV - T\Delta S$$

But E + PV can be replaced by H.

$$\Delta G = H - T\Delta S$$

or We can replace $E - T\Delta S$ with A [see Eq. (4.20)]

$$\Delta G = A + PV \text{ (Gibbs – Helmholtz Equation)}$$

Pressure and Temperature Co-efficients of Free energy

The free energy change of an ideal gas which is undergoing isothermal reversible or irreversible change can be denoted by

$$\Delta G = n\ RT\ \ln \frac{P_2}{P_1} = 2.303\eta\ RT \log \frac{P_2}{P_1} \qquad .....(4.22)$$

Spontaneity of a Reaction

Gibb's free energy can be used to determine the nature of a reaction i.e., spontaneous or non-spontaneous

If $\Delta G < 0$ (The reaction is spontaneous)

$\Delta G > 0$ (The reaction is non-spontaneous)

$\Delta G = 0$ (The reaction is at equilibrium)

Clausius - Clapeyron Equation

The changes in pressure of a two phase system for a single component with temperature is given by equation.

$$\log \frac{P_2}{P_1} = \frac{\Delta H_V}{2.303\ R}\left[\frac{1}{T_1} - \frac{1}{T_2}\right]$$

or $$\log \frac{P_2}{P_1} = \frac{\Delta H_v (T_2 - T_1)}{2.030\ RT_1T_2} \qquad .....(4.23)$$

where ΔH_V = Molar heat of vapourisation of liquid.

This equation is used to calculate the mean heat of vapourisation of a liquid if it's vapour pressure at two different temperatures is available. It is also helpful in the development of some colligative properties.

Problems

1. Calculate the maximum work done in ergs when one mole of an ideal gas expands from 10 liter to 20 liters at room temperature.

   Solution : Data given

   V_1 = 10 liters and V_2 = 20 liters.

   R = 1.98 cal. deg^{-1} $mole^{-1}$.

Equation for maximum work

$$W_{max} = 2.303 \text{ nRT} \log \frac{V_2}{V_1}$$

$$= 2.303 \times 1 \times 298 \times 1.98 \log \frac{20}{10}$$

$$= 409 \text{ calories.}$$

It can be converted to ergs.

$$W_{max} = JH = 4.2 \times 10^7 \times 409$$

$$= 1.72 \times 10^{10} \text{ ergs.}$$

2. Calculate the maximum work done in isothermal reversible expansion of 2 moles of an ideal gas from 1 to 5 liters at room temperature.

Solution : Data given

$$P_1 = 5 \text{ and } P_2 = 1$$

$$\text{Equations for } W_{max} = 2.303 \text{ nRT} \log \frac{P_1}{P_2}$$

$$= 2.303 \times 2 \times 1.98 \times 298 \times \log 5.$$

$$= 1908 \text{ cal.}$$

3. Calculate work done when 2 moles of H_2 expands from 15 to 50 liters at room temperature.

Solution : Data given

$$V_1 = 15, V_2 = 50.$$

$$\text{Equation for } W_{max} = 2.303 \text{ nRT} \log \frac{V_2}{V_1}$$

$$= 2.303 \times 2 \times 1.98 \times 298 \log \frac{50}{15}$$

$$= 1830 \text{ calories.}$$

4. Calculate the entropy change [ΔS] accompanying the vaporization of 1 mole of water in equilibrium with its vapour at 25 °C. In this reversible isothermal process, the heat of vaporization [ΔH_v] required to convert the liquid to vapour state is 12,500 cal/mole.

Solution : Data given

$$\Delta H_v = 12{,}500 \text{ cal/mole.}$$

Equation for entropy change

$$\Delta S = \frac{\Delta H_v}{T}$$

$$= \frac{12500}{298} = 41.94 \text{ cal/mole deg.}$$

5. A heat engine works between 130 °C and 42 °C. Calculate the efficiency of engine.

Solution : Data given

Temperature of hot reservoir = T_2 = 130 °C.

Temperature of cold reservoir = T_1 = 42 °C.

Equation of

$$\text{Efficiency} = \frac{T_2 - T_1}{T_2}$$

$$T_2 = 130\ ^\circ C = 273 + 130 = 403\ ^\circ K$$

$$T_1 = 42\ ^\circ C = 273 + 42 = 315\ ^\circ K$$

$$\text{Efficiency} = \frac{403 - 315}{403} = \frac{88}{403}$$

$$= 0.2183 = 21.84\%$$

6. A steam engine operates between the temperature of 397 °K and 298 °K.

(a) What is theoretical efficiency of the engine ?

(b) If the engine supplied units 1000 cal of heat Q_2. What is the theoretical work in ergs ?

Solution : Data given

(a) $T_1 = 298\ ^oK$

$T_2 = 397\ ^oK.$

Equation for efficiency

$$= \frac{T_2 - T_1}{T_2}$$

$$= \frac{397 - 298}{397} = 0.2493 \text{ or } \cong 25\%$$

(b) $W = 1000 \times 0.25 = 250$ cal.

$= 250 \text{ cal} \times 4.184 \times 10^7 \text{erg/cal.}$

$= 10.46 \times 10^9$ ergs.

7. A gas expands by 2 liters against a constant pressure of 1.2 atm at 25 °C. What is work done by system in joules ?

(1 atm= 1.013×10^6 dyne/cm^2)

$W = P \Delta V$

$= 1.2 \times 1.013 \times 10^6 \times 2000$

$= 2.43 \times 10^9$ ergs or 243 joules.

CHAPTER 5

Rheology

Rheology

Rheology is a branch of science which deals with the deformation of materials or matter under the influence of stress. The term *rheology* has its origin from the Greek "rheo" means flow and "logos" means science. So the definition can further be simplified as "*The science which deals with the flow of fluid type preparations*". In pharmaceutical and related research and technology, rheology helps in measuring the ease of pouring from bottle, extrusion of semisolid dosage forms after squeezing the tube, capability to spread on the surface of skin on application of pressure, passage through syringe needle.

In the recent years, the fundamental principles of rheology have been used in the study of paints, inks, doughs, road building materials, cosmetics, dairy products etc. Rheology is involved in the mixing and flow of materials, their packaging into containers and their removal prior to use etc.

To understand the concept of rheology we need to know definitions of basic terms which will be a part of our further discussion.

Viscosity ***(η)*** : It is the property of the body to resist the flow. It is denoted by Eta (η). Units are poise (S.I system) (or) C_p (10^{-2} poise).

The viscosity of water is around 1 C_p. The mathematical expression for viscosity will be discussed in the coming sections.

Shear Stress : It is denoted by 'F', and given by F'/A. In simple terms it is defined as force applied per unit area required to bring about flow. Unit is dyne/cm^2.

Rate of Shear : It is denoted by "G". It is the velocity gradient dv/dr between two planes of a body that are separated by an infinitesimally small distance. Unit is cm^{-1}.

To understand the terms in a better way just consider the Fig. 5.1.

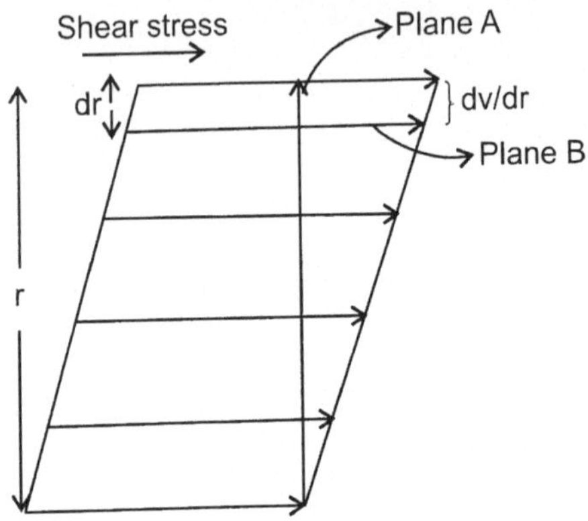

Fig. 5.1 Velocity gradient between parallel plants of a material.

The top plane A moves with greater velocity than the plane B which is separated by a distance dr. In more general terms, for any point in a layer that is separated by a distance dr from the upper plane the rate of shear is given by dv/dr.

Broadly all fluids can be classified as *newtonian fluids* and *non newtonian fluids*.

1. Newtonian Fluids

These are the fluids in which there is direct proportionality between shear stress and shear rate.

$$F \alpha \frac{dv}{dr} \qquad .....(5.1)$$

Taking the proportionality constant as η, the above equation becomes

$$F = \eta \frac{dv}{dr}$$

where, $$F = \frac{F'}{A}$$

So we can write $$\frac{F'}{A} = \eta \frac{dv}{dr}$$

So, $$\text{viscocity} = \eta = F/G \qquad .....(5.2)$$

in which $F = \frac{F'}{A}$ and $G = \frac{dv}{dr}$

mathematically the viscosity of a body is shear stress divided by shear rate.

So all bodies which statisfy Eq. (5.2) are called newtonian fluids.

E.g. : Water, True Solutions, Dilute Suspensions and Emulsions.

Fluidity : It is denoted by phi (ϕ). It is the reciprocal of viscosity.

$$\phi = \frac{1}{\eta}$$

So the bodies with less viscosity have high values of fluidity and vice-versa.

The other types of viscosities include :

(a) ***Kinematic Viscosity :*** It is denoted by (υ). Mathematically, when newtonian viscosity is divided by density gives Kinematic Viscosity.

$$\upsilon = \frac{\eta}{\rho}$$

Units – Stoke (S) and the centistoke (C_s)

(b) ***Relative Viscosity :*** It is denoted by (η_r). It is ratio of viscosity of the dispersion (η) to that of solvent (η_o).

Relative Viscosity,

$$\eta_r = \frac{\eta}{\eta_o}.$$

(c) ***Specific Viscosity :*** It is denoted as (η_{sp}).

Specific Viscosity is obtanied by substracting one from relative viscocity.

$$\eta_{sp} = \frac{\eta - \eta_o}{\eta_o}$$

(d) ***Reduced Viscosity :*** It is defined as ratio of specific viscosity to the concentration (C).

Reduced Viscosity

$$\eta_{red} = \frac{\eta_{sp}}{C} \qquad (\text{C in g/100 cm}^3)$$

(e) ***Intrinsic Viscosity :*** The Y-intercept obtained by extrapolating the curve obtained by taking reduced viscocity on Y-axis and concentration (C in g/100 cm^3) on x-axis. It is denoted by [η]. It is used in calculating approximate molecular weights of polymers. According to Mark-Houwink equation $[\eta] = KM^a$. K and a are constants of polymer solvent system and M is molecular weight. The details are given in unit colloids.

2. Non-Newtonian Fluids

Many pharmaceutical preparations does not obey Eq. (5.2) for the value of viscosity varies with varying shear rate. So one needs to take into consideration the apparent viscosites of these bodies at particular shear rates. The graphical representation of various Non-Newtonian fluids are denoted by curves b, c, d in Fig. 5.2.

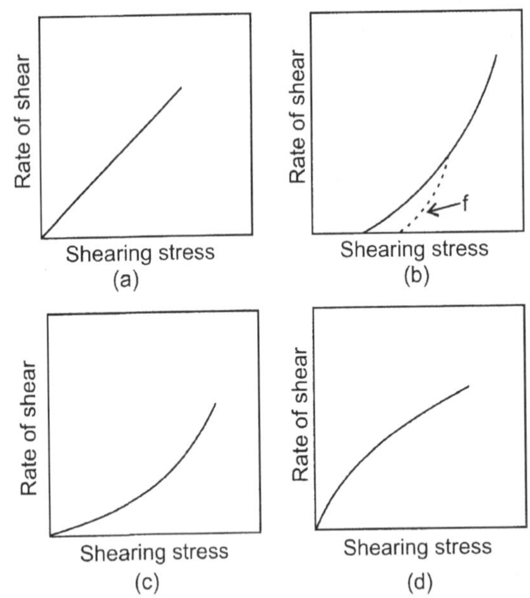

Fig. 5.2 Flow Curves of Newtonian and Non-Newtonian Fluids. (a) Newtonian (b) Plastic flow (c) Pseudoplastic (d) Dilatent flow

(a) ***Plastic Flow :*** The curve for plastic flow intersect to the axis of shear stress at some point without passing through origin. This indicated that a certain amount shear stress is required before the body begins to flow. If straight part of the curve extrapolated to the axis it is called yield point or yield value. The viscosity of these bodies is given by the equation

$$U = \frac{F - f}{G}$$

where U = plastic viscosity, f = yield value (or) Bingham yield value; G = rate of shear

Materials which show this type of behaviour are termed as Bingham bodies.

(b) ***Pseudoplastic Flow :*** This type of flow is represented by curve C in Fig. 5.2. The curve passes through origin and this implies that the molecules start disentangling immediately after the application of shear stress. The slope of the curve at any point is obtained by drawing a tangent to the curve intersecting the x-axis.

Slope of curve increases in ascending direction. The apparent viscosity at any shear rate is obtained by taking reciprocal value of slope. It can be clearly observed that the apparent viscosity decreases as the shear rate increases until a constant value is reached.

This type of curve fits in to the Eq.

$$F^N = \eta' G \qquad .....(5.3)$$

where F is shear stress, A is proportionality constant. The value of n indicates the type of flow.

N = 1 (Newtonian flow)

N < 1 (Psuedoplastic flow)

N > 1 (Dilatant flow)

Eq. (5.3) *is also called as Power Law Equation.* To find the individual values one needs to further simplify the Eq. (5.3) by applying logarithms.

$$\log G = N \log F - \log \eta' \qquad .....(5.4)$$

Eq. (5.4) can be compared to a straight line y = c + mx.

A plot of log G against log F results in a straight line with slope η' and log F as Y-intercept. A large number of pharmaceutical products like liquid dispersions of tragacanth, methylcellulose and gums shows this type of flow.

(c) ***Dilatant Flow :*** This type of behaviour is represented by curve d in Fig. 5.2. The behaviour of molecules which contributes this type of flow is exactly opposite to that of psuedoplastic flow. The slope of curve decrease with increasing shear stress and hence viscosity increases with increasing shear stress. The 'n' value is more than one for this type of flow. *These systems are also called as shear thickening system.* Suspensions with more than 50% of suspended particles, show dilatant flow properties. Explanation of dilatant flow behavior is as follows :

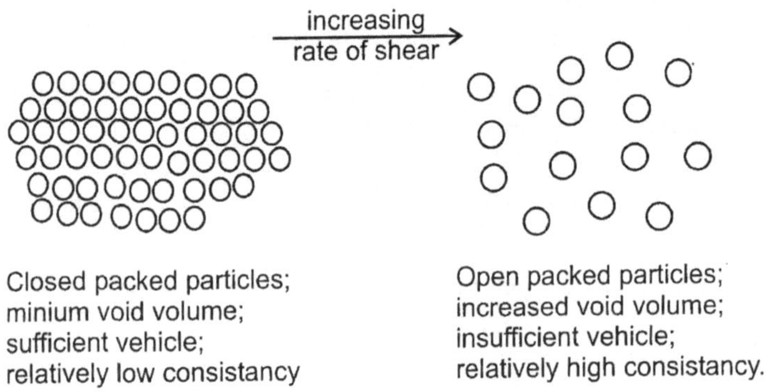

Mechanism which Contributes to Rheological Behaviour

The decrease in the apparent viscosity with increasing shear rates in plastic and psuedoplastic types of flow is due to disentangling of aggregates of dispersed particles of the system which contributes for the typical behaviour.

When shear stress values are reduced, the molecules get entangled and the curve falls to the left side of ascending curve as shown in Fig. 5.3. The psuedoplastic substances are also called as shear thinning systems as the viscosity of the bodies reduces with increasing shear stress.

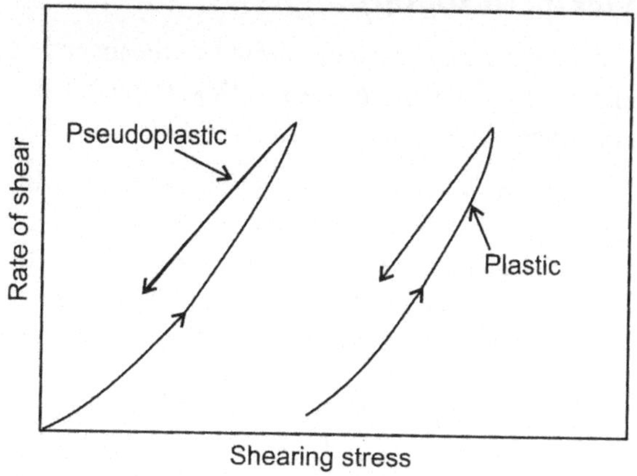

Fig. 5.3 Thixotopic curves of pseudoplastic and plastic bodies.

The curve or loop shown in Fig. 5.3 is *called thixotropic curve*, and the systems exhibiting this sort of curves are known as thixotropic systems. Thixotropy may be defined as "*an isothermal and comparatively slow recovery, on standing of a material, of a consistency lost through shearing*". In a newtonian system the down-curve is super-imposed on the up-curve. In case of pseudoplastic systems the down-curve falls to left side of up-curve. The curves obtained by the thixotropic materials are highly dependent on the changes in rate of shear and duration of time involved, at a particular rate of shear. Fig. 5.4 shows the rheograms of Bingham substance which are subjected to constant shear rate for time t_1 and t_2 seconds.

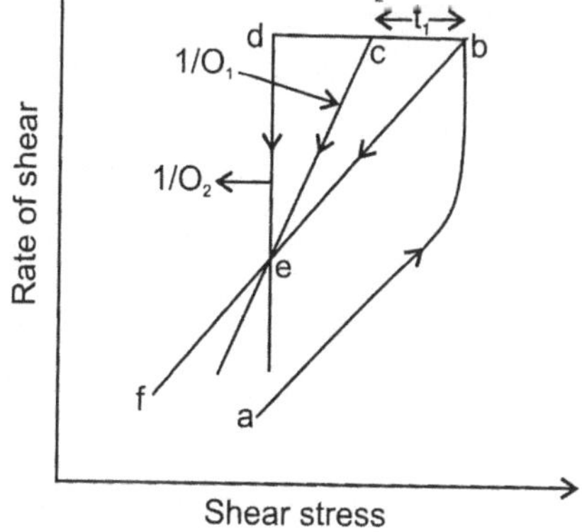

Fig. 5.4 Structural deformation of Thixotropic bodies.

Measurement of Thixotropy

The measure of area of hysteresis loop formed by the up and down curves in a thixotropic materials gives the value of thixotropic break down. This value can be obtained by using a planimeter.

In the rheogram shown in Fig. 5.4 the sample is applied with a constant shear rate for t_1 seconds results in formation of hysteresis loop abce. Similarly applying the shear rate for t_2 seconds results in formation of abcde. This behaviour can be used for calculating thixotropic coefficient, B, which indicates the rate of break down with time at constant shear rate.

$$B = \frac{U_1 - U_2}{\ln \frac{t_2}{t_1}} \qquad (5.5)$$

where U_1 and U_2 are the plastic viscosities, t_1 and t_2 are the time duration.

The other suggested method used for calculating thixotropic co-efficient M, which indicates loss in shear stress per unit increase in shear rate, is obtained from

$$M = \frac{(U_1 - U_2)}{\ln\left({}^{v_2}\!/\!{}_{v_1} \right)}$$

where, U_1 and U_2 are plastic viscosities, V_1 and V_2 are maximum shearing rates. The value M will depend on the rate of shear chosen.

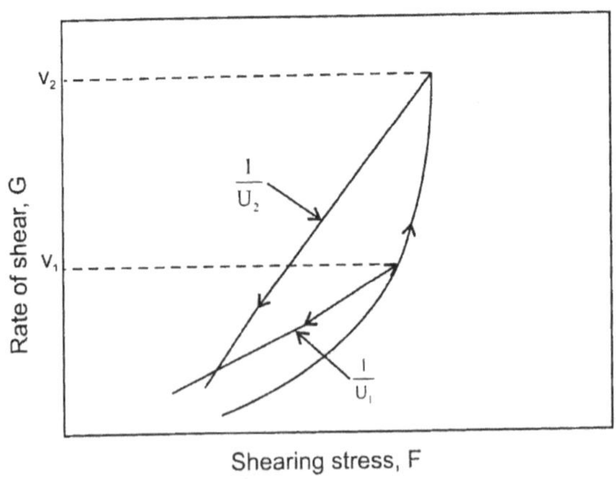

Fig. 5.5 Structural breakdown of plastic bodies.

Bulges

In case of concentrated aqueous magma (gel) of bentonite (10-15% w/w) produces a *hysteresis loop* with a characteristic bulge in the up-curve as shown in Fig. 5.6. This may be due to the arrangement of crystalline plates of bentonite in the form of "house-of-cards structure" that causes the swelling of bentonite magmas. This three-dimensional structure result in a bulged hysteresis loop as observed in Fig. 5.6.

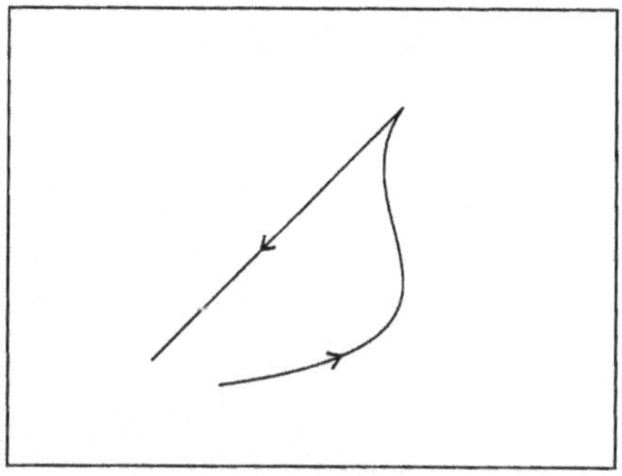

Fig. 5.6 Rheogram of bentonite magma.

Spurs

The gel formulations containing procaine pencillin gel shows a typical rheogram with a characteristic spur-like protrusion. The spur represents a sharp point of structural breakdown at low shear rate. The structure demonstrates a high yield or spur value, γ, that traces out a bowed up-curve when the three-dimensional structure breaks in the viscometer, as observed in Fig. 5.7.

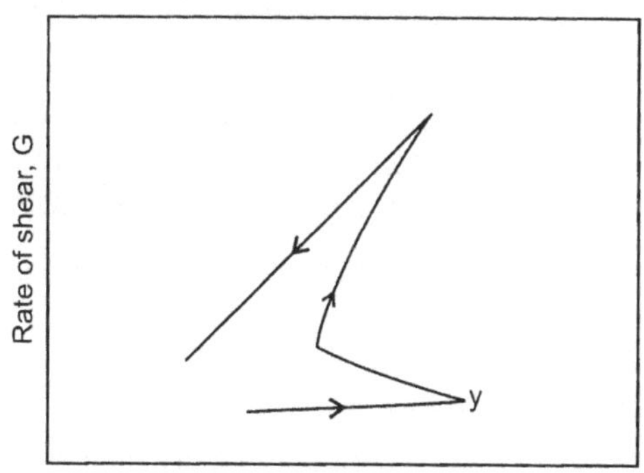

Fig. 5.7 Rheogram of procaine pencillin.

Negative Thixotropy (or) Antithixotropy

Generally thixotropic systems are shear thinning i.e., with a decrease in consistency in the down curve. But some materials like magnesia magma (1-10%) showed deviation from the suggested behaviour as shown in Fig. 5.8. The down curve falls to the right of up curve and it continously thickened and finally reached equilibrium at which the up and down curves overlapped each other. After reaching equilibrium the system was found to have gel-like property and showed greater suspendability. When allowed to stand, however, the material returned to its sol-like properties.

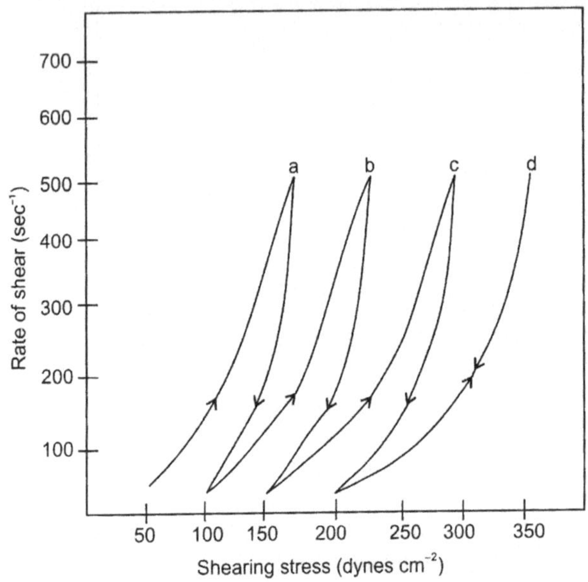

Fig. 5.8 Rhegram of antithixotropic materials.

Rheopexy

Rheopexy is a phenomenon in which solid substance forms a gel more readily when shaken gently or sheared. The system exists in gel state at equilibrium unlike antithixotropic substances which exists in sol form.

Magnesia magma and clay suspensions may show a negative rheopexy, analogons to negative thixotropy.

Thixotropy in Formulations

Various pharmaceutical dosage forms like suspensions, creams, gel, emulsions show thixotropic behaviour, which helps in easy spreadability and pourability from the containers.

For example, consider gel preparation stored in a lamitube.

The gel does not start flowing as we open the cap and invert the tube. It only starts flowing upon the application of pressure. The reason behind this is nothing but thixotropy (i.e., shear thinning).

The same principle also applies for suspensions. At rest they have high viscosity and does not allow the particles to settle down rapidly, whereas upon shaking its viscosity gets reduced and can be easily removed from the container. Thixotropy has yet another good applicability in case of procaine penicillin G in water (40-70% w/v). The structural breakdown that occurs when it passes through the syringe needle helps in easy flowability. After the injection, it restores its consistency and forms a depot at the site of injection which helps in maintaining the sustained levels of drug in the body.

Thixotropy is a time dependent phenomenon. The effects of aging should be studied so as to avoid inadequate formulation.

Viscosity Measurements

The selection of an appropriate viscometer is necessary in successful determination of viscosity. This selection depends on the type of system whose viscosity is to be determined. In the case of newtonian systems, where the shear rate is proportional to shear stress a single point viscometer can be used. It include :

(a) Capillary viscometer
(b) Falling sphere viscometer

For the measurement of viscosity in case of on non-Newtonian bodies a multipoint viscometers are used. These viscometers act at different shear rates to get the entire consistency curve. These include :

(a) Cone and plate viscometer
(b) Cup and bob viscometer

Capillary Viscometers

To determine the viscosites of the newtonian fluids capillary viscometers are mainly used. These type of viscometers act under the influence of gravity. These viscometers can be divided in to 2 types :

(a) Ostwald viscometer or U-tube viscometer
(b) Suspended level viscometer

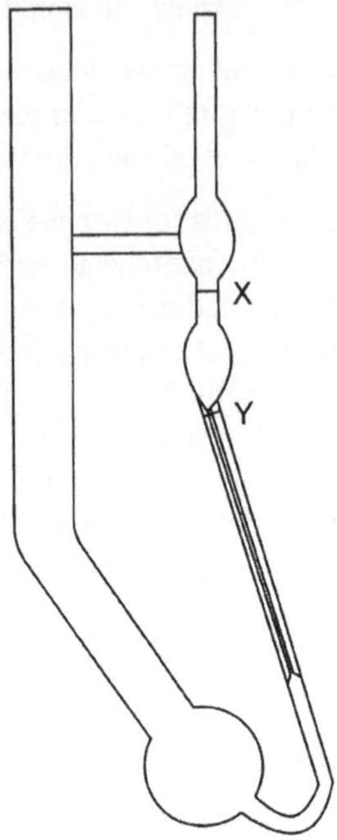

Fig. 5.9 Ostwald-Cannon-Fenske viscometer.

Ostwald Viscometer

Principle

In this the liquid is made to flow between two points X and Y as shown in Fig. 5.9. The time required for the flow is noted. The same procedure is repeated for both known sample (whose viscosity is known, generally water) and unknown sample (whose viscosity is to be determined).

The equation that governs the flow of liquids through capillary is Poiseuille's equation.

$$\eta = \frac{\pi r^4 t \, \Delta \rho}{8 l V} \qquad .....(5.6)$$

ΔP = Pressure head, dyne/cm^2.

r = radius of inside capillary (cm)

t = time of flow

l = length of capillary

V = volume of liquid flowing.

In the above Eq. (5.6). π, l, V, r are all constants. So these can be replaced by K. The pressure head Δp depends on the density of liquid being measured. So Eq. (5.6) can be written as

$$\eta_1 = K\, t_1\, \rho_1$$

Where subscript 1 denotes the material under study whose viscosity is to be determined.

Similarly, $\eta_2 = K\, t_2\, \rho_2$. [for standard].

Equating K values in both equations we get

$$\frac{\eta_1}{\rho_1\, t_1} = \frac{\eta_2}{\rho_2\, t_2}$$

$$\frac{\eta_1}{\eta_2} = \frac{\rho_1\, t_1}{\rho_2\, t_2} \qquad \text{.....(5.7)}$$

Eq. (5.7) is used for calculating the viscosity of unknown liquids. This viscometer is more suitable for liquids of low viscosity.

Falling Sphere Viscometer

It consists of glass tube, which is positioned vertically. The sample whose viscosity is to be determined is placed in the glass tube. A glass (or) steel ball is dropped into liquid as soon as the sample reaches equilibrium with that of temperature of outer jacket. The tube and jacket are then inverted, which effectively places the ball at the top of the inner glass tube.

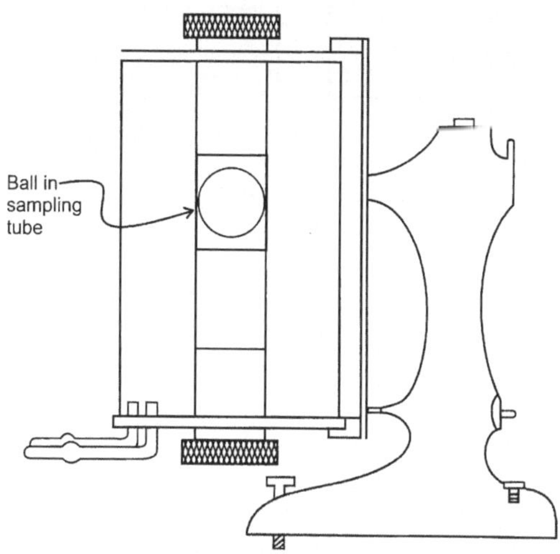

Fig. 5.10 Hoeppler falling ball viscometer.

The viscosity of fluid or liquid is directly related to the time taken by the ball to move between the two points as shown in Fig. 5.10.

Mathematically,

$$\eta = t\,(S_b - S_f)\,B. \qquad .....(5.8)$$

where,

t = time taken by the ball between two points, S_b and S_f – specific gravities of ball and fluid.

B = constant for a particular ball supplied by the manufacturer. For accurate results one should use largest possible diameter ball.

Reliable viscocity values ranging from 0.5 – 20,000 poise, depending on the nature ball can be obtained by using Hoeppler falling ball viscometer. For best results a ball whose t > 30 seconds should be used.

Cone and Plate Viscometer

In this the sample in placed in the center of plate which is then raised into a position under the cone. This can be easily understood from the Fig. 5.11.

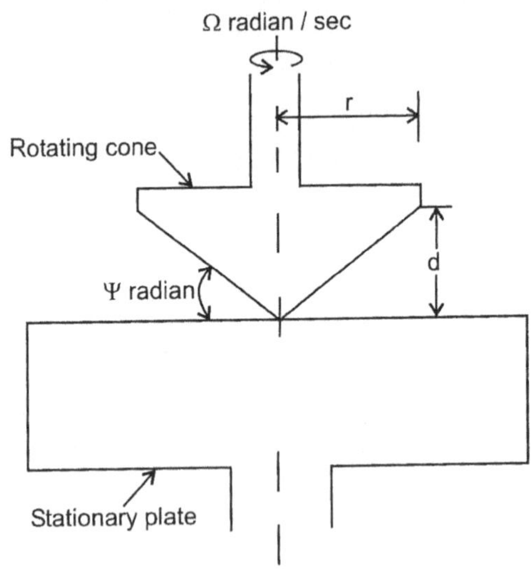

Fig. 5.11 Constant shear rate conditions in the cone and plate viscometer.

The sample is sheared in the narrow gap between the stationery plate and rotating cone. The speed of cone can be varied using variable - speed motor. The rate of shear in rpm is increased and decreased by a selector dial and the viscous traction (or) torque produced on the cone is read on the indicator scale. A plot of rpm (rate of shear) V_s scale reading (shearing stress) may thus be constructed. The Ferranti-Shirley viscometer is an example of a rotational cone and plate viscometer available commercially. The measuring unit of the apparatus/principle is shown in Fig. 5.11.

The Brook field viscometer (Searle type) is popular in quality-control laboratories.

Mathematical equation for calculating viscosity of Newtonian liquids,

$$\eta = C\left(\frac{T}{v}\right) \qquad .....(5.9)$$

C = Instrument constant

T = Torque reading

v = Speed of cone in rpm

for plastic systems it is given by

$$U = C\left(\frac{T - T_f}{v}\right) \qquad .....(5.10)$$

and the yield value is given by

$$f = C_f \times T_f$$

where,

T_f = Torque at the shearing stress axis. f (or) yield value is the product of C_f and T_f where C_f is an instrumental constant.

Cup and Bob Viscometer

This belongs to the category of rotational viscometers. It consists of a cup for holding the sample. The bob is positioned at an appropriate height as shown in Fig. 5.12.

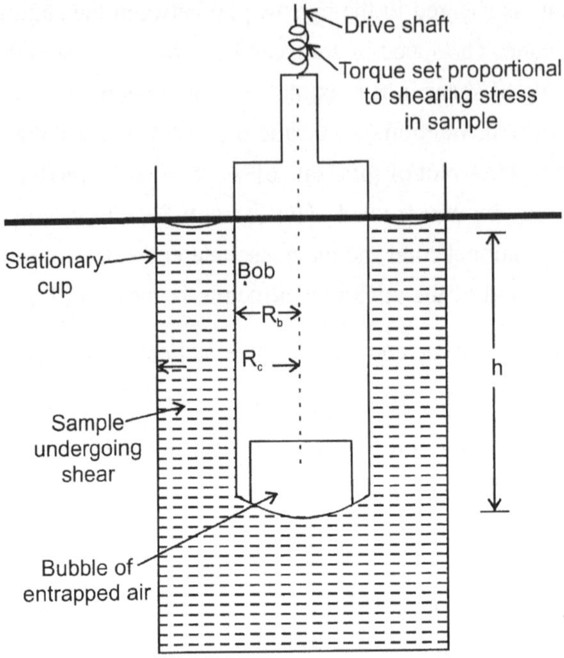

Fig. 5.12 Cup and Bob viscometer.

Sample under study is placed between the gap of cup and bob. Now either the cup or bob is made to rotate and the torque resulting from the viscous drag is measured by a spring or sensor in the drive attached to the bob.

The various instruments available differ mainly in – whether the torque set up in the bob results from the cup or from the bob being caused to revolve. Examples include :

- In the Coutte type of viscometer, the cup is rotated.
- The MacMichael viscometer,
- The Rotovisco viscometer.
- The stormer instrument etc.

The number of resolutions in (rpm) represents the rate of shear and the torque is represented by shearing stress respectively.

Apparent viscosity of a pseudoplastic system

$$\eta = K_V \left(\frac{W}{V}\right) \quad .....(5.11)$$

where,

V = rpm (or) shear rate

η = Apparent viscosity of liquid

W = Weight placed on hanger (gm)

K_V = Constant for instrument

In stormer instrument a weighed sample is placed on the hanger, and the time for the bob to make 100 revolutions is recorded by the operator. This data is converted in rpm. The whole procedure is repeated with increasing weights. A rheogram can be constructed using rpm values and weight added. We can also convert the rpm values and weight values to shear rate and shear stress values by using appropriate constants. This viscometer is not suitable for the systems with viscosity below 20 cps.

The equation for plastic viscosity when employing the Stormer viscometer

$$U = K_V \left(\frac{W - W_f}{V}\right) \quad .....(5.12)$$

in which U, is plastic viscocity in poises.

W_f is yield value intercept in grams.

The yield value of a Bingham body is obtanied by the use of expressions

$$f = K_f \times W_f$$

in which K_f is instrument constant.

Plug Flow : Cup and Bob viscometer suffers from disadvantage of plug flow, which is due to variable shear stress accross the sample i.e., the values of shear stress of the sample close to bob may be sufficiently higher than the yield value but the shear stress of the sample close to the inner wall of cup may be below the yeild value. This results in formation of solid plug and hence erratic values of viscosity. To avoid this largest bob that fits in to cup should be chosen. The plug flow is important in the flow of pastes and concentrated suspension through an orifice e.g., the extrusion of toothpaste from a tube.

Viscoelasticity

Viscoelastic measurements are based on the mechanical properties of materials that exhibit both viscous properties of liquids and elastic properties of solids. As many of the pharmaceutical products belongs to semisolids one must consider the oscillatory and creep measurements.

The instruments which are used for measuring the viscosity cause deformation in the arrangement of material. So, viscoelasticity is designed instead not to destroy the structure. This helps in knowing the intermolecular and interparticle forces.

For a Newtonian fluid of semisolid nature

$$\eta = \frac{F}{G}$$

But according to Hooke's law a solid material can be characterized by elasticity. So,

$$E = \frac{F}{\gamma} \quad .....(5.13)$$

where,

E = Elastic Modulus (dyne.cm^{-2})

F = Stress (dyne cm^{-2})

γ = Strain (dimension less)

Using a mechanical model, a viscous fluid may be represented as movement of a piston in a cylinder (or) dashpot filled with a liquid, as seen in Fig. 5.13. An elastic solid is modeled by movement of Hooke's spring. The combination of both Dashpot and spring in series is called as Maxwell unit. A combination of dashpot and spring in parallel is called Voigt element as seen in Fig. 5.14.

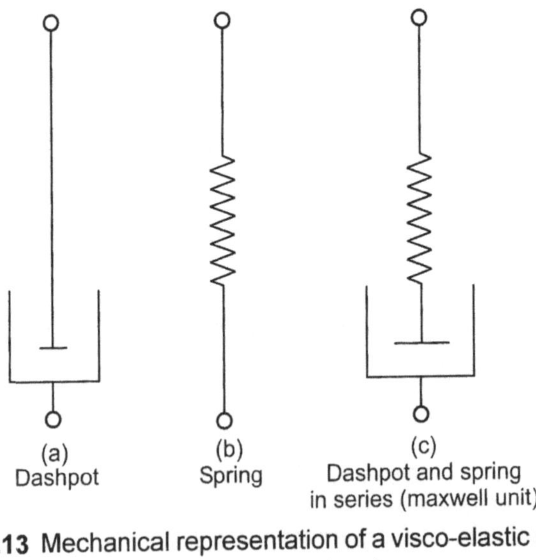

Fig. 5.13 Mechanical representation of a visco-elastic material using a dashpot and spring.

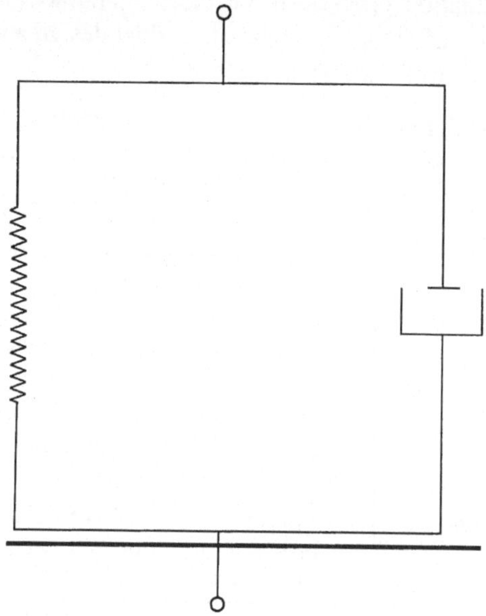

Fig. 5.14 Dashpot and spring in parallel as a mechanical model (Voigt element).

Applications

Viscosity of a sample is an important physical parameter in pharmaceutical industry and research. It is used as quality control tool for evaluation of flow properties of various dosage forms such as ointments, emulsions, suspensions and capsule manufacturing. Cellulose derivatives like sodium carboxy methyl cellulose, hydroxy propyl methyl cellulose etc., are widely used to increase viscosity. In designing equipment in productions operations such as mixing, filling into bottles, flow through pipes etc; the knowledge of viscosity of liquid is helpful. Viscosity can also be used to confirm the structure of certain compounds.

Polymer solutions may be used in ophthalmic preparations, as wetting solution for contact lens and as tear replacement solution (dry eye syndrome). Both natural (e.g., dextran) and synthetic (e.g., polyvinyl alcohol) are used. The rheological properties of suppositories at rectal temperatures can influence the release and bioabsorption of drugs from suppositories, particularly those having fatty base. One study indicated the rheological properties as a function of the temperature of mineral oil-water emulsions with triethanolamine stearate (TEAs). The rheology is important in cosmetics, granulation process in the tablet manufacturing, suspending agent. A summary of the major areas of product design and processing in which rheology is useful are given in Table 5.1.

Table 5.1 Use of Rhelogy in pharmaceutical area.

Pharmaceutical Area	Use of Rheology
1. Processing	Production capacity of the equipment processing efficiency
2. Solids	Flow of powder in tablet/capsule manufacturing, packagability of powdered or granular solids.
3. Fluids	Mixing, particle size reduction, passage through orifices, fluid transfer, physical stability etc.
4. Quasisolids	Spreading and adherence on the skin, removal from tubes, release of the drug from base etc.

Problems

1. The viscosity of given sample was measured using an Ostwald viscometer and found to have viscosity of 0.403 cp at 25 °C. Its density at 25 °C is 0.877 g/cm^3 · Compute the kinematic viscosity of given sample at 25 °C.

   Solution : Data given

   $\eta = 0.403$ cp and $\rho = 0.877$ g/cc

   Equation for kinematic viscosity

   $$\frac{\eta}{\rho} = \frac{0.403}{0.877}$$

   $$= 0.4595 \text{ Centistokes.}$$

2. The viscosities of water and acetone were determined with the help of capillary viscometer and found to have 0.8904 cp and 0.313 cp respectively. Compute the realtive viscosity of acetone.

   Solution : Data given

   Viscosity of accetone : 0.313 cp

   Viscosity of water : 0.8904 cp.

Equation for relative viscosity

$$\eta_{rel} = \frac{\text{Viscosity of acetone}}{\text{Viscosity of water}}$$

$$= \frac{0.313}{0.8904} = 0.3515 \text{ [dimensionless]}$$

3. A plastic material has shown the yield value of 1700 dynes cm^{-1}. If the rate of shear was 130 sec^{-1}, when shearing stress was 4700 dynes cm^{-1}, calculate U, the plastic viscosity of given sample.

Solution : Data given

$F = 4700$ dynes cm^{-1},

$G = 130$ Sec^{-1},

$f = 1700$ dynes cm^{-1}

Equation for plastic viscosity

$$U = \frac{(F - f)}{G}$$

$$= \frac{4700 - 1700}{130} = \frac{3000}{130} = 23.07 \text{ poise.}$$

4. The viscosity of a 2% W/V solution of a given sample (MW = 26,000) is 150 cps. The water is ordinarily used as a standard for viscosity of liquids and is 0.8904 cp at 25 °C.

Calculate the relative viscosity, specific viscosity and reduced viscosity of given sample.

Solution : Data given

Viscosity of water $= \eta_o = 0.8904$ cp,

Viscosity of sample $= \eta = 150$ cps,

Concentration = 2% W/V.

Equation for relative viscosity

$$\eta_{rel} = \frac{\eta}{\eta_o}$$

$$= \frac{150}{0.8904} = 168.46 \text{ [dimensionless]}$$

Equation for specific viscosity

$$\eta_{sp} = \frac{\eta - \eta_o}{\eta_o}$$

$$= \frac{150 - 0.8904}{0.8904} = 167.46 \text{ [dimensionless]}$$

Equation for reduced viscosity

$$\eta_{red.} = \frac{\eta_{sp}}{C}$$

$$= \frac{167.46}{2} = 83.73$$

5. The time flow for water through Ostwald viscometer was found to be 60 sec and liquid A is 25 sec. If densities of water and liquid A at 25 °C are 1.0 and 0.787 gm/cc respectively, calculate the viscosity of liquid A.

Soultion : Data given

t_1 = 25 sec, t_2 = 60 sec

ρ_1 = 0.787 g/cc, ρ_2 = 1 g/cc.

η_2 = 1.002 cp.

Equation for viscosity

$$\eta_1 = \frac{\rho_1 \, t_1}{\rho_2 \, t_2} \times \eta_2$$

$$\eta_1 = \frac{0.787 \times 25}{1 \times 60} \times 1.002$$

$$= 0.3285 \text{ cps.}$$

CHAPTER 6

Diffusion and Dissolution

Diffusion is a process which involves the mass transfer of individual molecules of a substance brought about by random molecular motion. It mainly depends on concentration gradient of the substance or drug under study.

The study of diffusion is very important in knowing passage of gases, drug, water vapour and excipients through the walls of packing. It also helps in studying the release of drug entity from the ointments, gels, suppository bases and permeation of these molecules through the skin.

The passage of matter through a barrier or membrane may occur by simple molecular permeation or by movement through the pores. Both the processes mentioned above require the dissolution of drug entity in the bulk of membrane or in the solvent-filled pores of membrane. Molecular diffusion or permeation through nonporous media depends on dissolution of the permeating molecules in the bulk membrane.

The process of diffusion depends on many variables like concentration gradient, size and shape of diffusing molecules, area of membranes involved in the process, type of membrane and affinity of diffusing molecules to the membrane. The relation will be dealt in detail in the later part of our discussion.

Dialysis : It is the separation process based on unequal rates of passage of solutes and solvent through microporous membranes, carried out in batch or continous mode. The apparatus used is called dialysis.

For example hemodialysis is used in kidney malfunction to get rid off metabolic waste products from blood.

Osmosis : It is the passage of solvent across a membrane which is semipermeable in nature. Osmosis is a greek term "Osmos" means to "push". If we consider a pure solvent and a solution separated by a membrane which selectively allows the passage of solvent molecules and not solute molecules, then the solvent molecules will slowly diffuse through the membrane. In terms of concentration gradient osmosis is exactly opposite to diffusion process as in diffusion the flow of molecules will be from higher concentration to lower concentration, whereas in osmosis the molecules move from lower concentration to higher concentration as shown in the Fig. 6.1(a) and 6.1(b).

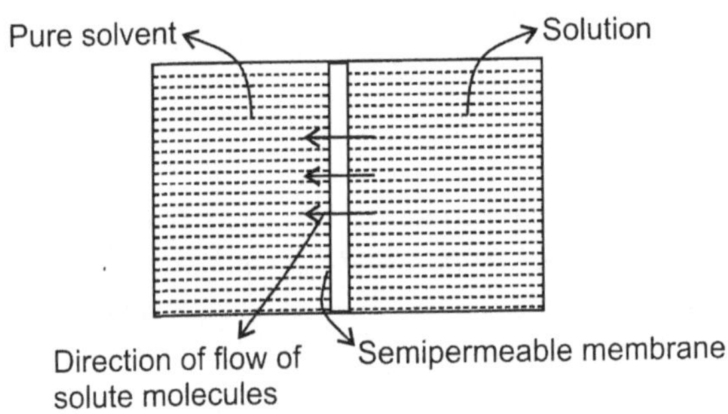

Fig. 6.1(a) Diffusion process.

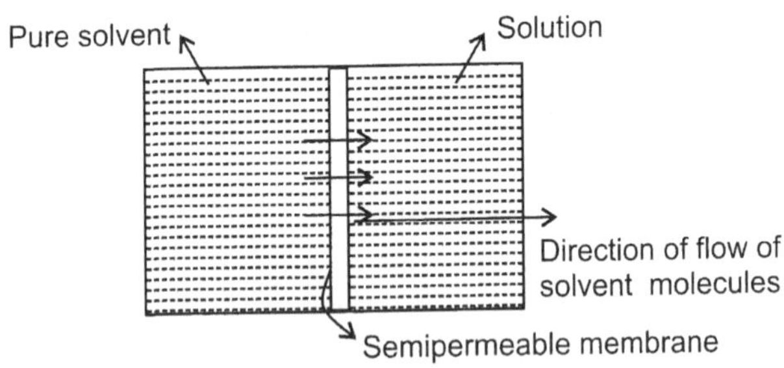

Fig. 6.1(b) Osmosis process.

Ultrafiltration : This is the separation of sol particle and macromolecules from a liquid medium by filtration through an ultrafilter. It involves the use of hydraulic or gas pressure to force the solvent molecules through the membrane. While microporons membrane prevents the passage of large solute molecules.

Ultrafiltration is used in the pulp and paper industry and in research to purify albumin and enzymes. A membrane is a film separating the phases, and material passes by passive, active or facilitated transport across the film.

Laws of Diffusion

Fick's First Law

The amount of material (M) flowing through a unit cross-sectional area (S) of a membrane in unit time (t) is denoted by the term flux, J.

So mathematically

$$J = \frac{dM}{S.dt} \quad .....(6.1)$$

In terms of concentration gradient we can say that

$$J \propto -\frac{dc}{dx} \quad .....(6.2)$$

where, $\frac{dc}{dx}$ is the concentration gradient.

The negative sign indicates that diffusion process occurs in a direction opposite to that of increasing concentration. Thus, flux is always a positive quantity.

The Eq. (6.2) can be equated by placing a constant.

So $$J = -D\frac{dc}{dx} \quad .....(6.3)$$

where, D is the diffusion coefficient of solute molecule with units cm^2/sec. The concentration c is expressed in g/cm^3 and x is given in cm. The units of J are g cm^{-2} sec^{-1}. The value of D depends mainly on concentration gradient and apart from this other parameters like temperature, pressure, nature of solvent, nature of solute, membrane properties also affect the value. Equation (6.3) is known as Fick's first law.

Fick's Second Law

This emphasizes on variation of the solute concentration at the barrier (or) membrane with time. According to this law the change in the concentration of the solute with time $\left(\frac{dc}{dt}\right)$ is equal to the change in flux with distance $\frac{dJ}{dx}$.

So mathematically,

$$\frac{dc}{dt} = \frac{-dJ}{dx} \qquad \text{.....(6.4)}$$

But $$J = -D\frac{dc}{dx} \qquad \text{[From Eq. (6.3)]}$$

Substituting in Eq. (6.4)

$$\frac{dc}{dt} = D\frac{d^2c}{dx^2} \qquad \text{.....(6.5)}$$

Eq. (6.5) represents the Fick's second law in one direction x. For the changes in the concentration along x, y and z axis the Eq. (6.5) can be generalized as below.

$$\frac{dc}{dt} = D\left(\frac{d^2c}{dx^2} + \frac{d^2c}{dy^2} + \frac{d^2c}{dz^2}\right) \qquad \text{.....(6.6)}$$

Measurement of Diffusion

Generally diffusion cells are used for carrying out the measurement of diffusion.

A diffusion cell consists of two chambers as shown in Fig. 6.2 (a).

(a) Donor chamber (b) Receptor chamber

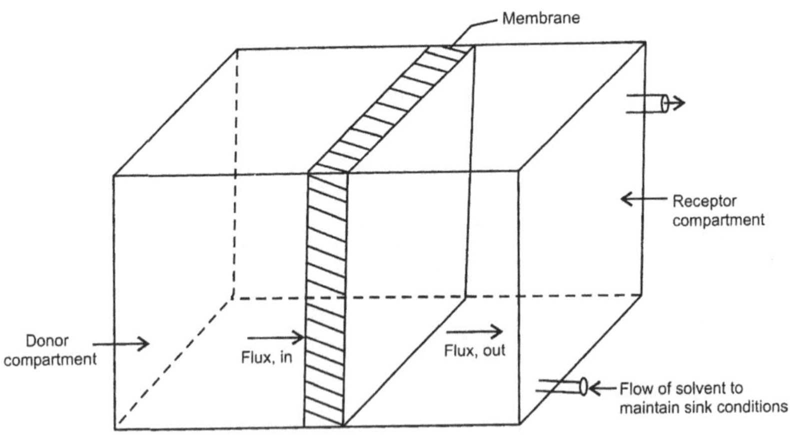

Fig. 6.2 (a) Diffusion cell.

The two chambers are separated by a membrane through which diffusion takes place.

The receptor chamber has sampling port which is used in taking out samples and replacing it again with same quantity of fresh solvent. The receptor chamber's temperature is maintained at $37^{o} \pm 0.5$ °C using a water jacket. The stirrer helps in mixing the contents thoroughly. Generally Teflon-coated magnetic beads are employed for stirring.

Concept of Steady State

As we have discussed earlier that diffusion is basically a mass transfer process. So the mass transfer from the donor compartment to receptor compartment takes place till the concentration of diffusant remains constant in both compartment with respect to time, but obviously not the same in the two compartments. This state is referred to as steady state. During the steady state if we consider any plane perpendicular to direction of flow the change in rate of concentration becomes zero.

So the Eq. (6.5) of Fick's second law becomes

$$\frac{dc}{dt} = D\,\frac{d^2c}{dx^2} = 0 \qquad .....(6.7)$$

The Eq. (6.7) demonstrates that since D is not equal to zero, $\frac{d^2c}{dx^2} = 0$.

So from this we can say that at steady state the concentration (c) versus distance (x) graph gives a straight line.

Let us consider a membrane of thickness 'h' that separates two compartments as shown in Fig. 6.2 (b).

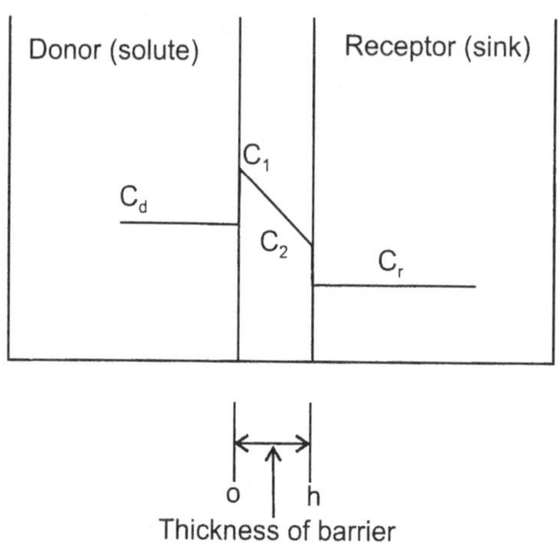

Fig. 6.2 (b) Concentration gradient of diffusant.

From the Ficks law we can state that

$$\frac{dM}{sdt} = \frac{D(C_{d1} - C_{r1})}{h} \qquad .....(6.8)$$

The partition coefficient of the diffusant is the ratio of concentration in lipid phase to concentration in aqueous phase.

So,

$$K = \frac{C_{d1}}{C_d} = \frac{C_{r2}}{C_r} \qquad .....(6.9)$$

$$\Rightarrow C_{d1} = KC_d \text{ and } C_{r2} = KC_r$$

Substituting in Eq. (6.8) we will get,

$$\frac{dM}{dt} = \frac{S\,D\,KC_d}{h}(C_d - C_r)$$

If sink conditions are maintained Cr $\cong$ 0

$$\frac{dM}{dt} = \frac{S\,D\,KC_d}{h}$$

In the Eq. (6.10) the terms $\frac{DK}{h}$ in which D represents diffusion coefficient $\left(\frac{cm^2}{sec}\right)$, K (partition coefficient) and h (thickness in cm) can be replaced by constant P.

i.e.,

$$P = DK/h \ (cm/sec) \qquad .....(6.10)$$

So the Eq. (6.10) will becomes

$$\frac{dM}{dt} = PSC_d$$

P is called as permeability coefficient. It has unit of linear velocity $\left(\frac{cm}{sec}\right)$. During steady state one can obtain the value of J (apparent flux) by plotting a graph of M Vs t.

where, M = amount of drug permeated through unit area,

T = time taken for permeation.

The other values can be calculated by using following equations :

$$P = \text{permeability coefficient} = \frac{J_{ss}}{C_d}.$$

When amount of drug permeated through skin is plotted against time the curve of Fig. 6.3 is convex to the time axis in the early stage and then becomes linear. Early stage (non-steady-state) and at later time it becomes steady state. When the steady state portion of the line extrapolated to the time axis the point of intersection is known as lag time. t_L. Mathematically

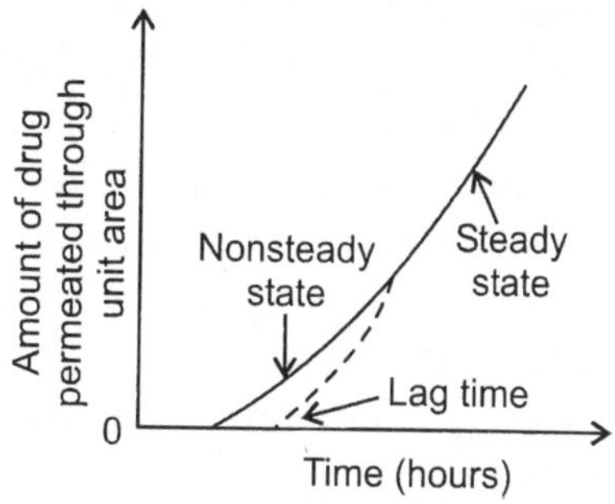

Fig. 6.3 Drug permeation curve.

The log time, $t_L = \frac{h^2}{6D}$ in which D is diffusivity combining the permeability Eq. (6.10) one can calculate partition coefficient.

$$\text{Partition coefficient} = K = \frac{Ph}{D}.$$

Lag time (t_L) is the time required for the diffusant to establish a uniform concentration gradient in the membrane. Graphically it is obtained by extrapolating the steady state curve to x-axis as represented in the Fig. 6.3.

Dissolution Studies

Dissolution is a process of mass transfer from the solid into the solvent. It is an important quality control parameter. When any solid dosage form is introduced into a beaker of water the following stages are involved before the drug gets into solution completely.

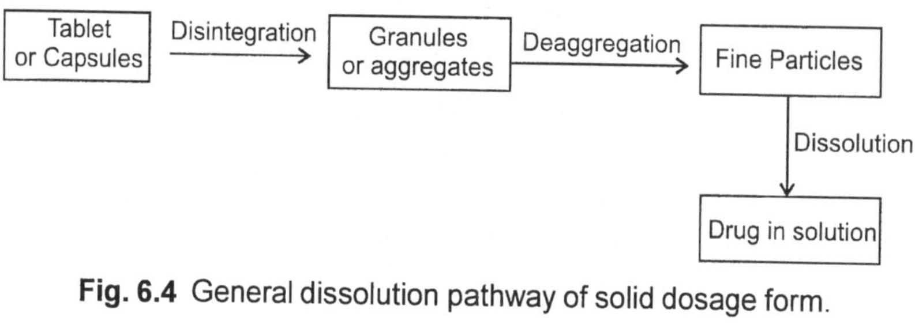

Fig. 6.4 General dissolution pathway of solid dosage form.

The rate at which the dissolution process takes place is quantified by Noyes and Whitney (1897) and may be written as

$$\frac{dM}{dt} = \frac{DS}{h}(C_1 - C_2) \quad .....(6.11)$$

where M is mass solute, t is time, h is thickness, S is surface area of exposed solid, D is diffusion coefficient of the solute in solution, C_1 refers to the solubility of solid (or) concentration of drug at the surface of solid and C_2 refers to concentration of drug in solution. Dissolution testing was made official in USP XVIII in 1970. It also recognizes dissolution testing as a tool for quality control. Dissolution plays a very important role in making the active ingredient available to the body. The dissolution had its origin with a simple beaker type apparatus. The official apparatus used for dissolution testing include:-

(a) Rotating Basket Apparatus (USP Apparatus 1)

It comprises of a round bottomed beaker generally made of glass and having a capacity of 1000 ml. The cylindrical basket is made up of 22 mesh and is attached to a motor with the help of a shaft. The speed of shaft can be adjusted as per requirement. This entire system is immersed in a water bath whose temperature in maintained at 37 $\pm$ 0.5°C as shown in the Fig. 6.5. All the metal parts used are made of stainless steel 316. The basket is held at a distance of 2 cm above from the bottom of vessel.

This is generally used for solid dosage forms

(b) Rotating Paddle Apparatus (USP Apparatus 2)

It consists of rotating paddle usually coated with an inert material.

Vessel: cylindrical,

Height: 160-210 mm

Inside diameter: 98-106 mm

Nominal capacity: 1000 mL (sides are flanged at the top)

Shaft: positioned so that its axis is not more than 2 mm at any point from the vertical axis of the vessel and rotates smoothly and without significant wobble.

Materials of Construction: Shaft and blade are a single entity that may be coated with a suitable inert coating.

Blade position: the distance between the inside bottom of the vessel and the blade is maintained at 25 +/- 2 mm during the test. The blade passes through the diameter of the shaft so that the bottom of the blade is flush with the bottom of the shaft. This is generally used for solid dosage forms

(c) Reciprocating cylinder type (USP Apparatus 3)

Reciprocating cylinder moves upward and downward through a total distance of 9.9- 10.1 cm.

Materials of Construction: stainless steel, type 316 or equivalent.

Generally used for extended release dosage forms

(d) Flow-Through Cell (USP Apparatus 4)

Materials of Construction: composed of inert and transparent mounted vertically with a filter system (prevents escape of undissolved particles from the top of cell). Tube connections are made up of polytef tubing with 1.6-mm diameter flanged-end connections.

Cell Assembly: Cell diameters are 12 and 22.6 mm and the cell assembly is fixed using a clamp mechanism and two O-rings.

(e) Paddle over disk (USP Apparatus 5)

Vessel: cylindrical.

Height: 160-210 mm

Inside diameter: 98-106 mm

Nominal capacity: 1000 mL (sides are flanged at the top)

Shaft: positioned so that its axis is not more than 2 mm at any point from the vertical axis of the vessel

Materials of Construction: Shaft and blade are a single entity that may be coated with a suitable inert coating. Disk assembly is stainless steel.

Blade Position: the distance between the surface of the disk assembly and the blade is maintained at 25 +/- 2 mm during the test.

The disk assembly holds the system flat and is positioned such that the release surface is parallel with the bottom of the paddle blade.

Used for transdermal delivery systems

Use paddle and vessel from Apparatus 2 with a stainless steel disk assembly to hold the transdermal on the bottom of vessel. The temperature is generally maintained at 32°C during the study

(f) Cylinder type apparatus *(USP* Apparatus 6)

Vessel: cylindrical

Height: 60-210 mm

Inside diameter: 98-106 mm

Nominal capacity: 1000 mL (sides are flanged at the top)

Shaft: positioned so that its axis is not more than 2 mm at any point from the vertical axis of the vessel

Materials of Construction: Cylinder stirring element type 316 stainless steel

Cylinder Position: distance between the inside bottom of the vessel and the cylinder is maintained at 25 +/- 2 mm during the test.

Similar to Apparatus 1 except replace the basket shaft with a stainless steel cylinder element.

Used for transdermal delivery system and temperature is generally maintained at 32°C during the study

(g) Reciprocating Holder (USP Apparatus 7)

Used for transdermal delivery systems and also a variety of dosage forms

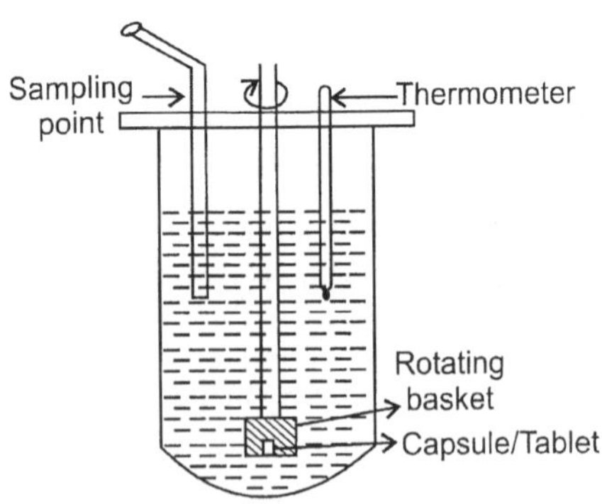

Fig. 6.5(a) USP dissolution apparatus I.

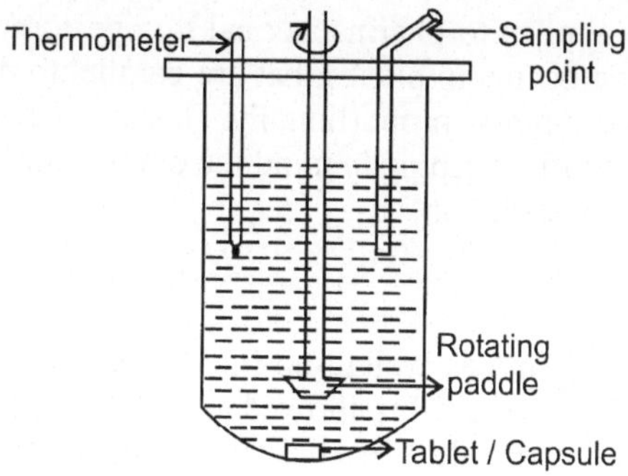

Fig. 6.5(b) USP dissolution apparatus II.

USP apparati

Apparatus 1 (baskct)

Apparatus 2 (paddle)

Apparatus 3 (reciprocating cylinder)

Apparatus 4 (flow-through cell)

Apparatus 5 (paddle over disk)

Apparatus 6 (cylinder)

Apparatus 7 (reciprocating holder)

Hixson–Crowell Cube Root Law

In the Noyes-Whitney equation no term regarding the area of the dosage form is mentioned, assuming that it is constant. So the Hixson - Crowell Cube Root law is introduced, on the basis of assumption that Arca (A) = K $M^{2/3}$, where, K is a constant which comprises of shape and density factor. M is the mass of undissolved drug. The final equation is given by

$$M_0^{1/3} - M^{1/3} = Kt. \qquad .....(6.12)$$

where,

M_o = Initial mass of drug taken.

M = Mass of undissolved drug.

K = Cube Root rate constant incorporating surface-volume relation.

T = Time taken

Eq. (6.12) is known as the *Hixson-Crowell cube root law.*

This expression applies to pharmaceutical dosage forms like tablets, where the dissolution occurs in planes that are parallel to drug surface if the tablet dimensions diminish proportionally. This model has been used to describe the release profile keeping in mind the diminishing surface of the drug particles during dissolution.

Problems

1. A sample of granules weighting 0.65 g having surface area of 0.32 m^2 (0.32×10^4 cm^2) is allowed to dissolve in 500 ml water at 25 °C. After first minute 0.76 g has passed into solution. If solubility C_s of the drug is 20 mg/ml. D/h in Noyes-Whitney equation to Fick's first law may be reffered to as a dissolution rate constant K. Calculate the dissolution rate constant.

   Solution : Data given

   Weight of granules : 0.65 g

   Surface area of granules = 0.32 m^2.

   Solubility C_s of drug = 15 mg/ml.

   Equation $$\frac{dM}{dt} = \frac{DSC_s}{h}.$$

   $$\frac{dM}{dt} = \frac{760 \text{ mg}}{60 \text{ sec}} = 12.67 \text{ mg/sec.}$$

   So, $$12.67 = K \times 0.32 \times 10^4 \text{ cm}^2 \times 15 \text{ mg/cm}^3$$

   $$12.67 = K \times 4.8 \times 10^4 \text{ cm}^3$$

   $$K = 2.6395 \times 10^{-4} \text{ cm/sec.}$$

2. As given in example 1 above, the diffusion layer thickness is estimated to be 6×10^{-3} cm. Compute D the diffusion coefficient, using relation $K = \frac{D}{h}$.

   Solution : Data given.

   $$K = 2.63 \times 10^{-4} \text{ cm/sec.}$$

   $$h = 6 \times 10^{-3} \text{ cm}$$

   Equation for $$K = \frac{D}{h}$$

   So $$D = (2.63 \times 10^{-4} \text{ cm/sec}) \times (6 \times 10^{-3} \text{ cm})$$

   $$= 1.5 \times 10^{-6} \text{ cm}^2\text{/sec.}$$

CHAPTER 7

Colloids

Colloids [Gr., = glue like], a mixture in which one substance is divided into minute particles and dispersed throughout a second substance. *The dispersed system consist of particulate matter, known as the dispersed phase, distributed throughout a continuous or dispersion medium. The mixture is also called a Colloidal system, colloidal solution or colloidal dispersion.*

Graham Thomas (1861) classified the matter into two types, *crystalloids and colloids* on the basis of the ability of dissolved substances to diffuse into water across a semipermeable membrane. Crystalloids or crystalline substances such as sugar, urea, sodium chloride passed through membrane, while others or colloids like glue, gelatin and gum arabic did not. Familiar colloids include smoke, homogenized milk, fog and ruby-colored glass.

Colloidal systems or the colloidal dispersions are intermediate between true solutions (size less than 10 $\overset{o}{A}$ or 1nm) and suspension (size more than 2000 $\overset{o}{A}$ or 0.5 µm). When the diameter of the particles of a substance dispersed in a solvent ranges from about 1 nm (10 $\overset{o}{A}$) to 0.5 µm (2000 $\overset{o}{A}$), the system is termed as colloidal solution or colloid.

Colloidal particles are larger than molecules but too small to be observed directly with a microscope; however, their shape and sizes can be determined by electron microscopy. The colloidal particles may have different shapes and sizes. The more extended the particle, the greater its specific surface and the greater attractive forces. A colloidal particles in a friendly environment, unrolls and exposes maximum surface area. Under adverse conditions, it rolls up and reduces its exposed area. Some important shapes are shown in Fig. 7.1.

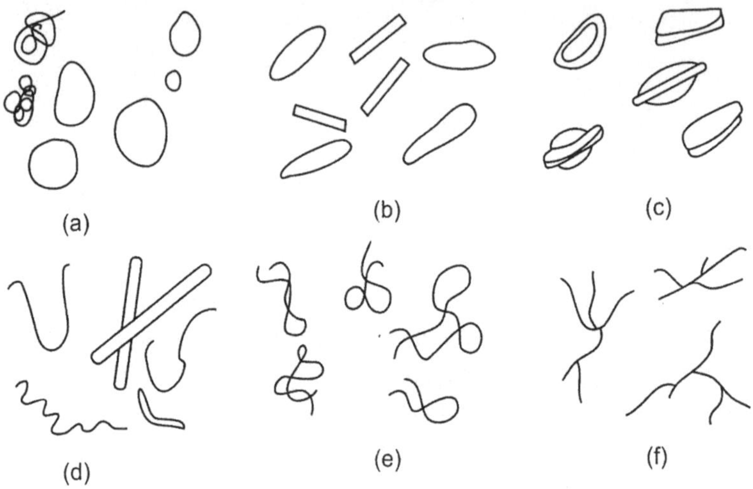

Fig. 7.1 Some shapes that may be assumed by colloidal particles: (a) spheres and globules (b) short rods and prolate ellipsoids (c) oblate ellipsoids and flakes (d) long rods and threads (e) loosely coiled threads (f) branched threads.

Purification of Colloids : The Colloidal dispersion may contain soluble or insoluble impurities. Insoluble impurities can be removed by filtration method. Many hydrosols contain low molecular-weight, water soluble impurities. Salt may create the problem since it may tend to coagulate such dispersions. These dissolved impurities of small molecular size are removed by means of membrane with pore openings smaller than the colloidal particles.

The purification of sols can be accomplished by three methods :

(a) Dialysis

(b) Electrodialysis

(c) Ultra filtration

(a) ***Dialysis :*** Mostly membranes in current use consist of cellulose nitrate prepared from collodion, cellulose acetate, synthetic polymers, animal membrane or those made up of parchment paper and cellophane sheet, are available in a variety of shapes, gauges and pore sizes. Because of their size, colloidal particles may be separated from molecular particles, the technique of separation, known as dialysis, uses a semipermeable membrane, the pore size of which will prevent the passage of colloidal particles but will permit small particles or molecules such as urea, glucose, sodium chloride etc.

The principle of dialysis is illustrated in Fig. 7.2 which shows that at equilibrium, the colloidal material retained in compartment A, while subcolloidal material is distributed equally on both the side of membrane. By continually removing the liquid in compartment B, we will get pure colloid in compartment A.

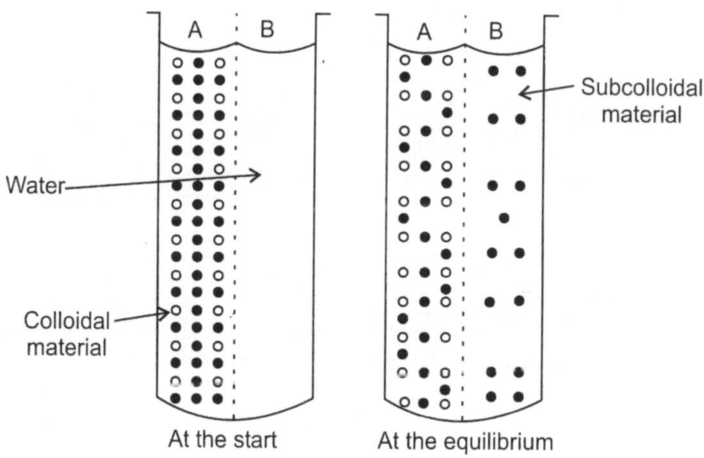

Fig. 7.2 Removal of electrolytes from colloidal material by diffusion.

Dialysis can be carried out by batch process or continuous process as shown in Fig. 7.3 and Fig. 7.4.

In the batch process the sol is placed inside a cellophane sac dipping in water. The small solute molecules diffuse out into the water while the colloidal material remains trapped inside because of its size. The batch process is illustrated in Fig. 7.3.

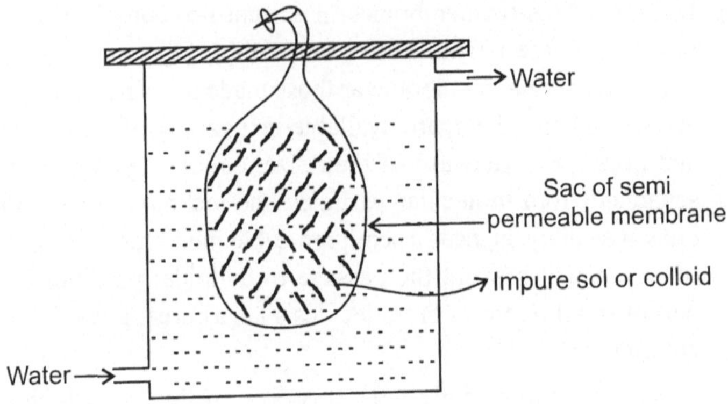

Fig. 7.3 Batch process dialyser.

In the continuous process a cellophane tube is placed in water and from one side colloidal solution is added and pure colloidal solution is collected from other end as shown in Fig. 7.4.

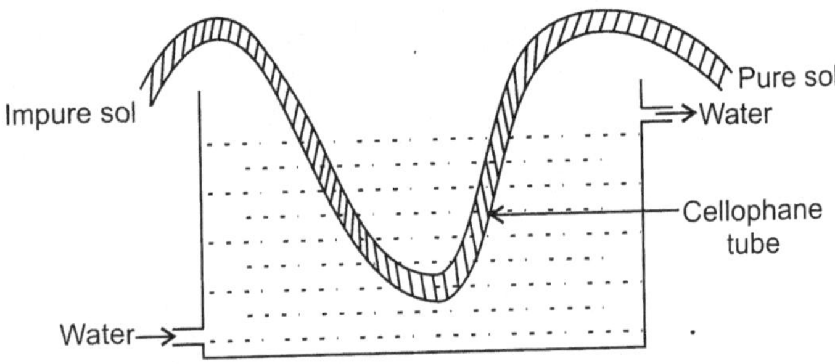

Fig. 7.4 Continuous process dialyser.

The process of removing ions (or molecules) from a sol by diffusion through a semipermeable membrane is called dialysis.

(b) ***Electrodialysis :*** If the low molecular-weight impurities to be removed are electrolytes, dialysis is carried out under the influence of electric field; the dialysis can be speeded up by applying an electric potential to the sol which produces electrolysis. For electrodialysis an electrodialyzer as shown in Fig. 7.5 is used. It consists of three compartments with two membranes supported by screens. Under the influence of the applied potential, anions migrate from the solution into the anode compartment while cations migrate into the cathode compartment.

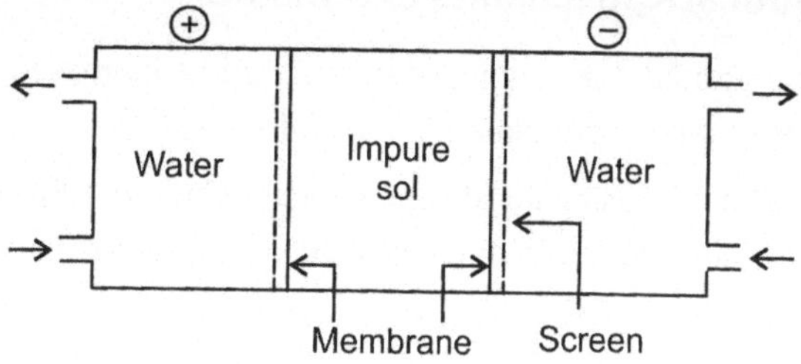

Fig. 7.5 Electrodialysis.

(c) ***Ultrafiltration :*** Solution can pass through an ordinary filter paper. When a sol is placed in a compartment closed by a dialysis membrane and pressure is applied, the liquid and small molecules are forced through membrane while the colloidal particles are retained. This process is called ultrafiltration as shown in Fig. 7.6.

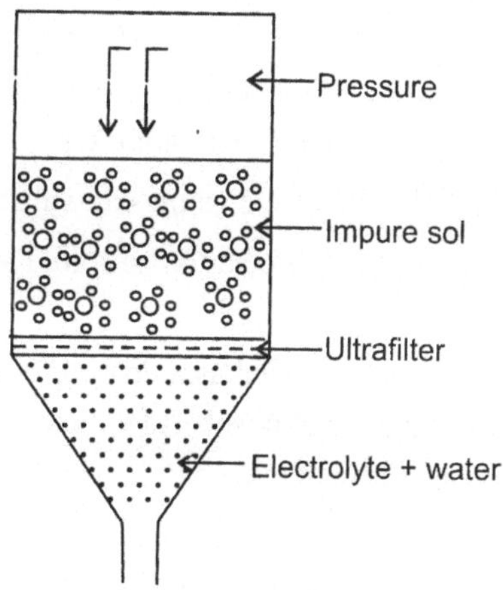

Fig. 7.6 Ultrafiltration.

Ultrafiltration is a slow process. The pressure difference required to push the dispersion medium through ultrafilter is provided by the gas pressure applied on sol side or by suction on the filter side. The membrane is supported by fine wire screen.

Dialysis occurs in our body i.e., *in vivo*. The ions and small molecules pass readily from the blood, through natural semipermeable membrane, to the tissue fluid. The colloidal components of blood remain within capillary system. This principle is utilized in the artificial kidney.

Pharmaceutical Applications of Colloids

- Some colloidal dispersions show unusual or increased therapeutic properties when formulated in the colloidal state.

  Ex : Colloidal silver chloride (germicidal), Colloidal silver iodide and silver proteins are effective germicides and do not cause irritation.

  Colloidal copper has been used in the treatment of cancer, colloidal gold as diagnostic agent for paresis and colloidal mercury for syphilis.
- Colloidal sulphur shows better and faster absorption than coarse dispersion of sulphur.
- Solubility of some drugs is improved by using colloidal systems containing surface active agents.

  Ex : Solubility of sulfonamides.
- Proteins are important natural colloids and are found in various parts of body like component of muscle, bone and skin.
- Naturally occurring plant molecules such as starch and cellulose that are used as pharmaceutical adjuncts.
- Hydroxyethyl starch is used as plasma substitute.
- Surface active agents (association colloids) are used to improve the stability of drugs.
- Synthetic polymers are used as a coating material for solid dosage form to protect it from atmospheric moisture and degradation under acid conditions of the stomach.
- In the formulation of new drug delivery systems colloids are used in targeting the drugs to specific body organs.

Classification of Dispersion Systems

The dispersion systems are classified as molecular dispersion, colloidal dispersion and coarse dispersion on the basis of particle size of the dispersed phase. Molecular dispersion is also called as true solution and coarse dispersion is called as suspension.

A comparative properties of molecular dispersion, colloidal dispersion and coarse dispersion are given in the Table 7.1.

Table 7.1 A comparison of various types of dispersions.

Sr.No	Property	Molecular Dispersion	Colloidal Dispersion	Coarse Dispersion
1.	Size	Less than 1.0 nm	1nm to 0.5 μm	Greater than 0.5 μm
2.	State	Monophasic (Homogeneous)	Biphasic (Heterogeneous)	Biphasic (Heterogeneous)
3.	Visibility	Invisible in electron microscope	Not resolved by ordinary microscope	Visible under microscope
4.	Appea-rance	Clear	Clear	Opaque
5.	Settling	Does not settle under gravity	Does not settle under gravity	Settles under gravity
6.	Filteration	Pass through ultrafilter or perchment membrane	Do not pass through semipermeable membrane	Do not pass through normal filter paper
7.	Diffusion	Rapid diffusion	Diffusion slowly	No diffusion
8.	Brownian Motion	Particles have constant kinetic motion	Particles shows Brownian motion	Particles shows negligible motion
9.	Scattering of light	Do not scatter light. Tyndall effect not observed	Shows scattering of light. Tyndall effect observed.	Shows scattering of light. Tyndall effect observed.
10.	Examples	Oxygen moleculco, ordinary ions glucose etc	Silver sol Natural and Synthetic sols	Emulsions suspensions, Red Blood cells

Types of Colloidal Systems

Ostwald classified the colloidal dispersions on the basis of the affinity or interaction between the dispersed phase and dispersion medium. According to this classification, colloidal dispersions are divided into three groups :

(a) Lyophilic Colloids

(b) Lyophobic Colloids

(c) Association Colloids

(a) ***Lyophilic Colloids :*** Lyophilic sols are those in which the dispersed phase exhibits a definite affinity for the medium or the solvent. It is also called *solvent-loving*. If the dispersion medium is water, the system is said to be hydrophilic.

Ex : Dispersion of starch, gum and protein in water.

The dispersed particles may be hydrophilic or lipophilic (such as rubber and polystyrene). Dispersion of rubber or polystyrene can be prepared in organic solvents such as benzene is referred as lyophilic sol. When water is used as dispersion medium, the dispersions are referred as hydrophilic colloids. These colloids are thermodynamically stable. These sols are ususally obtained simply by dissolving the material in the solvent being used. They may or may not have charge.

(b) ***Lyophobic Colloids :*** Lyophobic colloids are composed of materials that have little attraction for dispersion medium. These are also called as solvent-hating systems. This is primarily due to the absence of a solvent sheath around the particles. They generally consist of inorganic particles dispersed in water.

Ex : Dispersion of gold, iron hydroxide, sulphur, arsenous sulphide, silver iodide in water.

These are stable because of the presence of a charge on particles. The like charges on particles keep them away from each other and no coalscence of particles takes place. These dispersions are thermodynamically unstable. When water is used as a dispersion medium, the systems are termed as hydrophobic dispersions.

(c) ***Association colloids or Amphiphilic :*** Organic compounds which contain large hydrophobic moieties together with strong hydrophilic groups in the same molecule are said to be amphiphilic. Amphiphilic or surface active agents, are characterized by having two distinct regions of opposing solution affinities within the same molecules or ions. In water, at low concentrations surface active agents exist individually as monomers having subcolloidal size. When concentration increases monomers aggregate themselves and form micelles. Each micelle may contain 50 or more monomers. The concentration of monomer at which micelles form is termed the critical micelle concentration or CMC. The surface active agents are represented as

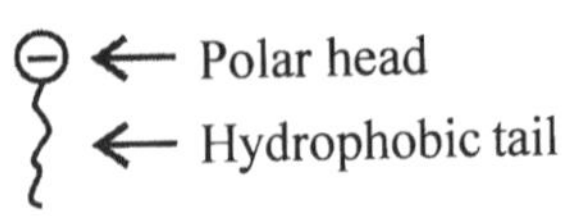

Some probable shapes of micelles are shown in Fig. 7.7.

Below the CMC, the surfactants are adsorbed at air-water interface. In the case of amphiphiles in water, the hydrocarbon chains face inward into the micelles to form their own hydrocarbon environment. Aggregation also occurs in nonpolar liquids. In this case the orientation of the molecules is now reversed, with the polar heads facing inward and hydrocarbon chains are associated with the continuous non polar phase as shown in Fig. 7.7

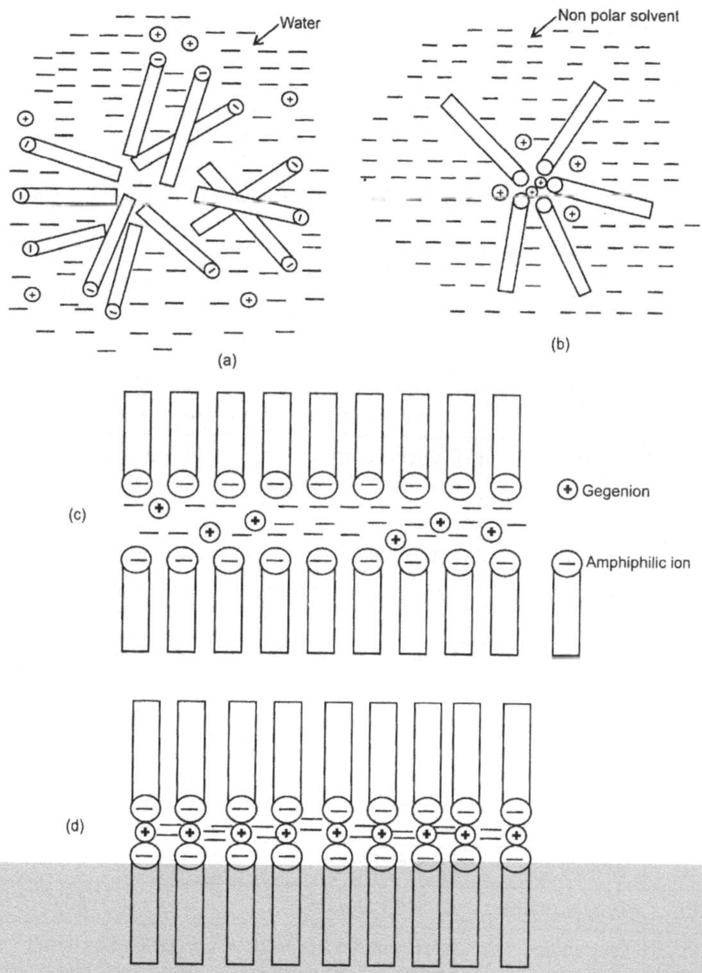

Fig. 7.7 Some probable shapes of micelles : (a) spherical micelle in aqueous-media, (b) reversed micelles in non-aqueous media, (c) Laminar micelle, formed at higher amphiphile concentration, in aqueous media.

Amphiphiles may be anionic (sodium lauryl sulphate); cationic (cetyl trimethyl ammonium bromide); nonionic (polyethylene lauryl ether); or ampholytic or Zwitterionic (dimethyl dodecyl ammonio-propane sulfonate).

A certain numbers of the sodium ions are attracted to the surface of micelle, reducing the over all negative charge. These bound ions are termed as gegenions. In the pharmaceutical preparations mixture of two or more amphiphiles are used.

Characteristics of Lyophobic and Lyophilic Sols : Some important features of lyophobic and lyophilic sols are given in Table 7.2.

Table 7.2 Characteristics of Lyophobic and Lyophilic sols.

Sr.No.	Property	Lyophobic Sols	Lyophilic Sols
1.	Ease of preparation	Easily not obtanied	Easily obtanied
2.	Visibility	Detected with an ultra microscope	Cannot detected by ultra microscope
3.	Charge	Particles carry a characterstic charge	May or may not carry charge
4.	Hydration	Particles usually poorly hydrated	Particles are heavily hydrated
5.	Electrophoresis	Shows electrophoresis	May or may not show electrophoresis
6.	Effect of electrolytes	Addition of electrolyte cause coagulation	Large concentration of electrolyte required for coagulation.
7.	Viscocity	Viscocity is almost same as dispersion medium.	Viscocity is higher than dispersing medium.
8.	Reversibility	Irreversible	Reversible
9.	Stability	Less stable	More stable
10.	Tyndall effect	Exhibit Tyndall effect	Show no Tyndall effect
11.	Preparation	Not prepared by direct mixing with the medium.	Prepared by direct mixing with dispersion medium.

Methods of Preparation of Colloidal Sols

There are two basic methods of forming a colloid; reduction of larger particles to the colloidal size and condensation of smaller particles (e.g., molecules) into colloidal particles. Some substances are easily dispersed in solvent to form a colloid. This dispersion is called peptization. The particle size of colloidal solution is intermediate to true solutions and suspensions. To get such particles mechanical methods or electrical methods can be employed. These methods fall into two categories.

Methods of Preparation of Colloids

(a) **Dispersion Method :** In which larger or macro sized particles are broken down to colloidal size.

(b) **Aggregation Method :** In which subcolloidal particles are built up by aggregating ions/molecules. *This method is also called condensation method.*

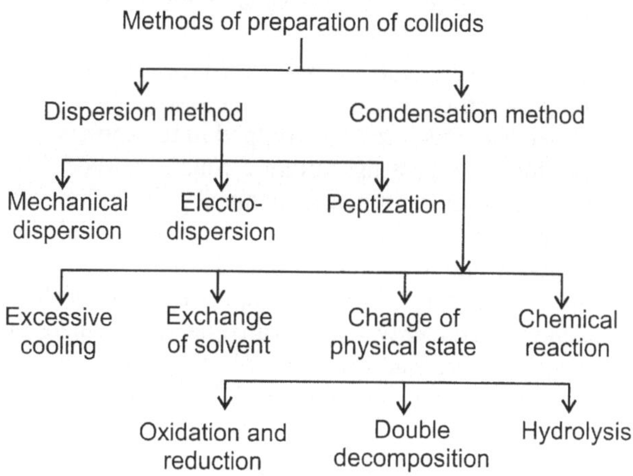

(a) ***Dispersion Method :*** In this method the bulk material is dispersed in given medium.

1. *Mechanical dispersion using Colloidal Mill :* Coarser particles of a substance are broken into colloidal size by grinding them between two discs having a narrow clearance. The solid alongwith the liquid dispersion medium is fed into a colloid mill. The solid particles are ground down to colloidal size and form sol. The discs are made to rotate in opposite directions with high speed as shown in Fig. 7.8.

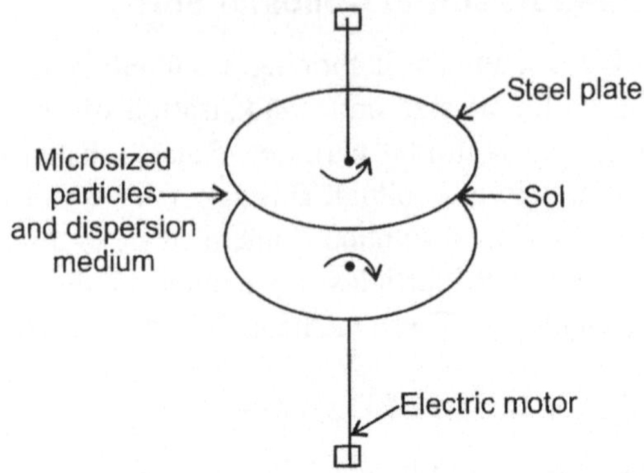

Fig. 7.8 A colloidal mill.

Examples of preparation of sol by this method includes : preparation of Indian ink which is prepared by grinding lamp black with medium and stabilized by stabilizing agents. Colloidal sulphur is made by grinding sulfur with sucrose or lactose.

2. *Electro Dispersion - Bredig's Arc Method :* It is used for preparation of hydrosols of metals e.g., gold, platinum and silver. The metal rods are dipped in the solvent and an arc is produced by passing current through the rods. The water is kept at lower temperature by placing the entire system in ice/ water bath. Deionised water with trace of alkali (KOH) is added in the vessel containing solvent. The intense heat of spark across the electrodes vaporises some of the metal that condenses under water. This arc liberates particles of colloidal size which are readily absorbed by the medium giving a colloid suspension as shown in Fig. 7.9.

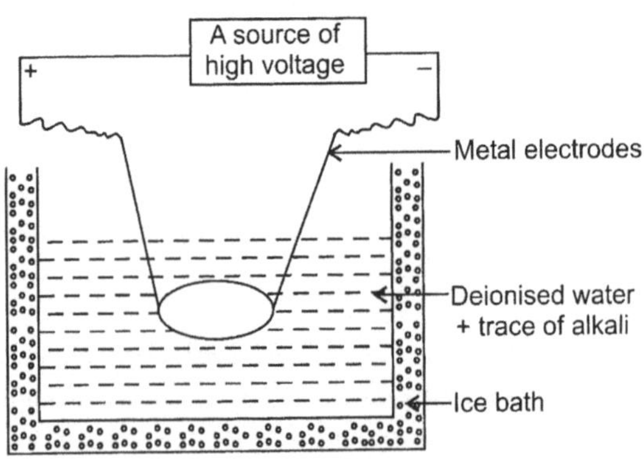

Fig. 7.9 Bredig's arc method.

Non-metal solutions can be made by suspending coarse particles of the substance in the dispersion medium and applying an arc between electrodes.

3. *Peptization :* Peptization is inverse of coagulation. In a freshly precipitated ionic solid, small quantities of electrolytes specially common ions are incorporated to stabilize the system, this stabilizing agent is known as peptizing agent, which prevent the coagulation of particles.

Example : A freshly prepared precipitate of ferric hydroxide (Fe (OH_3)) is peptized by addition of ferric chloride ($FeCl_3$) as shown in Fig. 7.10. Similarly silver chloride Ag^+ Cl^- can be converted into a sol by adding hydrochloric acid (Cl^- being common ion).

Milk is a colloidal dispersion of oil in water. As oil is a hydrophobic substance, casein in milk serves as peptizing agent. Milk coagulates by the addition of common salt.

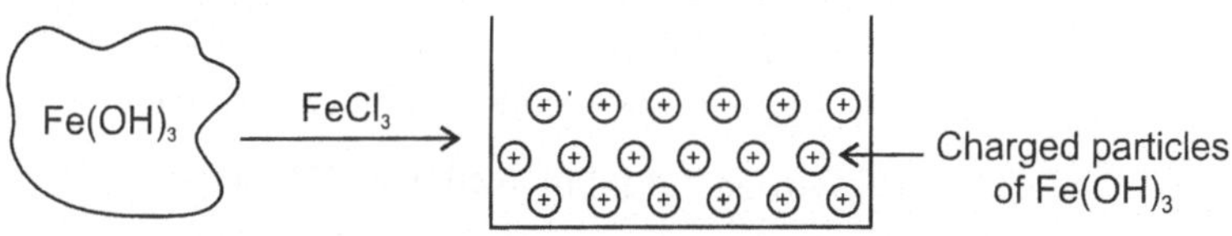

Fig. 7.10 Peptization.

(b) ***Condensation Methods*** **:** In this method, particles of subcolloid range are made to aggregate or condense into particles of colloidal range. Generally chemical reactions are involved in this method and performed by :

1. *By Excessive Cooling :* Colloidal solution of ice in organic solvents like chloroform, ether are formed below 0 °C, a solution of water in these solvents. On excessive cooling the solubility decreases and fine colloidal particles of ice are formed.

2. *By Solvent Exchange :* Change of solvent will lower the solubility of solute.

   Ex : Sulfur, phosphorous first dissolved in alcohol and adding excess of water to it, result formation of hydrosol of these substances. This can be illustrated as given in Fig. 7.11. Resin sol is also prepared by this method.

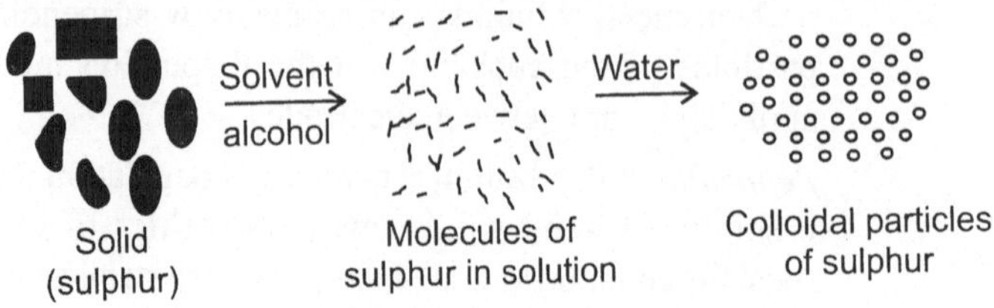

Fig. 7.11 Change of solvent method .

3. *Change of Physical State* : Change in physical state results in formation of sol e.g., sulphur and phosphorus vapours when passed through the dispersion medium containing stabilizer yields a colloid.
4. *Chemical Methods* : Chemical reactions may be used for the preparation of lyophobic sols.
   (i) *Double decomposition* : Arsenic sulphide sol can be prepared by passing a slow stream of hydrogen sulphide gas through a dilute solution of arsenious oxide.

   This is carried out till the yellow color attains to sol.

   $$As_2O_3 + 3H_2S \rightarrow \underset{\text{Yellow color}}{As_2S_3\ (Sol)} + 3\ H_2O$$

   Excess hydrogen sulphide removed by boiling the solution which may otherwise lead to precipitation.

   (ii) *Oxidation* : A sol of sulphur is produced by passing hydrogen sulphide into a solution of sulphur dioxide.

   $$2\ H_2S + SO_2 \rightarrow 2\ H_2O + S\ (\text{Sulphur sol})$$

   Oxidizing agent bromine or nitric acid can be used for this purpose.

   $$H_2S + Br_2 \rightarrow 2\ HBr + S$$

   (iii) *Reduction* : The colloids of metals such as gold, silver, lead, platinum can be prepared by reducing the metal salts with reducing agents like tannic acid, formaldehyde.

   $$Ag\ NO_3 + \text{Tannic acid} \rightarrow Ag\ sol$$

   $$Au\ Cl_3 + \text{Tannic acid} \rightarrow Au\ sol$$

(iv) *Hydrolysis* : Sols of hydroxides of iron, aluminium can be prepared by hydrolysis of salts of given metals.

Ferric hydroxide sol can be prepared by addition of ferric chloride sol in boiling water.

$$FeCl_3 + 3H_2O \rightarrow Fe\,(OH)_3 + 3\,HCl$$

The HCl can be removed by dialysis.

Optical Properties of Colloids

The study of optical properties will be useful in obtaining information regarding the shape, size, structure and molecular weight of colloids.

(i) The Faraday - Tyndall Effect : When a beam of light is directed at a colloidal sol some of the light may be absorbed, some is scattered and remainder transmitted through the sample. Due to the light scattered the sol appears turbid, this phenomenon is known as Tyndall effect.

This scattering of light, illuminates the path of the beam in the colloidal dispersion. The illuminated beam or cone formed by the scattering of light by the sol particle is referred as Faraday - Tyndall effect.

When a strong beam of light is passed through the dispersion colloid, its path becomes visible, due to scattered light. This scattered beam is called as Tyndall beam. The beam is rendered visible against black background.

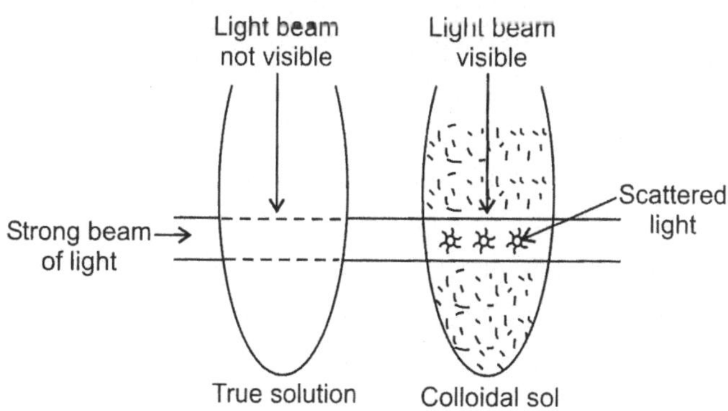

Fig. 7.12 Tyndall effect.

This Tyndall effect can not observed in true solutions since ions or solute molecules are too small to scatter light. Ultramicroscope is used for the study of Tyndall effect.

(ii) ***Electron Microscope :*** In this microscope beam of electrons is focussed by electric and magnetic field on to a photographic plate. This focussed beam is allowed to pass through sol particles. With this instrument, one can get a picture of the actual particles under observation i.e. the size, shape and structure of sol particles and viruses and bacteria. The radiation source is a beam high-energy electrons having wavelengths in the region of 0.1 Å. With the microscope it is possible to get a picture of the an individual particles showing a magnification of the order of 10,000.

(iii) ***Light Scattering :*** Light scattering measurements are useful in estimating particles size, shape and interactions, particularly of dissolved macromolecular materials as the turbidity depends on the size of the colloidal material. This property is widely used for determining the molecular weight of colloids. Scattering may be described in terms of turbidity, τ, the fractional decrease in intensity due to scattering as the incident light passes through 1 cm of solution.

The turbidity of a solution is given by the expression

$$I = I_0 \exp^{-\tau l} \qquad .....(7.1)$$

where I_0 = Intensity of the incident beam.

I = Intensity of the transmitted light.

l = Length of sample = 1 cm.

τ = Turbidity

At a given concentration of dispersed phase, the turbidity is proportional to the molecular weight of the lyophilic colloid.

The turbility can be calculated from the intensity of light (scattered). The molecular weight of colloid can be calculated from the equation derived by Debye in 1947.

$$HC/\tau = 1/M + 2\,BC \qquad .....(7.2)$$

Where, C is concentration of solute, τ is the turbility in cm^{-1}, M is average molecular weight, and B is an interaction constant.

H, is an optical constant for a particular system depending on the value of refractive index that changes with concentration and the wavelengths of light used.

A plot of HC/τ against concentration results in straight line with slope 2B. The intercept on HC/τ axis is 1/M allowing the molecular weight to be calculated.

Kinetic Properties of Colloids

Kinetic properties of colloidal dispersions plays an important role in study of –

(a) Stability of system

(b) Molecular weight of given sample

(c) Transport of kinetics of colloidal particles.

Several properties that relates to the motion of the particles. The motion may be thermally induced (Brownian movement, diffusion, osmosis); gravitationally induced (sedimentation) or applied externally (viscosity) and electrically induced.

(a) ***Brownian Motion :*** Colloidal particles are subject to random collisions with the molecules of the dispersion medium with the result that each particle shows eratic motion. The eratic motion, (upto about 2 μm diameter) of particle are observed under a microscope. The eratic motion seen is referred to as Brownian motion after Robert Brown (1827) who first observed this phenomena.

The velocity of particles increases with decreasing particle size. Increasing viscosity of the medium decreases and finally stops the Brownian movement.

(b) ***Diffusion :*** Diffusion process is a direct result of Brownian movement. Diffusion occurs spontaneously from a region of higher concentration to one of lower concentration until the concentration of the system is uniform throughout. Diffusion can be expressed by Fick's first law.

This property can be useful to determine the molecular weight of polymers by using a relationship,

$$D = \frac{RT}{6\pi\eta_o N} \sqrt[3]{\frac{4\pi N}{3m\bar{\nu}}} \qquad .....(7.3)$$

where, D = Diffusion coefficient of the polymer

R = Gas constant

T = Absolute temperature

η_o = g of dispersion medium

N = Avogadro's number

M = Molecular weight

$\bar{\nu}$ = Partial specific volume

(c) ***Osmotic Pressure :*** Osmotic pressure is mostly useful in measurement of molecular weight range of about 10^4 to 10^6.

The Van't Hoff equation, π = cRT can be used to calculate molecular weight of colloid.

Replacing C with Cg/M in above equation.

$$\pi = \frac{C_g}{M} RT \qquad .....(7.4)$$

This equation can be written :

$$\frac{\pi}{C_g} = RT\left(\frac{1}{M} + BC_g\right)$$

in which B is a constant for any particular solvent/solute system and depends on degree of interaction.

(d) ***Sedimentation :*** Consider a spherical particle of radius r, density ρ falling in liquid of density ρ_o and viscosity η_o. The velocity V of sedimentation is given by Stoke's law :

$$V = \frac{2r^2(\rho - \rho_o)g}{9\,\eta_o} \qquad .....(7.5)$$

If the particles are only subjected to the force of gravity then, the lower size limit of particles obeying stoke's equation is about 0.5 μm. A stronger force than gravity is needed for colloidal particles to sediment. This can be accomplished by high speed centrifuge or ultracentrifuge. In a centrifuge, g is replaced by $\omega^2{}_x$, where ω is angular velocity and x is the distance of the particle from centre of rotation, so equation can be written as

$$V = \frac{2r^2(\rho - \rho_o)\omega_x^2}{9\eta_o} \quad .....(7.6)$$

(e) ***Viscosity :*** Viscosity is an expression of the resistance to flow of a system under and applied stress. Viscosity of a colloidal dispersion is affected by many factors like shape, size of particles, molecular weight of particles, affinity of particles to the medium etc.

Einstein developed an equation of flow applicable to colloidal dispersions of spherical particles :

$$\eta = \eta_o (1 + 2.5\ \phi) \quad .....(7.7)$$

where η_o = viscosity of dispersion medium
η = viscosity of dispersion
ϕ = volume fraction of particles

Several viscosity coefficients may be defined by rearranging Eq. (7.7).

- Relative viscosity = $\eta_{rel} = \dfrac{\eta}{\eta_o} = 1 + 2.5\ \phi$ .....(7.8)

- Specific viscosity = $\eta_{sp} = \dfrac{\eta}{\eta_o} - 1$

$$= \frac{\eta - \eta_o}{\eta_o} = 2.5\ \phi$$

$$\frac{\eta_{sp}}{C} = 2.5 \text{ or } k \quad .....(7.9)$$

where, C = Particles in grams per 100 ml of dispersion.
k = intrinsic viscosity

The η at various concentrations can be determined and knowing η_o, η_{sp} can be calculated from given equation. When η_{sp}/C is plotted against C and the line is extrapolated to infinite dilution the intercept is K, (Fig. 7.13). This constant K, commonly known as intrinsic viscosity [η] used to calculate the approximate molecular weight.

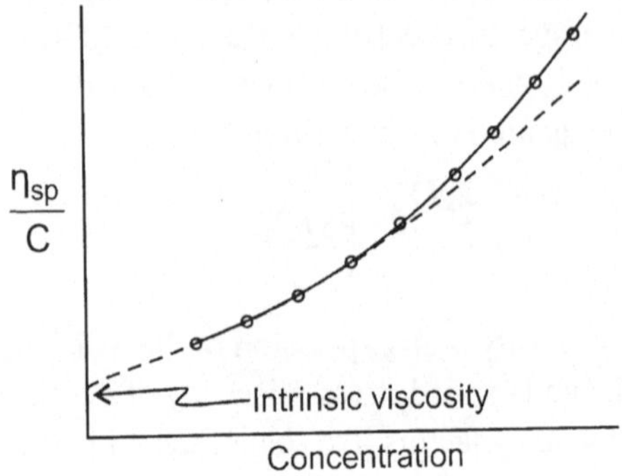

Fig. 7.13 Viscocity data for molecular weight determination.

The approximate molecular weight can be calculated by using *Mark - Houwink equation*

$$[\eta] = KM^a \qquad .....(7.10)$$

where K and a are constants.

$[\eta]$ = intrinsic viscosity determined from plot as shown in Fig. 7.13.

Constant K and a are characteristics of a particular polymer-solvent system. From this the molecular weight can be calculated.

Electrical Properties of Sols

The important property of colloidal dispersion is that all the suspended particles possess either a positive or negative charge. Aggregation of particles can be prevented by mutual forces of repulsion between similarly charged particles and it also prevents settling under the action of gravity. This gives stability to the solution.

(a) ***Electric Double Layer :*** The electrical double layer study has been outlined in interfacial phenomenon (Chapter no. 14) along with *Zeta and Nernst potential.* Zeta potential has an application in predicting the stability of the dispersion system.

(b) ***Electrokinetic Phenomena :*** The colloidal solution consists of particles that generally possess a charge on their surfaces. The movement of a charged surface with respect to an adjacent liquid phase. There are four main electrokinetic phenomena :

(a) Electrophoresis or cataphoresis.
(b) Electro-osmosis
(c) Sedimentation potential
(d) Streaming potential

(a) ***Electrophoresis :*** It involves the moment of a charged particles through a liquid under the influence of an applied potential difference. The movement of sol particles under an applied electric potential is called electrophoresis or cataphoresis. If electrical potential is applied across platinum electrodes dipping in a hydrophilic sol as shown in Fig. 7.14. The dispersed particles migrate towards the positive electrode, they carry a negative charge, if they move towards negative electrode, they are positively charged. Thus one can determine whether the particles of sol carry positive or negative charge. Ex : As_2S_3 sol migrated to positive electrode, indicating particles are negatively charged.

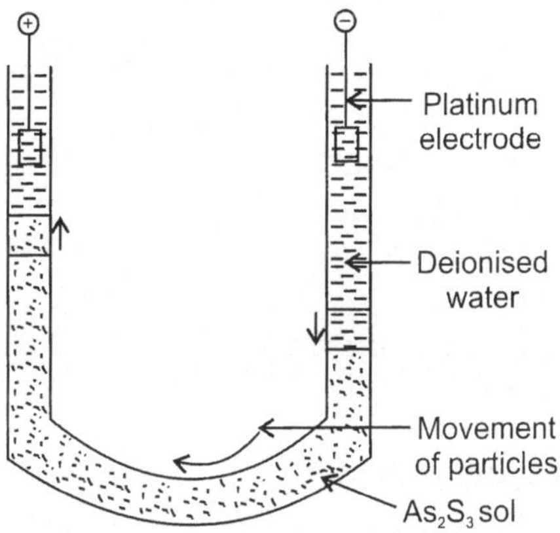

Fig. 7.14 Electrophoresis/cataphoresis of a sol.

The electrophoresis is applied for removal of smoke from chimney gases, impurities, painting of metal parts of motor cars with colloidal pigments etc.

(b) ***Electro-osmosis :*** *The movement of the dispersion medium under the influence of applied potential is known as electro-osmosis.* In electro-osomosis liquid moves through a plug or membrane across which a potential is applied. The dispersed phase is stationary, the medium moves to the electrode with opposite sign. As shown in Fig. 7.15 a 'U' tube in which a plug (a negative colloid) is fixed. The two limbs of tube are filled with water to the same level.

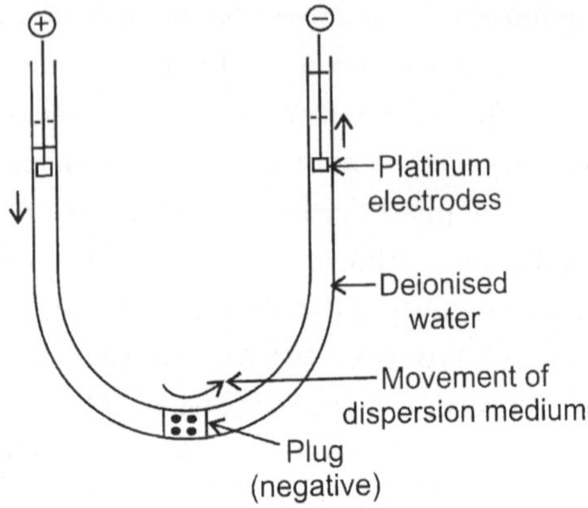

Fig. 7.15 Electro-osmosis.

When a potential is applied across electrodes immersed in water; the water level rises on cathode side. The movement of the medium indicates that the charge on medium is positive.

(c) ***Sedimentation Potential :*** This process involves the creation of a potential when particles undergo sedimentation. It is opposite to electrophoresis.

(d) ***Streaming Potential :*** Here the potential is created by forcing a liquid to flow through a plug or bed of particles.

Stability of Colloidal Systems

The main factor contributing in stability of lyophobic colloids is the electric charge present on it. Stabilization can be done by two ways : Providing the dispersed particles with an electric charge, and protective solvent sheath surrounding each particle specially for lyophilic sol. The stability of a lyophobic sol is due to the adsorption of +ve or –ve ions by dispersed particles. In the stable lyophobic sol all particles have same charge so there is repulsive forces between charged particles. If a charge is removed by any means, these particles aggregate or coalesce and settle down. This phenomena is called coagulation or precipitation of sol. Hence addition of small electrolyte to a lyophobic solution tends to stabilize the system.

Excess addition of electrolyte sometimes results in accumulation of opposite ions and reduces the Zeta potential below its *critical value* (critical value for oil hydrosol is about 40 millivolts). The critical zeta potential of a gold sol is nearly zero, suggests that particles require minute charge for stabilization. The precipitating power increases rapidly with the valance or charge of the ions, this statement is known as Schulze-Hardy rule.

If a small amount of hydrophilic colloid is added to a hydrophobic sol, it may coagulate. This is due to neutralisation of the charge on the hydrophobic colloidal particles as shown in Fig. 7.16.

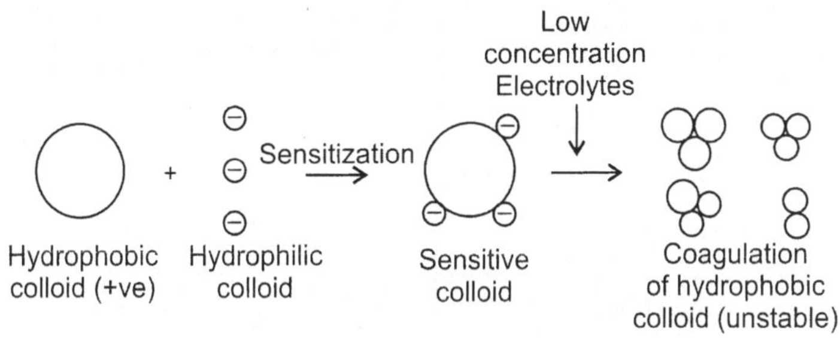

Fig. 7.16 Sensitization of hydrophobic colloid.

When large quantity of hydrophilic colloid added to hydrophobic colloid carrying opposite charge, the hydrophilic colloid gets adsorbed on hydrophobic particles forming a layer around it. The coagulation of particles is prevented due to the layer. This phenomenon is known as protection and the colloid that helps to stabilize the hydrophobic colloid is called protective colloid. The phenomenon is depicted in Fig. 7.17.

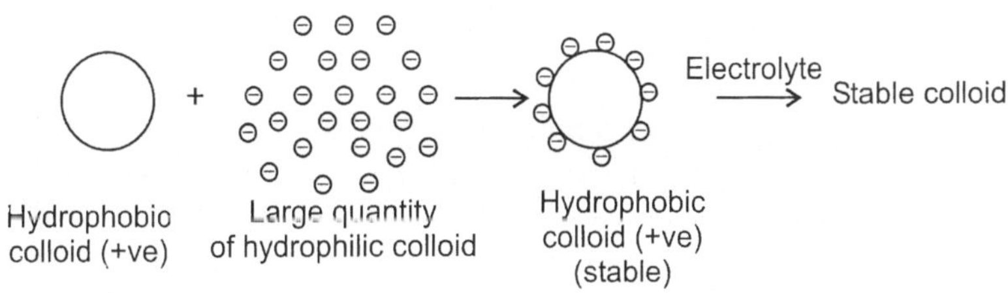

Fig. 7.17 Protective colloidal action.

Example of protective colloids : gelatin, gum acacia, tragacanth, etc.

The protective property of colloids is expressed in terms of *gold number*.

The gold number is the minimum weight in milligrams of a hydrophilic colloid (dry weight) required to prevent a colour change from red to violet in 10 ml of gold sol on addition of 1 ml of 10% sodium chloride sol.

The gold sol is hydrophobic colloid (red colour), can be stabilized by addition of protective colloid and prevent color change to violet.

Some examples of gold numbers of protective colloids are given in Table 7.3.

Table 7.3 Some protective colloid and their gold numbers.

Protective colloid	Gold number
Gelatin	0.005 – 0.01
Egg albumin	0.1
Acacia	0.1 – 0.2
Sodium oleate	1 – 5
Tragacanth	2

The protective colloids used in many preparations to stabilize the systems. Ex : In the preparation of ice cream, gelatin it is added.

Lyophobic colloids are thermodynamically unstable. The stability of dispersion is explained according to approach, known as the DLVO theory, the forces on colloidal particles in a dispersion are due to electrostatic repulsion and London-type van der Waal's attraction.

DLVO theory : The quantitative theory of the interaction between Lyophobic disperse particles was worked out by *Derjaguin and Landau in the USSR and by Verwey and Over beek in the Netherlands (1940) known as DLVO theory.*

This theory is useful to determine approximate amount of electrolyte required to precipitate or stabilize a colloid. When two particles approach each other closely, the attractive forces take over and cause them to adhere. Coagulation occurs as the particles aggregates into increasingly larger secondary particles or flocs. The electrostatic repulsion prevents particles from coagulation.

The forces on particles in dispersion are due to electrostatic repulsion and London-type Van der Waal's attraction. These forces result in potential energy of repulsion, V_R and attraction, V_A, between particles. As shown in Fig. 7.18 together with the curve for the composite potential energy, V_T.

Primary Minimum : When the particles are very close to each other, atomic orbitals overlap that leads to rise in potential energy and precipitation. The minimum potential, V_m, corresponds to a Zeta potential of about 50 mV for obtaining a kinetically stable colloidal system.

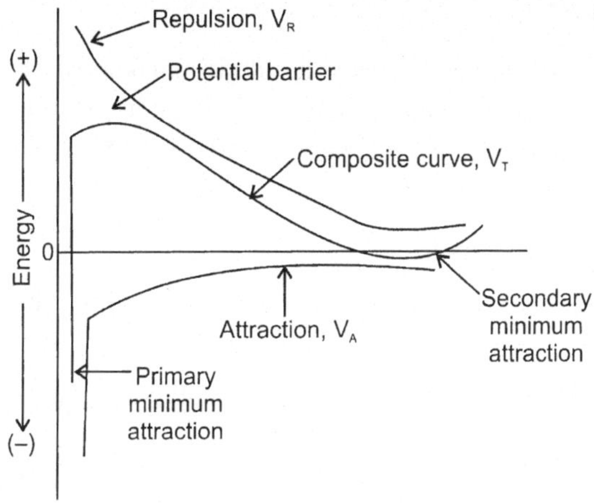

Fig. 7.18 Potential energy versus interparticle distance (angstroms) for particles in suspension.

Secondary Minimum : Here particles form aggregates due to attractive forces. From this principle, one can determine quantitatively the amount of electrolyte of a particular valence type required to precipitate a colloid.

Schulze-Hardy rule arranges ions in the order of their capacity to coagulate hydrophobic colloids, the *Hofmeister or lyotropic series* ranks cations and anions in order of coagulation of hydrophilic sols. According to this, anions or cations are arranged in a series as given below. Several anions of *Hofmeister series* in decreasing order of precipitating power are citrate, tartrate, sulfate, acetate, chloride, nitrate, bromide and iodide.

When negatively and positively charged hydrophilic colloids are mixed, the particles may separate from the dispersion to form a layer rich in the colloidal aggregates, known as a Coacervate and the phenomenon referred as *coacervation.*

Ex : Mixing of gelatin (+ve) and acacia (–ve) results coacervation.

Kraft Point : Is the temperature at which the solubility of the surfactant equals the CMC.

Cloud Point : Many nonionic, polyoxyethylated surfactant in solution shows a cloud point. It is the temperature, above which cloudiness suddenly appears, is known as *cloud point.*

Problems

1. Calculate the relative viscosity of given unknown sample. The time required for a volume of water to flow through capillary viscometer is 50 seconds and for unknown liquid is 415 seconds. The density of unknown liquid is 1.15 g/cm^3 and of water is 1.0 g/cm^3.

   Solution : Data given

   Time required to flow capillary tube for water is 50 second and for unknown liquid is 415 seconds.

   The density of water is 1.0 and unknown liquid is 1.15 g/cm^3.

   Equation for relative viscosity

   $$\eta_{rel} = \frac{t_2 \times \rho_2}{t_1 \times \rho_1} = \frac{415 \times 1.15}{50 \times 1.0} = \frac{477.25}{50}$$

   $$= 9.545.$$

2. Calculate the molecular weight of a given material if constant, $K = 4 \times 10^{-5}$, $a = 0.99$ and viscosity (intrinsic) = 2.41.

   Solution : Data given

   $$K = 4 \times 10^{-5},\ a = 0.99;\ [\eta] = 2.41$$

   Equation for molecular weight determination is

   Mark-Houwink equation

   $$[\eta] = KM^a$$

   $$2.41 = 4 \times 10^{-5} \times M^{0.99}$$

   $$\log (M) = 4.90$$

   $$M = \text{antilog } (4.90)$$

   $$= 67051$$

3. Compute the Zeta potential of the colloid from the given data. The mobility of given solution at 20 °C was observed to be 35×10^{-5} cm^2 volt^{-1} sec^{-1}.

   Solution : Data given

   Mobility of given solution = 35×10^{-5} cm^2 volts^{-1} sec^{-1}

Equation for zeta potential

$$\zeta = 150 \times V/E \text{ (mobility)}$$

$$= 150 \times (35 \times 10^{-5})$$

$$= 00525 \text{ volts}$$

$$= 52.5 \text{ millivolts.}$$

4. Calculate the ratio of concentration of diffusible ions at equilibrium as per Donnan membrane concept from given data. Concentration of anionic polyelectrolytes was 14.5×10^{-3} gm equivalent/mole and of penicillin was 4.10×10^{-3} mole/liter inside the sac at equilibrium.

   Solution : Data given

$$[D^-] = 4.10 \times 10^{-3} \text{ moles/liter}$$

$$[R^-] = 14.5 \times 10^{-3} \text{ gm equivalent/mole.}$$

Equation : Donnan membrane equilibrium.

$$\frac{[D^-]_0}{[D^-]_i} = \sqrt{1 + \frac{[R^-]_i}{[D^-]_i}}$$

$$= \sqrt{1 + \frac{14.5 \times 10^{-3}}{4.10 \times 10^{-3}}} = \sqrt{1 + 3.5365}$$

$$= \sqrt{4.53658} = 2.1299 = 2.123$$

or 2.123 to 1.

CHAPTER 8

Chemical Kinetics

The first milestone in the field of chemical kinetics was laid down by L. Wilhelmy (1850), while studying the inversion of sucrose in presence of acid. His finding included that the rate of the reaction at any instant was proportional to the amount of sucrose remaining unchanged at that instant. The study of kinetics further gained momentum with the contributions of A.V. Harcourt and W. Esson in the year 1867.

This branch of science mainly reveals the velocity of chemical reactions. The various factors which contribute to the rate of reaction include concentration, temperature, pressure and presence of catalyst.

All these factors directly or indirectly help the scientists in determining mechanism by which the reaction takes place.

This study helps a formulator in formulating a more stable drug preparation by choosing a suitable vechile or solvent or ingredients that will prevent or retard the degradation. Apart from the above mentioned applications this study also helps in deciding the routes of administration and storage conditions of various pharmaceutical dosage forms.

Rate of Reaction

The rate of a reaction gives an idea about the velocity or speed at which it occurs. The rate of a reaction is denoted by $\frac{\Delta c}{\Delta t}$ or $\frac{dc}{dt}$ for infinitesimal change in concentration and time parameters.

For Example

$$\underset{\text{Reactant}}{x} \rightarrow \underset{\text{Product}}{y}$$

The rate of above reaction is given by

$$= \frac{\text{change in concentration of x}}{\text{Time taken for the change}} \text{ or } \frac{\Delta [x]}{\Delta t}$$

The term ΔC or $\Delta(x)$ is a negative quantity since the concentration of reactant decreases as time proceeds. So,

$$\text{Rate} = \frac{-\Delta [x]}{\Delta t}$$

The rate can also be expressed in terms of change in concentration of products, which does not carry any negative sign.

Units - mol/liter.sec or mol/liter. min or mol/liter.hour

According to law of mass action, the rate of a chemical reaction is proportional to the product of molar concentration of reactants each raised to power of the number of molecules of substrate undergoing reaction.

For Example

$$ax + by + ... = \text{products..}$$

The rate of reaction is

$$\text{Rate} = \frac{-1}{a}\frac{d(x)}{dt} + \frac{-1}{b}\frac{d(y)}{dt} \text{ -----} + k[x]^a [y]^b$$

where K is the rate constant

Order of Reaction

The order of reaction is obtained by adding up all the powers of concentration in the rate law.

$$\text{Rate} = K[x]^a [y]^b$$

Over all order of reactions = a + b. The order of reaction with respect to x is *a* and with respect to y is *b*.

Based on the order of reaction a reaction can be classified as

- First order (a + b = 1)
- Second order (a + b = 2)
- Third order (a + b = 3)

and zero order reaction if the reaction proceeds independent of concentration terms.

We will discuss these reactions in detail in subsequent sections.

Consider an example of

$$(CH_3CO)_2 O + 2C_2H_5OH \rightarrow 2CH_3 CO_2 C_2H_5 + H_2O$$

The order of reaction with respect to $(CH_3 CO)_2 O$ is 1, with respect to C_2H_5OH is 2 and the over all order is 3.

Molecularity : It is the number of atoms, molecules or ions colliding simultaneously to give the products. Unlike the order of reaction it has only integral values.

Unimolecular Reaction : This reaction involves only one molecule.

Eg : Cis - Lactic acid → Trans - Lactic acid.

Bimolecular Reaction : This involves reaction between two molecules

Eg : $H_2 + I_2 \rightarrow 2HI$

Trimolecular Reaction : These reactions which involve more than two molecules and are rarely occur.

Mathematical Treatment

Zero Order Reaction : As discussed earlier a zero order reaction proceeds independent of concentration term of the reactants.

So

$$\frac{-dc}{dt} = K_o \qquad .....(8.1)$$

Where, K_o is specific rate constant

The Eq. (8.1) can be rewritten as

$$- dc = K_o\, dt$$

Integrating on both sides

$$-\int_{C_o}^{C_t} dc = K_o \int_{o}^{t} dt$$

$$\Rightarrow C_0 - C_t = K_0 t$$

$$\Rightarrow C_t = C_0 - K_0 t \qquad .....(8.2)$$

Where, C_0 is initial concentration of reactant, C_t is concentration of reactant at time t.

The Eq. (8.2) is in the form of $y = -mx + c$.

where, $y = C_t$, $x = t$, $c = C_0$. So by plotting values C_t on y-axis and corresponding values of time, t on x-axis, we obtain a straight line, with negative slope with magnitude equal to K_0.

The units of K_0 are moles/liter.sec.

Half-life : It is denoted by $t_{1/2}$. For a zero oder reaction $C_t = C_0 - K_0 t$. Half life is the time required by a reactant to reduce to half of its initial concentration.

$$\therefore \qquad C_t = \frac{C_0}{2} \qquad \text{[substituting in Eq. (8.2)]}$$

$$\Rightarrow \frac{C_0}{2} = K_0 t_{1/2} \text{ or } t_{1/2} = \frac{C_0}{2K_0}$$

First Order Reaction : In a first order reaction the rate of reaction is directly proportional to concentration of one of the reactants

So $$\frac{-dc}{dt} = K_1 C \qquad .....(8.3)$$

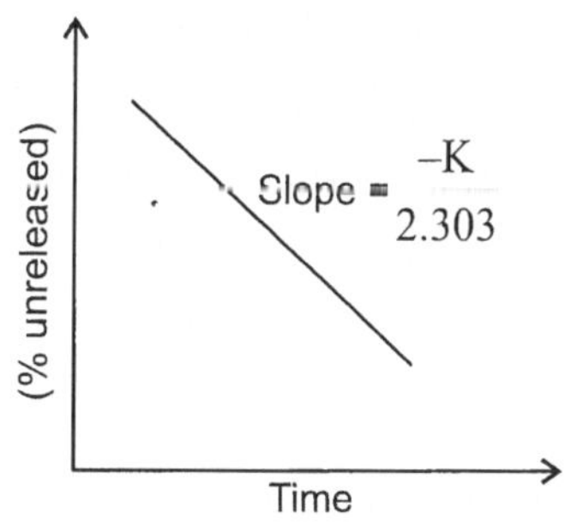

Fig. 8.1 A linear plot of log C verses time for first order reactions.

Rewritting Eq. (8.3), we get

$$-\int_{C_0}^{C_t} \frac{dc}{c} = K_1 \int_0^t dt$$

$$\ln \frac{C_o}{C_t} = K_1 t$$

$$\Rightarrow K_1 = \frac{2.303}{t} \log_{10} \frac{C_o}{C_t} \quad .....(8.4)$$

By plotting logarithmic values of % unreleased drug on y-axis and time on x-axis we obtain a straight line, whose slope $= \frac{-K_1}{2.303}$.

Hence we can obtain the value of first order rate constant (K_1). Unit : min^{-1} or Sec^{-1}.

Half-life : Substituting $C_t = \frac{C_o}{2}$ and $t = t_{1/2}$ in Eq. (8.4)

$$\Rightarrow K_1 = \frac{2.303}{t_{1/2}} \log_{10} \frac{C_o}{C_o/2}$$

$$\Rightarrow K_1 = \frac{2.303}{t_{1/2}} \log_{10} 2$$

$$\Rightarrow t_{1/2} = \frac{0.693}{K_1} \quad .....(8.5)$$

The half-life of a first order reaction can be calculated using Eq. (8.5).

Pseudo First Order Reaction : In some reaction the concentration of one of the reactant is maintained in excess compared to the concentration of other.

For example, in the below mentioned reaction

$$CH_3\,COOC_2H_5 + Na\,OH_{solution} \rightarrow CH_3\,COONa + C_2H_5OH$$

The rate of reaction depends on ethyl acetate which is present relatively in low concentration, where as $NaOH_{solution}$ is present in excess quantity. So this falls under the category of pseudo first order reaction.

i.e. $$\frac{-dc}{dt} = K_2\,[C]\,[\text{constant}]$$

or $$\frac{-dc}{dt} = K_1\,[C]$$

Hence the rate depends on the concentration of one reactant, *although* we have two reacting species. *These reactions are termed as pseudo first order reactions.*

Second Order Reactions : In second order reactions the rate of reaction depends on the concentration terms of two reactants raised to power one.

Consider two reactants A and B.

$$A + B \rightarrow \text{Products}$$

The rate of reaction can be written as

$$\frac{-dA}{dt} = \frac{-dB}{dt} = K_2\,[A]^1\,[B]^1 \quad \text{.....(8.6)}$$

where, K_2 is second order rate constant. For the sake of simplicity consider,

$$2\,A \rightarrow \text{products}$$

The rate of above reaction is

$$\frac{-dA}{dt} = K_2\,[A]^2 \quad \text{.....(8.7)}$$

Let 'a' be the initial concentration of reactant at t = 0, and x is the concentration of reactant in time t.

The Eq. (8.7) becomes

$$\frac{dx}{dt} = K_2\,[a - x]^2 \quad \text{.....(8.8)}$$

Now Eq. (8.8) can be integrated, using conditions x = 0 at t = 0, x = x at t = t.

$$\int_0^x \frac{dx}{(a-x)^2} = K_2 \int_0^t dt$$

$$\left(\frac{1}{a-x}\right) - \left(\frac{1}{a-o}\right) = K_2\,t$$

$$\frac{x}{a(a-x)} = K_2 t \quad \text{.....(8.9)}$$

$$K_2 = \frac{1}{at}\left(\frac{x}{a-x}\right) \quad \text{.....(8.10)}$$

The above equation in general case equals to

$$K_2 = \frac{2.303}{t(a-b)} \log \frac{b(a-x)}{a(b-x)} \qquad .....(8.11)$$

when two different reactants a, b are taken.

The Eq. (8.9) is in the form of a straight line whose slope equals K_2 when $\frac{x}{a(a-x)}$ is taken on y-axis and t on x-axis. On the similar lines Eq. (8.11) can be represented in the form of a straight line with $\log \frac{b(a-x)}{a(b-x)}$ on y-axis and time on x-axis. The slope of the straight line equals $\frac{(a-b)}{2.303} K$.

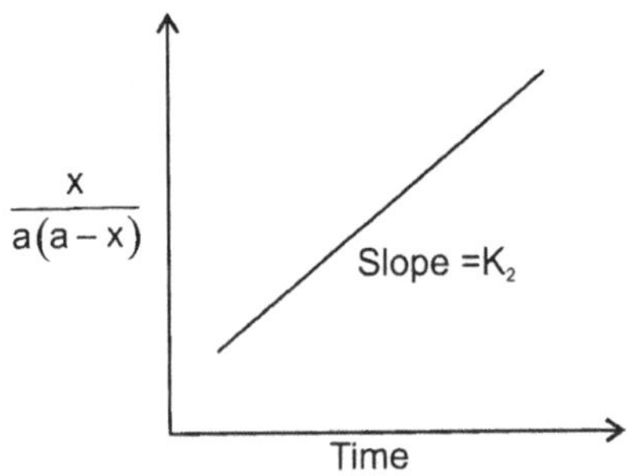

Fig. 8.2 A second order reaction plot when a = b.

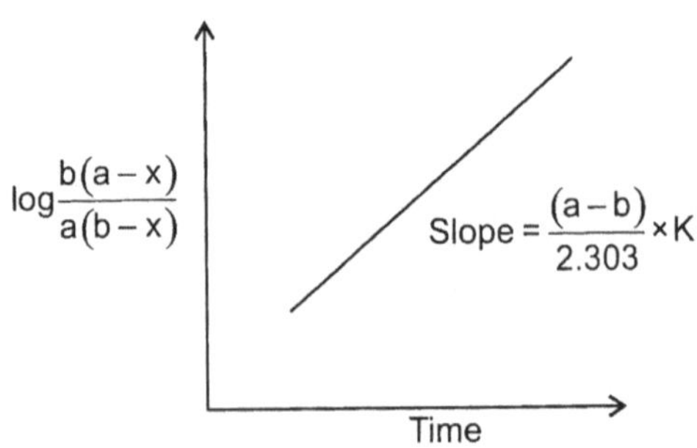

Fig. 8.3 A second order reaction plot when a ≠ b.

***Half-life of a Second Order Reaction :** It is the time required to reduce the concentration of reactant to half of its initial concentration.*

$$t = t_{1/2} \text{ and } x = \frac{a}{2}$$

Substituting it in Eq. (8.9)

$$K_2 = \frac{1}{at_{1/2}} \cdot \frac{a/2}{\left(a - \frac{a}{2}\right)}$$

$$\Rightarrow t_{1/2} = \frac{1}{ak_2}.$$

The second order is the inverse of product of initial concentration of reactants and rate constant.

$$\text{Units of } K_2 = \text{liter. mol}^{-1}.\text{sec}^{-1}$$

Determination of Order

(a) ***Substitution Method :*** In this method different initial concentrations of the reactant (a) are taken. The values of concentration (a – x) at regular intervals of time (t) were noted. These values a, (a – x) and t thus obtained from the experiment are substituted into the integrated rate equations for the first, second and third order. The equation that yields a constant value of K corresponds to the order of the reaction.

(b) ***Half-life Method :*** In this method half-life is determined as a function of concentration. The order is considered as unity if the half-life is independent of concentration. The Half-life of a reaction is inversely proportional to the concentration term raised to the power (n – 1), where n = order of reaction.

So, $\text{half-life} \ \alpha \ \frac{1}{[A]}$ (for 2nd order reaction)

$\text{half-life} \ \alpha \ \frac{1}{[A]^2}$ (for 3rd order reaction)

For a ηth order reaction.

$$\text{half-life} \ \alpha \ \frac{1}{[A]^{n-1}}$$

If two different reactions are run at different initial concentrations, a_1 and a_2, the half lives $t_{\frac{1}{2}(1)}$ and $t_{\frac{1}{2}(2)}$ are related as follows :

$$\frac{t_{\frac{1}{2}(1)}}{t_{\frac{1}{2}(2)}} = \frac{(a_2)^{n-1}}{(a_1)^{n-1}} = \left(\frac{a_2}{a_1}\right)^{n-1}$$

or in logarithmic form finally we will get

$$n = \frac{\log\left(t_{\frac{1}{2}(1)} / t_{\frac{1}{2}(2)}\right)}{\log(a_2/a_1)} + 1$$

The rate and half life equations are given in Table 8.1.

(c) ***Graphical Method :*** As seen earlier for first order reaction the rate reaction is

$$\ln \frac{C_o}{C_1} = k_1 t$$

(or)

$$\ln (C_t) = \ln (C_o) - kt$$

$$y = C - mx.$$

So for the values of two variables $\ln \frac{C_o}{C_1}$ (vs) t if, we obtain a straight line then the corresponding reaction is said to be first order. If a curve is obtained then the reaction is not a first order reaction.

For second order similarly we plot for values of $\frac{1}{(a-x)}$ versus t.

The line obtained has equation

$$\frac{1}{(a-x)} = kt + \frac{1}{a}$$

$$y = mx + c.$$

In case if we get a curve for values of $\frac{1}{(a-x)}$ versus t then it is not a second order reaction.

If straight line obtained then it is second order reaction. When a plot of $\frac{1}{(a-x)^2}$ aganist t produces a straight line, with all reactants at the same initial concentration, the reaction is third order.

(d) ***Ostwald's Isolation Method :*** This method is generally useful for determining the order of complex reaction whose rate is influenced by more than two ingredients.

Lets consider the reaction

$$A + B + C \rightarrow \text{products}$$

The order of reaction with respect to three reactants is given by

$$n = n_A + n_B + n_C$$

n_A is determined by taking B and C in excess concentration. Similarly n_B is determined by taking A and C in excess and so can be determined n_C.

(e) ***Van't Hoff's Differential Method :*** The rate of a reaction of nth order is directly proportional to the concentration term raised to n^{th} power.

$$\frac{-dc}{dt} = KC^n$$

For two experiments with different initial concentration we can write the rate of reactions as

$$\frac{-dc_1}{dt} = KC_1^n \quad .....(8.12)$$

$$\frac{-dc_2}{dt} = KC_2^n \quad .....(8.13)$$

Applying log to both equations

$$\log\left(\frac{-dc_1}{dt}\right) = \log K + n \log C_1 \quad .....(8.14)$$

$$\log\left(\frac{-dc_2}{dt}\right) = \log K + n \log C_2 \quad .....(8.15)$$

Subtracting Eq. (8.15) from Eq. (8.14) we get,

$$n = \frac{\log\left(\frac{-dc_1}{dt}\right) - \log\left(\frac{-dc_2}{dt}\right)}{\log C_1 - \log C_2}$$

So, in order to calculate the value of n, one should plot the values of concentration and time on y-axis and x-axis respectively.

The slope $\frac{-dc}{dt}$ is found by drawing tangent at a given time internal.

Table 8.1 Rate and half-life equations.

Order	Integrated rate equation	Half-life equation	Units of k
0	$C' = Kt$	$t_{1/2} = \frac{a}{2k}$	moles/liter.sec
1	$\log \frac{C_o}{C_t} = \left(\frac{k}{2.303}\right) t$	$t_{1/2} = \frac{0.693}{k}$	min^{-1} or sec^{-1}
2	$\frac{x}{a(a-x)} = kt$	$t_{1/2} = \frac{1}{ak}$	liter/moles.sec
3	$\frac{x(2a-x)}{a^2(a-x)^2} = 2Kt$	$t_{1/2} = \frac{3}{2}\,\frac{1}{a^2k}$	$moles^2liter^2$/time

Complex Reactions : These are reactions which include more than one step. These are broadly classified into three types

(a) ***Reversible Reaction***

$$A + B \underset{K_{-1}}{\overset{K_1}{\rightleftharpoons}} C + D$$

(b) ***Parallel or side Reactions***

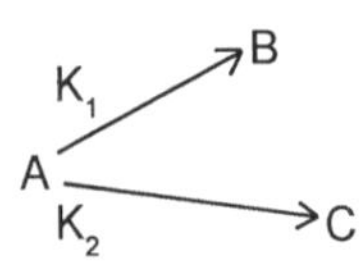

(c) ***Series or Consecutive Reactions***

$$A \xrightarrow{K_1} B \xrightarrow{K_2} C.$$

(a) ***Reversible reactions***

In a reversible reaction that invloves first-order process for forward and reverse reaction

$$A \underset{K_r}{\overset{K_f}{\rightleftharpoons}} B$$

The rate law is given by

$$\log \frac{A_o - A_{eq.}}{A - A_{eq.}} = \frac{(K_f + K_r)}{2.303}\, t$$

which corresponds to a straight line intersecting at zero and having slope $\frac{(K_f + K_r)}{2.303}$.

(b) ***Parallel reactions***

In case of parallel or side reactions prednisolone is well known example. It degrades to give acidic and neutral steroid products.

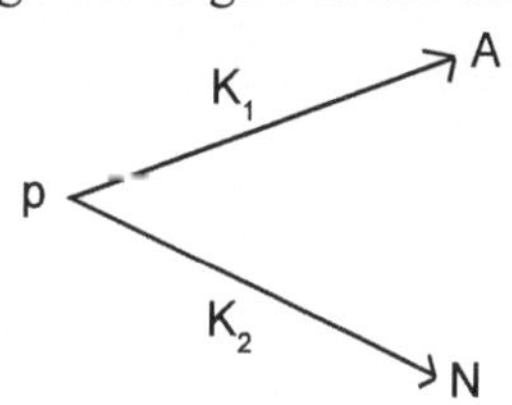

P denotes prednisolone, A denotes *acid product* and N for *neutral product*. The corresponding rate equation is

$$\frac{-dp}{dt} = K_1P + K_2P = KP$$

where, $K = K_1 + K_2$. So the above equation is integrated to give

$$\ln\left[\frac{P_o}{\rho}\right] = Kt.$$

The individual concentration of A and N can be found by

$$A = \frac{K_1}{K} P_o (1 - e^{-kt})$$

$$N = \frac{K_2}{K} P_o (1 - e^{-kt})$$

So, the plot of A or N against $(1 - e^{-kt})$ yields a straight line from which rate constants can be obtained.

$$K_1 = \text{Slope} \times \frac{K}{P_o}.$$

The value of K_2 is obtained by subtracting K_1 from K.

(c) Series or Consecutive Reactions : It is the case when two first order reactions occur consecutively, thus

$$A \xrightarrow{K_1} b \xrightarrow{K_2} C.$$

The rate equations with respect to each substance are

$$\frac{-dC_A}{dt} = K_1 C_A$$

$$\frac{-dC_B}{dt} = -K_1C_A + K_2C_{B.}$$

$$\frac{-dC_C}{dt} = K_2 C_B.$$

At t = 0, $C_A = [A_o]$ and $C_B = 0$, $C_C = 0$. Up on integration of the above equation, we obtain

$$C_A = CA_o e^{-K_1t}$$

$$C_B = \frac{C_{Ao}K_1}{(K_2 - K_1)} [e^{-K_1t} - e^{-K_2t}]$$

$$C_C = C_{Ao} [1 + \frac{1}{(K_1 - K_2)} (K_2e^{-k_1t} - K_1e^{-K_2t})$$

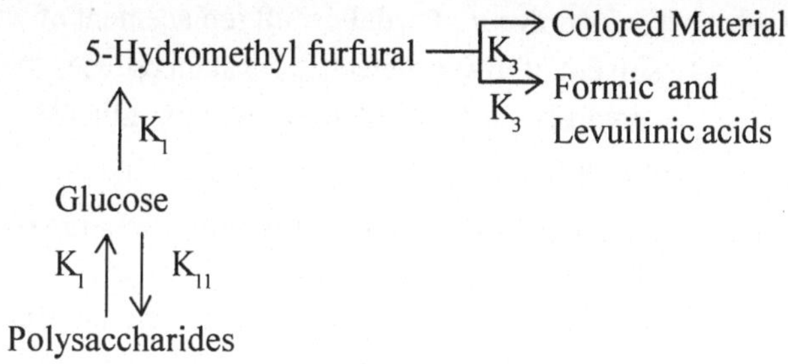

The above given reaction of glucose involves complex, reversible, parallel and consecutive types.

Degradative Pathways

Decomposition of active ingredient in pharmaceutical dosage forms can occurs through several phathways i.e., hydrolysis, oxidation-reduction, racemization, decarboxylation, ring cleavage and photolysis. Most frequently encountered are hydrolysis and oxidation-reduction.

(A) Hydrolysis : Many pharmaceuticals contain ester or amide functional groups which undergo hydrolysis in solution. Examples of drugs are – Anesthetics, antibiotics, vitamins and barbiturates.

(i) ***Ester hydrolysis :*** Hydrolysis of an ester into a mixture of an acid and alcohol involves rupture of a covalent linkage as given below.

$$\underset{\text{Ester}}{R_1-\overset{\overset{O}{||}}{C}-OR} + H^+ + OH^- \rightarrow \underset{\text{Acid}}{R_1-\overset{\overset{O}{||}}{C}-OH} + \underset{\text{Alcohol}}{HOR}$$

Majority of hydrolysis reactions takes place in presence of a catalyst [catalysts are mineral acids, alkalies or acids etc]. Examples of drugs degrade through ester hydrolysis are procaine, atropine, methyl p–aminobenzoate etc.

Methods to enhance the stability of pharmaceuticals undergoing ester hydrolysis are –

(a) *pH :* If physiologically permissible, the pH of a formulation should be as close as possible to its pH of optimum stability.

(b) *Type of Solvent* : Partial or full replacement of water with a solvent of lower dielectric constant reduces the velocity of hydrolysis. Ex : ethanol, glycols, glucose, mannitol solutions.

(c) *Complexations* : Complex formation, example – caffeine with benzocaine decreases the velocity of reaction. Similarly caffeine complexes with local anesthetics such as procaine, tetracaine, can reduce the velocity of hydrolytic degradation.

(d) *Surfactants* : It has been observed that nonionic, cationic and anionic surfactants stabilize the drug against hydrolysis. A 5 % sodium lauryl sulphate (anionic) causes 18-fold increase in the half life of benzocaine.

(e) *Modifications of chemical structure* : Certain substitutes added to the alkyl or acyl chain of aliphatic or aromatic esters decreases the hydrolytic rate.

(ii) ***Amide Hydrolysis :*** Pharmaceutical compounds containing amide group can undergo hydrolysis. In the amide hydrolysis acid and amine are formed as given below;

$$\underset{\text{Amide}}{R-\overset{\overset{\displaystyle O}{\|}}{C}-\overset{\overset{\displaystyle H}{|}}{N}-R_1} + H_2O \rightarrow \underset{\text{Acid}}{R-\overset{\overset{\displaystyle O}{\|}}{C}-OH} + \underset{\text{Amine}}{H_2N-R^1}$$

Similar methods are used to protect compound from amide hydrolysis, as given under ester hydrolysis.

(B) ***Oxidation-Reduction :*** A number of pharmaceutical compounds undergo oxidative reaction includes vitamins, steroids, antibiotics, epinephrine etc. These reactions are mediated either by free radicals or by molecular oxygen.

Common form of oxidation is autoxidation; and is defined as the reaction of any material with molecular oxygen. This may be given as follows:

$$A:B \rightarrow A^{\cdot} + B^{\cdot}$$

$$CH_3:CH_3 \rightarrow 2\,CH_3^{\cdot}$$

These are free radicals and are highly unsaturated and readily takes electrons from other substances causing oxidation. Autoxidation may be described as follows:

Initiation

$$RH \xrightarrow[\text{light,heat}]{\text{activation}} R^{\cdot} + (H^{\cdot})$$

Propagation

$$R^{\cdot} + O_2 \rightarrow RO_2^{\cdot}$$

$$RO_2^{\cdot} + RH \rightarrow ROOH + R^{\cdot}$$

Hydroperoxide decomposition

$$ROOH \rightarrow RO^{\cdot} + O^{\cdot}H$$

Termination

$$RO_2^{\cdot} + x \rightarrow \text{Inactive products}$$

$$RO_2^{\cdot} + RO_2^{\cdot} \rightarrow \text{Inactive products}$$

The initiation of oxidation reactions can be produced by the thermal decomposition by light. Many oxidations are catalyzed by hydrogen and hydroxyl ions. Oxygen concentration is important in autoxidation process. Examples of drugs undergoing oxidative degradation are prednisolone, morphine, epinephrine, isoamyl nitrite.

Rancidity, which can affect nearly all oils and fats, causes typical off-flavors, due to the autoxidation of unsaturated fatty acids present in fat or oil.

Methods to protect drug from oxidation includes - oxygen content, use of antioxidants (oil soluble and water soluble example Sodium sulphate, sodium meta bisulphate, sodium bisulphate, ascorbic acid, thiourea, thioglycolic acid, propyl gallate, BHT, BHA, Lecithin etc), use of chelating agent (examples – EDTA, citric acid, tartaric acids); adjustment of pH, use of solvent etc.

(C) ***Photolysis :*** Decomposition of drugs due to absorption of radiant energy in the form of light. If the molecules absorbing the radiation take part themselves, in the main reaction, the reaction is said to be a photochemical one. Ex : chlorpromazine hydrochloride, hydrocortisone, prednisolone and methyl prednisolone etc.

(D) ***Racemization :*** An optically active substance loses its optical activity without changing its chemical composition. The biological effect of the dextro form can be considerably less than the levo form. Ex. Levo-adrenaline is 15 to 20 times more active than dextro-adrenaline. Solutions of levo-adrenaline form a racemic mixture of equal part of levo, and dextro adrenaline having pharmacological activity half than pure levo compound.

Influence of Temperature on Drug Decomposition

Arrhenius was the pioneer, who studied the effects of temperature on decomposition of drug. The rate of a reaction doubles with every 10° rise in temperature.

Arrhenius equation illustrates the effect of temperature on reaction rate.

$$K = Ae^{-Ea/RT}$$

where K = Specific rate constant

A = Frequency factor or Arrhenius factor.

E_a = Activation energy.

R = Ideal gas constant (1.987 cal/mol.deg).

T = Absolute temperature

Taking logarithm on both sides

$$\log K = \log A - \frac{E_a}{2.303\ RT} \quad .....(8.16)$$

Frequency factor (A) is the product of the number of collisions and probability of collisions which give a reaction product.

Activation energy (E_a) is the minimum energy that a molecule should possess so as to produce the product.

Estimation of K : The value of K can be found out by conducting the experiment at different temperatures. The concentration values at different time points is calculated and graph is ploted for concentration Vs time. From the slope of line one can calculate the value of K.

Estimation of Activation Energy and Arrhenius Factor : As stated above one can get values of K at different temperatures. Let the value of $K = K_1$ at temperature t_1 and $K = K_2$ at temperature t_2.

So Eq. (8.16) can be written as

$$\log K_1 = \log A - \frac{E_a}{2.303\ RT_1} \qquad .....(8.17)$$

$$\log K_2 = \log A - \frac{E_a}{2.303\ RT_2} \qquad .....(8.18)$$

Substracting Eq. (8.17) and Eq. (8.18) yield

$$\log \frac{K_2}{K_1} = \frac{E_a}{2.303\ R}\left(\frac{T_2 - T_1}{T_2\ T_1}\right) \qquad .....(8.19)$$

Now substitute the value of E_a in the equation to obtain value of A.

We can also estimate the value of E_a from the slope of line obtained by drawing the values of log K on y-axis and $\frac{1}{T}$ on x-axis as given in Fig. 8.4.

$$\text{Slope} = \frac{E_a}{2.303\ R}$$

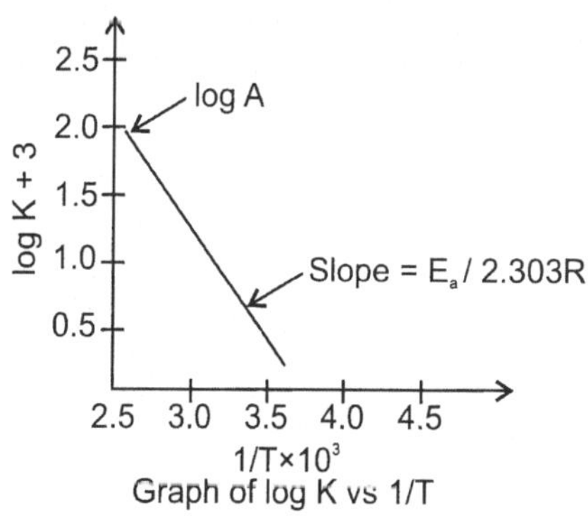

Fig. 8.4

Accelerated Stability Testing

A pharmaceutical dosage form is a combination of various chemicals, so the chances of degradation of active ingredient are very high. According to the guidelines the dosage form should contain active ingredient not less than 90% through out the shelf-life period. In the past pharmaceutical companies used to observe formulations for years so as determine the shelf life. This process was time consuming and tedious. With advancement in branch of kinetics, the shelf life of a dosage form can be predicted with in months based on the *Accelerated Stability Reports*. These studies are designed to increase the rate of chemical degradation and physical change of a drug product by using exaggerated storage conditions as part of the formal stability testing program. This data helps to evaluate the impact of short time excursions outside the label storage conditions, as might occur during shipping. The results of accelerated studies are not always predictive of physical changes and potency.

Table 8.2 Recommended storage conditions.

Study	Intended Storage Conditions of Finished Products			
	Room Temperature (General case)	**Refrigerator**	**Freezer**	**Minimum time period covered by data at submission**
Long Term	25°C/60% RH	–	–	6 Months
	30°C/65% RH	5 °C	–20°C	12 Months
Intermidiate	30°C/65% RH	–	–	6 Months
Accelerated	40°C/75% RH	25°C/60%RH	–	6 Months

Recommended Storage Conditions are given in Table 8.2. Under accelerated stability studies the dosage form is kept at higher temperatures like 40 °C, 50 °C, 60 °C, 70 °C. Samples are collected at regular intervals and analysed for the active drug content. From the data obtained the graphs are plotted as given in Fig. 8.5 and Fig. 8.6. As given in Fig. 8.5, the K values can be obtained.

The values of K are plotted against temperature so as to obtain a straight line. From the straight line one can find K at 25 °C by extrapolation as shown in Fig. 8.6.

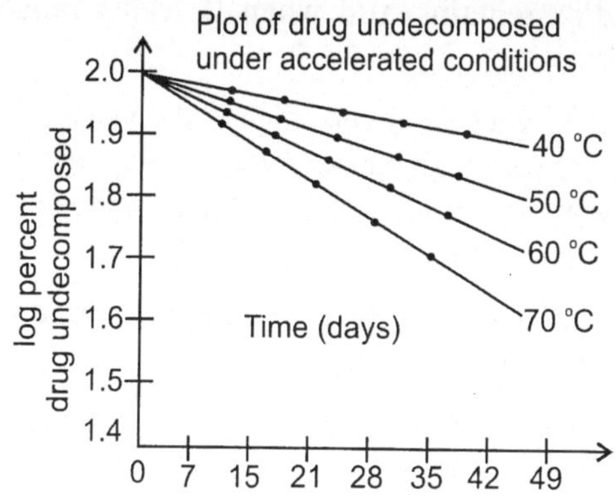

Fig. 8.5

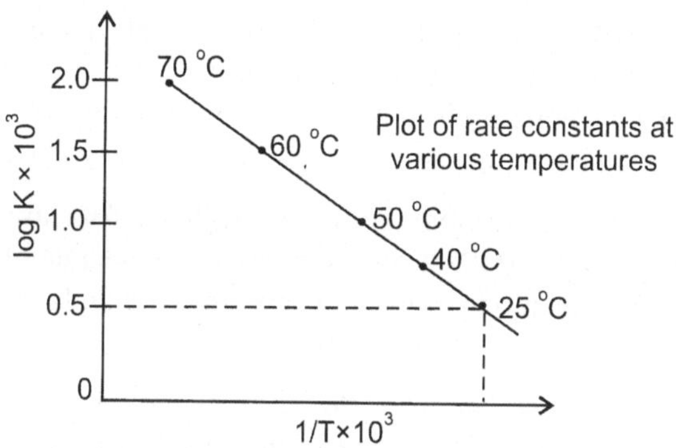

Fig. 8.6

Stability Testing of Medicinal Products : If a medicinal product is sufficiently stable at room temperature for longer storage period then it can be marketed. In case the product degrades at room temperature then manufacturer indicates the storage temperature that takes care of the product till its ultimate use.

Pharmaceutical companies try to predict the rate of degradation at room temperature by using the data obtained at several elevated temperatures. This infact saves time and delays that occur in the formulation of a drug.

The major limitations of Arrhenius plot are -

(a) These are only pertained to temperature dependent chemical reaction.

(b) These studies remain valid when E_a value ranges between 10-30 Kcal/mole.

The rate of reaction is very high if the value is less than 10 Kcal/mole and very high temperatures are required if the value is above 30 Kcal/mol. Studies at these higher temperatures become irrelevant at ambient storage conditions.

(c) When order of reaction changes during the period of study, the results obtained may be erratic.

Keeping these limitations in mind one cannot expect success in all types of dosage forms.

(d) Generally solution type of dosage form give satisfactory results, but suspensions which are non homogenous in nature may not provide linear arrhenius plot. The differences in the solubility of several solid phases which exist in the suspension at elevated temperatures invalidate the usual arrhenius plots. In case of tablets, higher temperatures lead to changes in quantity of moisture in product which inturn influence the stability of product.

Modern methods such a high-performance liquid chromatography (HPLC) helps in measuring the rate of formation of degradation products even in very small amounts (less than 1% of parent compound).

Manufacturers are interested in finding out t_{90} or t_{95} which is the time required for the drug to decompose to 10% or 5%, respectively, of original potency. This can be obtained directly from the arrhenius plot.

Problems

1. A drug preparation was exposed to 45° C and the intensity of colour was measured. The absorbance was measured after four months and to have 1.202 at 500 mm. The initial absorbance was 1.457 at 500 mm. The reaction follows zero order, calculate reaction rate, K_o.

   Solution : Data given.

Initial absorbance	= 1.457 at 500 nm = A_o.
Absorbance after four months	= 1.202 = A_t.
Time in days	= 120 days = t.

Equation for reaction rate $= K_o = \dfrac{A_o - A_t}{t}$

$$= \frac{1.457 - 1.202}{120} = 0.002125 \text{ day}^{-1}.$$

2. A solution of drug contained 1200 units per ml when prepared. After 60 days it was analyzed and found to have 400 units/ml. Assuming the decomposition is first order, calculate half life, shelf life and rate of reaction.

Solutions : Data given

Initial concentration = 1200 units/ml

After 60 days concentration = 400 units/ml.

Equations for rate of reaction

$$K = \frac{2.303}{t} \log \frac{C_o}{C_t}$$

$$= \frac{2.303}{60} . \log \frac{1200}{400}$$

$$= \frac{2.303 \times 0.4786}{60}$$

$$= 0.01837 \text{ day}^{-1}.$$

Half life $= t_{1/2} = \dfrac{0.693}{K} = \dfrac{0.693}{0.01837} = 37.724$ days

Shelf life $= 0.152 \times t_{1/2} = 0.152 \times 37.724$

$= 5.7340$ days.

3. Calculate reaction rate and shelf life of the product that decomposes by first order. The half life of drug is 65 days.

Solution : Data given

$$t_{1/2} = 65 \text{ days.}$$

Equation for reaction rate

$$K = \frac{0.693}{t_{1/2}}$$

$$= \frac{0.693}{65} = 0.01066 \text{ day}^{-1}.$$

Shelf life $$t_{90} = \frac{0.105}{K}$$

$$= \frac{0.105}{0.01066} = 9.849 \text{ days.}$$

4. In one reaction the initial concentration was found to be 0.066 M. The concentration after a period of 24 hours was 5.20×10^{-2} mole/liter. Calculate reaction rate constant and the quantity of active constituent remaining undecomposed after 8 hours.

Solution : Data given

Initial concentrations = C_o = 0.066 M Time = t = 24 hr

Concentrations after time t = C_t = 0.052.

Equation for rate constant

$$K = \frac{2.303}{t} \cdot \log \frac{C_o}{C_t} = \frac{2.303}{24} \cdot \log \frac{0.066}{0.052}$$

$$= 0.09595 \times \log 1.2692$$

$$= 0.009892 \text{ hr}^{-1}.$$

Now C_o = 0.066, t = 8 hr , so C_t = ?

$$0.009892 = \frac{2.303}{8} \cdot \log \frac{0.066}{C_t}$$

$$\frac{8 \times 0.009892}{2.303} = \log \frac{0.066}{C_t}$$

$$0.03436 = \log \frac{0.066}{C_t}$$

$$\frac{0.066}{C_t} = \text{antilog } 0.03436 = 1.084$$

$$\therefore \qquad C_t = \frac{0.066}{1.084} = 0.06088$$

$$= 6.088 \times 10^{-2} \text{ moles/liter.}$$

5. In the saponification of ethyl acetate at 25 °C, the initial concentrations of ester and base were 0.01 M. The concentration of base remaining after 85 min was 0.00662 M. If the reaction follows second order reaction, calculate rate constant and half life of reaction.

   Solution : Data given

   Initial concentration = 0.01 M. = a

   Concentration after 85 mint, (a – x) = 0.00662 M

   Time = t = 85 mint, x = a – (a – x) = 0.00338 min.

   Equation for rate constant

$$K = \frac{1}{at}\frac{x}{(a-x)}$$

$$= \frac{1}{0.01 \times 85}\frac{0.00338}{0.00662}$$

$$= \frac{1}{0.85} \times 0.5105 = 0.6005 \text{ liter/mol.min.}$$

   Half life
$$t_{1/2} = \frac{1}{ak} = \frac{1}{0.6005 \times 0.01}$$

$$= 166.52 \text{ min.}$$

6. What expiration date should be assigned to the product showing following data.

   The initial concentration of drug decomposing according to first order kinetics is 84 units/ml. The specific rate constant K is found to be 3.05×10^{-5} hr^{-1} at room temperature. The experiment has shown that when concentrations of drug falls below 55 units per ml it is not sufficiently potent for use.

Solution : Data given

Initial concentrations = 84 units/ml = C_o

Specific rate constant = K = 3.05 × 10^{-5} hr^{-1}

Equations for time

$$t = \frac{2.303}{K} \log \frac{C_o}{C}$$

$$= \frac{2.303}{3.05 \times 10^{-5}} \log \frac{84}{55}$$

$$= \frac{2.303}{3.05 \times 10^{-5}} \log 1.52$$

$$= 3.5 \times 10^{4} \text{ hr}$$

$$= 4 \text{ years}$$

CHAPTER 9

Solutions of Non-electrolytes

Substance whose aqueous solutions does not conduct electricity are called as non-electrolytes. When a non-electrolyte is dissolved, it produces neutral molecules in the solution.

Examples of non-electrolyte substances include sugar, glycerol etc. A solution consists of solute (substance being dissolved) and solvent (substance dissolving the solute). Generally the concentration of solute is small and that of solvent is high. Concentration of solution is expressed in terms of grams/liter or moles/liter or gram.equivalent/liter. Based on the concentration we can divide solutions into two types.

(a) ***Dilute Solutions :*** The concentration of solute is relatively low.

(b) ***Concentrated Solutions :*** The concentration of solute is relatively high.

Colligative Properties of Solution

These are the properties which depend on the number of solute particles present in the solution, irrespective of whether they are molecules or ions. In Greek, colligative means collective.

The colligative properties which will be considered are:

1. Lowering of vapour pressure.
2. Elevation of boiling point.
3. Depression in freezing point.
4. Osmotic pressure.

1. Lowering of Vapour Pressure

Some solvent molecules have the tendency to escape into vapour state. *These molecules in vapour state exert pressure on the surface of solvent known as vapour pressure.* When a non-volatile solute is added to the solvent the vapour pressure of solvent gets reduced. This can be described qualitatively by visualizing solvent molecules on the surface of solvent, which normally could escape in to the vapour, being replaced by solute molecules which have little if any vapour pressure on their own.

Relatively lowering of vapour pressure

$$= \frac{P_o - P}{P_o}$$

where P_o = vapour pressure of pure solvent.

P = vapour pressure of solution.

According to Raoult's law the relative lowering of vapour pressure is directly proportional to the mole fraction of the solute present in dilute solution.

Mathematically,

$$\frac{P_o - P}{P_o} = \frac{n_1}{n_1 + n_2} \qquad .....(9.1)$$

where n_1 = moles of solute.

n_2 = moles of solvent.

$$\Delta P = P_o X_1 \qquad .....(9.2)$$

where X_1 = mole fraction of solute

The solutions which obey Raoult's law are called ideal solutions and solutions which deviate from Raoult's law are called Real or non-ideal solution. These deviations mainly come into play due to the cohesive and adhesive forces between the molecules. Cohesive forces exist between two solute or two solvent molecules. Adhesive forces exist between solute and solvent molecules. If adhesive forces dominate cohesive forces, then negative deviation occurs, as solvent molecules will less readily escape. On the other hand if cohesive forces dominate adhesive forces solvent molecules will escape more readily and vapour-pressure will be more than predicted by Raoult's law.

Examples

Negative Deviation : Mixture of choloroform and acetone.

Positive Deviation : Mixture of Benzene and ethyl alcohol, Chloroform and ethyl alcohol.

One can get better idea from the diagrams given in Fig. 9.1, 9.2 and 9.3.

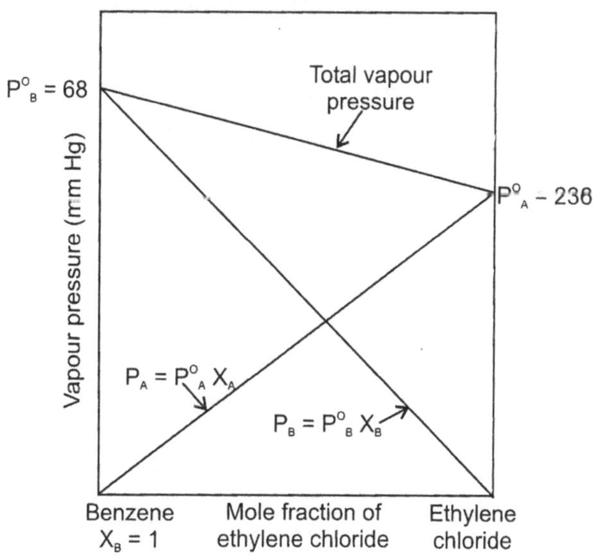

Fig. 9.1 Vapour pressure-composition curve for an ideal binary system.

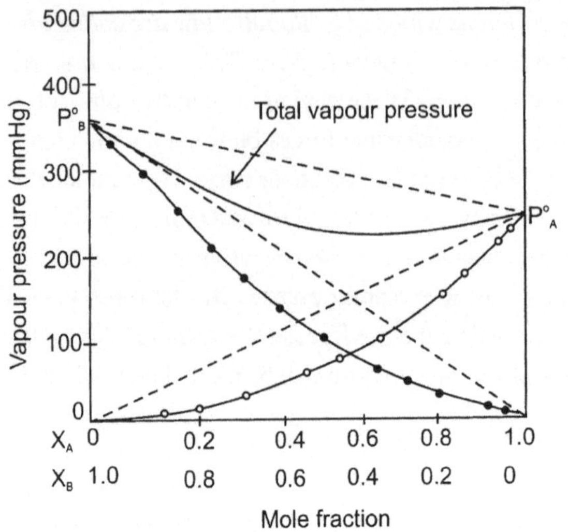

Fig. 9.2 Vapour pressure of a system showing negative deviation from Raoult's law.

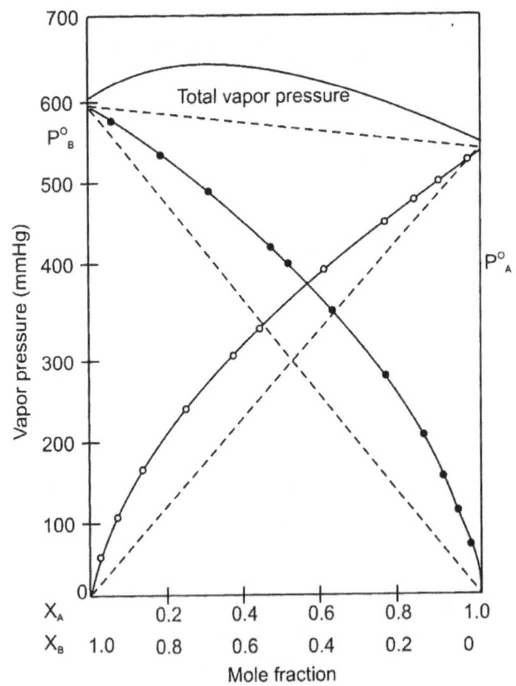

Fig. 9.3 Vapour pressure of a system showing positive deviation from Raoult's law.

Determination of the Vapour Pressure of Solutions

(a) ***Isopiestic Method :*** The word Isopiestic means equal pressure (Greek origin). In this method the solution whose vapour pressure is to be determined and solution containing standard solute are placed in separate beakers in a closed container as shown in Fig. 9.4. The vapour of the solution having higher pressure travels to the one having lower pressure until a constant weight is obtained.

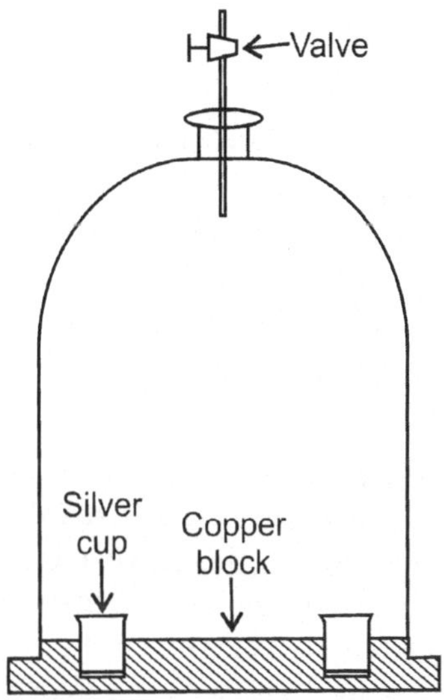

Fig. 9.4 Apparatus for the isopiestic method.

Here potassium chloride can be used in preparation of standard solution. Once, a constant weight is achieved then the solutions are analysed for their concentrations. From the standard literature values the vapour-pressure of the test solution can be calculated which is isopiestic with standard solution. The difference between the vapour pressure value of water at that temperature and vapour pressure value obtained gives the value of vapour pressure lowering of solution.

(b) ***Thermoelectric Method :*** It consists of combination of copper, magnesium, constantan arranged as shown in Fig. 9.5, which are in turn connected to a galvanometer for determining the relative vapour pressures of small amounts of liquids.

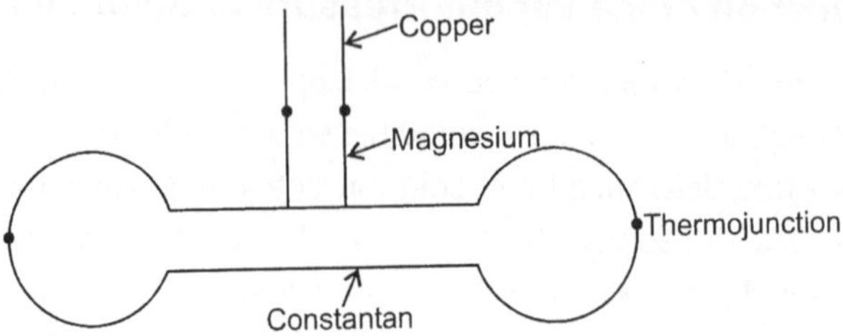

Fig. 9.5 Hill-Baldes apparatus for the thermoelectric determination of vapour pressure.

This apparatus was designed by Hill and Baldes, and it determines the change in potential as a solution of known vapour pressure and unknown evaporate in a chamber maintained at constant humidity. The lower of vapour pressure of the solution is then obtained from a standard curve of vapour pressure versus galvanometer readings of potential. It is widely used in measuring colligative properties of ophthalmic solutions.

2. **Elevation of the Boiling Point :** *A liquid starts boiling when the vapour pressure of liquid becomes equal to external pressure of 760 mm Hg.* (Fig. 9.6). When a non-volatile solute is added to solvent, its vapour pressure gets reduced and hence temperature of solution must be elevated to a value above that of pure solvent to reach the normal boiling point. This can be clearly seen in Fig. 9.6.

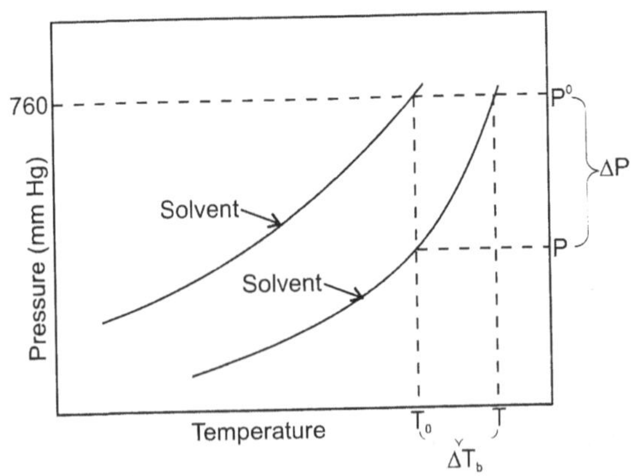

Fig. 9.6 Boiling point elevation of the solvent due to addition of a solute.

The elevation of the boiling point is shown in figure as

$$\Delta T_b = T - T_o$$

where ΔT_b = Elevation in boiling point.

T = Boiling point of solution

T_o = Boiling point of pure solvent

$\Delta T_b = K' \Delta P$ (Elevation in boiling point is directly proportional to vapour pressure lowering)

K' = constant

But from Raoult's law

$$\Delta P = P_o \times 2$$

Substituting in above equation

$$\Delta T_b = K' P_o X_2 \qquad .....(9.3)$$

But $$X_2 = \frac{n_2}{n_1 + n_2} \qquad .....(9.4)$$

In case of dilute solutions we can write Eq. (9.4) as

$$X_2 = \frac{n_2}{n_1} = \frac{w_2 / M_2}{1000 / M_1} = \frac{\frac{m}{1000}}{M_1} \qquad .....(9.5)$$

where, m is molality

M_1 = molecular weight of the solvent.

Now substituting Eq. (9.5) in Eq. (9.3), we can get,

$$\Delta T_b = \frac{K\, M_1}{1000} \times m \qquad .....(9.6)$$

or $$\Delta T_b = K_b\, m$$

where, K_b is molal elevation constant or ebullioscopic constant.

The molal elevation constant is the ratio of the boiling point elevation to the molal concentration in an extremely dilute solution in which the system is approximately ideal.

Determination of Boiling Point Elevation : It is determined by Cottrell Boiling Point Apparatus. In this weighed amount of solute is placed in solvent provided with and reflux condenser and thermometer. The vapour is forcefully sprayed over the bulb of thermometer to obtain an invariant equilibrium temperature. In the similar way boiling point of pure solvent is also found out.

3. ***Depression of Freezing Point :*** The freezing point of a solvent is defined as the temperature at which the solid and liquid forms of solvent co-exist in equilibrium at 760 mm Hg. At freezing point, vapour pressure of liquid is equal to vapour pressure of solid, in case these were not so, the form having the higher vapour pressure would change into that having the lower vapour pressure.

From Raoult's law we have learnt that a solution will have lower vapour pressure than that of its liquid solvent, it is obvious that solid solvent and solution cannot co-exist at the same temperature as solid solvent and liquid solvent; only at some lower temperature one can achieve the equilibrium between solution and solid solvent.

The freezing point depression of a solution can be quantitatively determined for ideal solutions by equations:

$$\Delta T_f = K_f \times m \qquad .....(9.7)$$

or

$$\Delta T_f = K_f \frac{1000\, w_2}{w_1 M_2}$$

$$K_f = \frac{RT_o^2 M_A}{1000 \Delta H_f} \qquad .....(9.8)$$

where, ΔT_f = Freezing point depression

K_f = Molal depression constant or Cryoscopic constant

m = molal concentration.

The above equation indicates that depression in freezing point is proportional to molal concentration of solute.

The value of K_f for water = $\frac{1.987 \times (273.1)^2 \times 18.02}{1000 \times 79.7 \times 18.02}$ =

1.86 deg Kg/mole

Determination of Freezing Point Lowering : There are two ways available for the determination of freezing point lowering.

(a) ***Beckmann Method :*** It consists of jacketed tube with a side arm through which the test material is introduced. A Beckmann thermometer that extends into test solution as shown in Fig. 9.7.

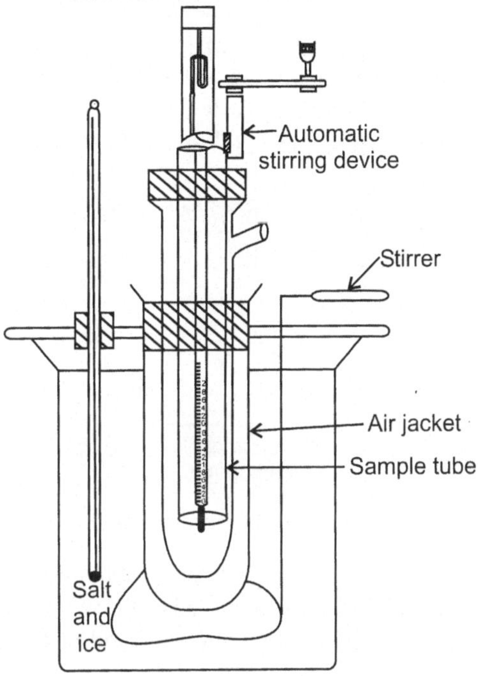

Fig. 9.7 Beckmann freezing point apparatus.

The stirring device shown in the Fig. 9.7 is operated either manually or automatically. The tube and jacket are supported in a vessel containing a cooling mixture of salt and ice. A known quantity of sample whose freezing point lowering is to be determined is placed in the apparatus, containing a specified amount of solvent. The freezing point of sample is obtained from thermometer.

(b) ***Equilibrium Method :*** In this method, the freezing point of pure solvent is determined by using Beckmann thermometer or a multijunction thermocouple and potentiometer. The entire process is carried out in a jacked tube or Dewar flask. Same procedure is carried out as given earlier and by placing solution (test sample). The difference in freezing points of the two systems can be determined within ± 0.00002 °C.

4. ***Osmotic Pressure :*** *Osmosis is the process which involves the transfer of solvent through the semipermeable membrane into solution.* It is a uphill process i.e., the diffusion takes place against the direction of concentration gradient. In a similar manner, if two solutions of different concentrations are separated by a membrane, the solvent will move from the solution of lower solute concentration to the solution of higher solute concentration. This diffusion of solvent through a membrane is called osmosis. The osmosis can be demonstrated as given in Fig. 9.8.

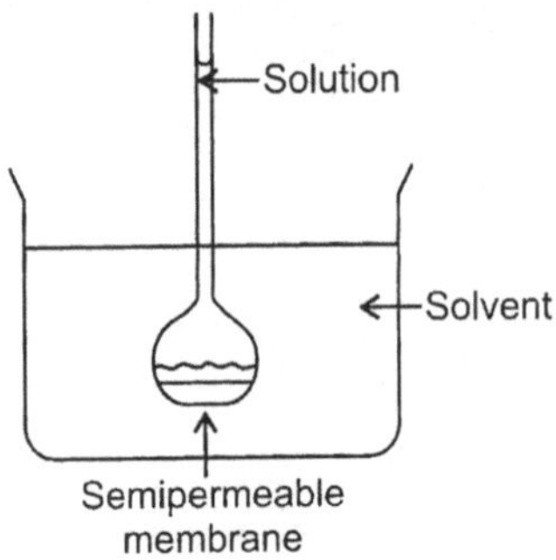

Fig. 9.8 Apparatus for demonstrating osmosis.

The activity or escaping tendency of the water molecules found in the solvent and solution separated by the semipermeable membrane is different. The activity which is related to the concentration of water which is higher in the pure solvent compartment. This difference in escaping-tendency gives rise to osmotic pressure of solutions. In the Fig. 9.8, the height of solution rises until the hydrostatic pressure exerted by the column of solution equals to osmotic pressure.

Osmotic pressure can be quantitatively determined by using osmometer as shown in Fig. 9.9. The equation involved is

$$\pi = h\rho g$$

where, π = osmotic pressure in (atm)

h = hydrostatic head

ρ = solution density

g = acceleration due to gravity

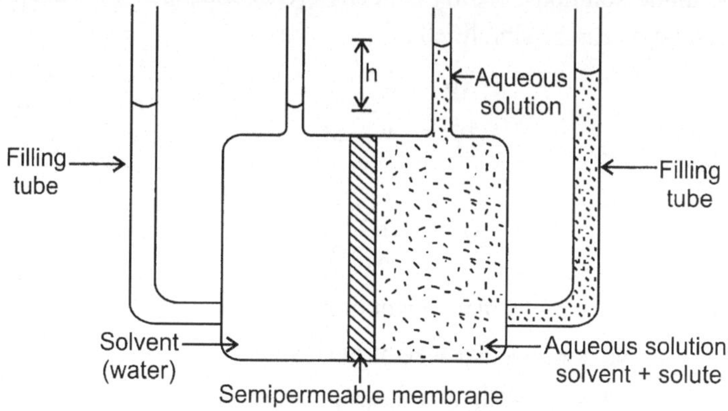

Fig. 9.9 Osmotic pressure osmometer.

Van't Hoff and Morse Equations for Osmotic Pressure : Van't Hoff recognised that osmotic pressure is directly proportional to concentration and temperature.

The equation suggested by Van't Hoff is as follows

$$\pi V = nRT \qquad .....(9.9)$$

where, π = osmotic pressure (atm)

V = volume in liters.

n = number of moles of solute.

R = Gas constant equal to 0.082 liter atm/mole degree.

T = absolute temperature

Morse and others have shown that when the concentration is expressed in molality rather than molarity $\pi V = nRT$, can be conveniently written as $\pi = RTm$, (where m = molality).

Molecular Weight Determination : Above discussed colligative properties can be used in calculating molecular weights of non-electrolytes that are present as solutes. In this section we will discuss the equations for arriving at molecular weight of dissolved non-electrolytes.

The equation for vapour pressure lowering is

$$\frac{P_1^0 - P_1}{P_1^0} = \frac{n_2}{n_1 + n_2} = \frac{w_2 / M_2}{w_1 / M_1 + w_2 / M_2} \qquad .....(9.10)$$

For dilute solutions, w_2/M_2 is negligible as compared to w_1/M_1, and entire equation can be simplified to

$$\frac{\Delta P}{P_1^0} = \frac{w_2/M_2}{w_1/M_1} \qquad .....(9.11)$$

or

$$M_2 = \frac{w_2 M_1 P_1^0}{w_1 \Delta P} \qquad .....(9.12)$$

where, M_2 = molecular weight of solute

M_1 = molecular weight of solvent

ΔP = lowering of vapour pressure

w_2 & w_1 = weights of solute and solvent respectively.

Using the equation of elevation in boiling point, molecular weight can be determined using equation

$$M_2 = K_b \frac{1000 w_2}{w_1 \Delta T_b} \qquad .....(9.13)$$

The molecular weight of organic substances soluble in molten camphor may be determined by observing the freezing point of mixture of the substance with camphor. This procedure, is known as Rast method, uses camphor because it has very large molal freezing-point depression constant, about 40°. Determination of molecular weight by freezing point method is more advantageous over boiling-point method, for its greater accuracy and precision. This is due to larger magnitude of freezing point depression compared to boiling point elevation.

For example; the molal elevation constant of water is 0.513° which is 3.5 times less than depression constant, i.e., 1.86°.

As discussed earlier, π = RTm for finding osmotic pressure. This can also written as π = RTc where c = molarity or moles/liter.

i.e.,

$$\pi = \frac{C_g RT}{M_2}$$

where M_2 = Molecular weight of solute

C_g = Concentration in grams/liter.

Problems

1. The vapour pressure of pure propellant 11 is 14.4 pounds/sqaure inch having molecular weight 137.4 at 21 °C and that of propelant 12 is 87.9 psi and molecular weight 120.9. A 50:50 mixture consits of 0.364 moles of propellant 11 and 0.414 mole of propellant 12. Calculate partial pressure of mixture of properlants and total vapour pressure of this mixture.

   Solution : Data given

Vapour pressure of propellant 11	= 14.4 psi
Molecular weight of propellant of 11	= 137.4
Vapour pressure of propellant 12	= 87.9 psi
Molecular weight of propellent 12	= 120.9

   Equation

   $$p_{11} = \frac{n_{11}}{n_{11}+n_{12}} p_{11}^{0} = \frac{0.364}{0.364+0.414} \times 14.4$$

   $$= 6.73 \text{ psi.}$$

   $$p_{12} = \frac{n_{12}}{n_{11}+n_{12}} p_{12}^{0} = \frac{0.414}{0.364+0.414} \times 87.9$$

   $$= 46.77 \text{ psi}$$

   The total vapour pressure of mixture is

   $$6.73 + 46.77 = 53.7 \text{ psi}$$

2. Compute relative vapour pressure lowering at 20 °C for a solution containing 184.2 gm of sucrose in 1000 g of water. Molecular weight of sucrose is 342.3 and that of water is 18.02 g/mole.

   Solution : Data given

   Solution of sucrose containing 184.2 gm of sucrose in 1000 gm of water.

   Molecular weight of sucrose is 342.3

   Molecular weight of water is 18.02

   $$\text{Moles of sucrose} = n_2 = \frac{w_2}{M_2} = \frac{184.2}{342.3} = 0.538$$

$$\text{Moles of water} = n_1 = \frac{w_1}{M_1} = \frac{1000}{18.02} = 55.5$$

Equation of relative vapour pressure lowering

$$\frac{\Delta p}{p_1^0} = X_2 = \frac{n_2}{n_1 + n_2}$$

$$\frac{\Delta p}{p_1^0} = \frac{0.538}{55.5 + 0.538} = 0.0096.$$

3. When 0.538 mole sucrose is added to1000 g of water at 20 °C, calculate vapour pressure if the vapour pressure of water at 20 °C is 17.54 mm Hg.

Solution : Data given

Sucrose = 0.538 mole in 1000 g of water at 20 °C

vapour pressure of water at 20 °C is 17.54 mm Hg.

Equation for vapour pressure

$$\Delta p = p_1^0 \; X_2 = p_1^0 \times 0.018 \times m$$

$$= 17.54 \times 0.018 \times 0.538$$

$$= 0.1698 \text{ mm} \simeq 0.17 \text{ mm}.$$

So the final vapour pressure is

$$17.54 - 0.17 \text{ mm} = 17.37 \text{ mm}.$$

4. Compute the molal elevation constant for the solvent water if a 0.350 m aqueous solution of a drug gave a boiling point elevation of 0.104 °C .

Solution : Data given

Concentration of drug in water = 0.350 m.

Elevation of boiling point = 0.104 °C

Equation for molal elevation constant

$$K_b = \frac{\Delta T_b}{m} = \frac{0.104}{0.350} = 0.2971 \text{ deg. Kg/mole.}$$

5. What is the freezing point of sucrose solution containing 3.52 g sucrose in 500 gm water ? Molecular weight of sucrose 342 and molal depression constant is 1.86.

Solution : Data given

Solution of sucrose contaning 3.52g in 500 g water.

Molecular weight of sucrose is 342.

Equation for freezing point depression

$$\Delta T_f = K_f m = K_f \frac{1000 w_2}{w_1 M_2}$$

$$\Delta T_f = 1.86 \times \frac{1000 \times 3.52}{500 \times 342}$$

$$= 0.038\ ^{o}C$$

Therefore, the freezing point of aqueous solution is 0.038 °C.

6. Calculate the freezing point depression of a 1.5 m solution of sucrose in water and depression constant is 2.1.

Solution : Data given

Molal depression = m = 1.5

Molal depression constant = K_f = 2.1

$$\Delta T_f = K_f \times m = 2.1 \times 1.5$$

$$= 3.15\ ^{o}C$$

7. Two gram of sucrose is dissolved in 100 ml of water at 25 °C. What is osmotic pressure of the solution ?

Solution : Data given

Two gram of sucrose in 100 ml water.

Molecular weight of sucrose = 342.

Temperature = 298 °K

$$\text{Mole of sucrose} = \frac{2.0}{342} = 0.0058.$$

Formula/equation for osmotic pressure

$$\pi V = \eta RT$$

$$\pi \times 0.1 \text{ liter} = 0.0058 \times 0.082 \times 298$$

$$\pi = 1.417 \text{ atm.}$$

8. Calculate molecular weight of sucrose if 20 gram of sucrose dissolved in 100 gm of water has a boiling point of 100.149 °C and $K_b = 0.51$.

Solution : Data given

Sucrose 20 gm in 100 gm water

Boiling point = 100.149 °C

Equation for molecular weight

$$M_2 = K_b \times \frac{1000 \times w_2}{w_1 \Delta T_b}$$

$$M_2 = 0.51 \times \frac{1000 \times 20}{100 \times 0.149}$$

$$= 684.5 \text{ g/mole.}$$

CHAPTER 10

Solutions of Electrolytes

In the earlier chapter we had a detailed discussion on non-electrolyte and their colligative properties. This section is oriented for electrolytes, which when dissolved in water produce charged particles known as ions. The charge of positive ions (cations) is equal to charge of negative ions (anions), thus the solution remains neutral inspite of the presence of charges.

$$K^+_{(solid)}\ Cl^-_{(Solid)} \xrightarrow{H_2O} K^+_{(solution)} + Cl^-_{(solution)}$$

These substances have the property to conduct electricity. When a molecule of KCl is dissolved in water it produces two charged particles. As colligative property depends on the number of particles, it is expected that osmotic pressure of solution would be twice that of a solution containing the same molal concentration of a non ionizing solute. Osmotic pressure data indicates that, the pressure is very nearly double that of solutions containing equimolar concentration of non-electrolyte. Similar relationship occured in vapour pressure lowering, elevation of boiling point and depression of freezing point in very dilute solutions where dissociation of electrolyte into ions is complete.

Van't Hoff defined a factor, i, which is the ratio of colligative effect produced by a concentration m, of electrolyte divided by the effect observed for the same concentration of nonelectrolyte. i.e.,

$$i = \frac{\pi}{\pi_0} = \frac{\Delta p}{\Delta p_0} = \frac{\Delta T_b}{(\Delta T_b)_0} = \frac{\Delta T_i}{(\Delta T_f)_0} \quad .....(10.1)$$

The subscript 'o' denotes non-electrolyte of the same concentration as electrolyte. The value of 'i' is equal to number of ions produced when electrolyte goes into solution (2 for KCl and NaCl, 3 for $CaCl_2$ etc).

As we increase the concentration of electrolyte the value of 'i' will decrease gradually, which can be attributed to interionic attraction between the positively and negatively charged ions, due to incomplete dissociation of the charges.

So we can conclude that Van't Hoff's factor holds good in case of very dilute solutions.

When a graph of i *vs* molality is plotted for electrolytes and noneletrolyte, as shown in Fig. 10.1, it is observed that non-electrolytes approach unity and strong electrolytes tends toward a value equal to the number of ions formed upon dissociation.

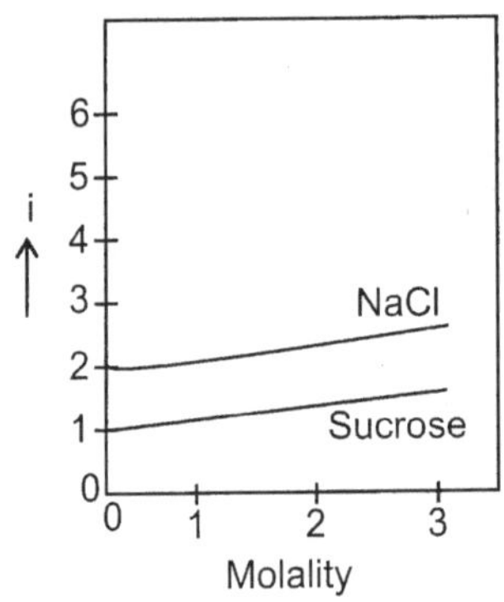

Fig. 10.1 Van't Hoff i factor of representative compounds.

Electrolytes can be classified into strong electrolytes and weak electrolytes.

Strong electrolytes include the solutions of strong acids, strong base and their salts. The extent of ionization is more and exists in the form of ions in solution.

Weak electrolytes include weak acids, weak bases, and their salts. Most of the organic acids, amines come under this category.

Conductivity of Electrolytes

It is the ability of electrolytes to conduct electricity in solution state. These solutions behave like metallic conductors and obey Ohm's law, except under abnormal conditions as very high voltages or with very high frequency currents.

According to Ohm's law.

$$I = E/R \quad .....(10.2)$$

where I = current that is flowing

R = resistance of conductor

E = electromotive force (EMF) applied or voltage.

Unit of resistance is Ohm.

From Ohm's law we can conclude that current flowing through a given conductor, under the influence of constant EMF is inversely proportional to the resistance; the quantity 1/R is a measure of the conducting power, and is called conductance (C); units "mhos" or ohm^{-1}.

The resistance of a conductor is directly proportional to length (l in cm) and inversely proportional to area (a in cm^2).

So mathematically,

$$R \propto l/a$$

i.e.,

$$R = \rho\, l/a \quad .....(10.3)$$

ρ is a constant, the specific resistance or resistivity of the conducting material. Units are Ohm. cm. It is also called as resistivity of conducting material.

Resistivity : It is the resistance in ohms of a specimen with 1 cm in length and 1 sq. cm in cross section. The inverse of resistivity is called specific conductance with units ohm^{-1}. cm^{-1}. Specific conductance is defined as "the conductance of one centimetre cube (CC) of a solution of an electrolyte". It is denoted by κ. Thus,

$$\kappa = \frac{1}{\rho} = \frac{1}{R} \times \frac{l}{A} \quad .....(10.4)$$

The conductivity power of all the ions produced by 1 gm equivalent of an electrolyte at any particular concentration may be evaluated by using two parallel electrodes, separated by 1 cm distance and a solution containing 1 gm equivalent to be placed between them. The conductance obtained by such system is called as equivalent conductance denoted by 'Λ' at the given concentration. The equivalent conductance at a concentration of C gram equivalent per liter is the product of specific conductance κ and volume V in cm^3 that contains 1 gm-equivalent of electrolyte at the dilution V.

$$\Lambda = \kappa V = \frac{\kappa \times 1000}{C} \text{ ohms}^{-1}\text{cm}^2\text{ eqvt}^{-1} \qquad .....(10.5)$$

where C is the concentration of solution in gram equivalent/liter.

Molar Conductance : It is denoted by 'μ' and is obtained by multiplying κ with volume in cubic centimeter containing 1 mole of electrolyte. Λ and μ are the same for univalent electrolytes as mole and gram equivalent are the same. Unit : Ohm^{-1} cm^2 $mole^{-1}$.

Theories of Electrolytic Dissociation

(a) ***Arrhenius theory***

Arrhenius came with his theory in 1887 explaining behaviour of electrolytic solutions and also regarding the enhancement in colligative properties. This theory can be successfully applied to weak electrolytes but failed for the strong electrolytes.

Arrhenius neglected the fact that ions in the solutions, being oppositely charged, tend to associate through electrostatic attraction. In dilute solutions, in which the strong electrolytes are assumed to be completely ionized, the interionic attractions become major factor and this effect is more pronounced as the concentration of electrolyte or the valence of the ions is increased.

In case of weak electrolytes the number of ions is not large enough to cause appreciable deviation from the theory.

Moreover if we consider a solid form of sodium chloride, sodium and chloride exist as ions, which are capable of conducting electric current in molten states. The addition of water dissolves the solid and separates the ions in solution.

(b) *Debye-Huckel Theory*

Debye-Huckel equation is applicable to very dilute solutions (about 0.02μ – 0.1 μ concentrations). The equation relates the activity co-efficient of a particular ion or the mean ionic activity co-efficient of an electrolyte to the valence of the ions, the ionic strength of the solution, and the characteristics of the solvent. According to the theory of Debye and Huckel, the activity coefficient γi of an ion of valence zi given by the expression.

$$\log \gamma i = -Azi^2 \sqrt{\mu} \qquad .....(10.6)$$

This equation measures the activity coefficient of an ion species upto an ionic strength μ of about 0.02.

Ionic strength (μ) relates the interionic attractions and activity coefficients. Mathematically,

$$\mu = \frac{1}{2} (C_1 z_1^2 + C_2 z_2^2 + ...C_n z_n^2)$$

or $$\mu = \frac{1}{2} \sum_1^n C_i z_i^2 \qquad .....(10.7)$$

It is the measure of intensity of the electrical field in a solution.

Equivalent Conductance of Strong and Weak Electrolytes

The value of Λ for a strong electrolyte increases on dilution, which is due to the decrease in hinderance from the neighbouring ions. As a results the ions can move faster in more dilute solution. In case of weak electrolytes the rate at which the Λ value increases is less as compared to strong electrolyte.

Kohlrausch, found that the equivalent conductance was a linear function of the square root of the concentration for strong electrolyte in very dilute solutions, as shown in Fig. 10.2.

$$\Lambda_C = \Lambda_o - b\sqrt{C} \qquad .....(108)$$

where Λ_C = equivalent conductance at concentration C.

Λ_o = equivalent conductance at infinite dilution.

b = constant and is the slope of the line for the strong electrolytes shown in Fig. 10.2

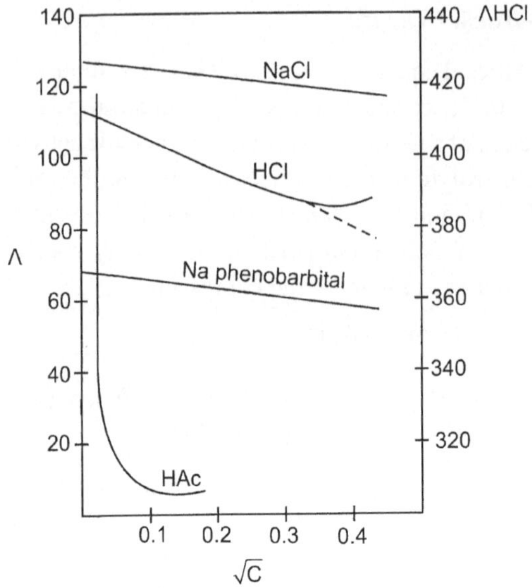

Fig. 10.2 Equivalent conductance of strong and weak electrolytes.

Conductometric Titrations

These are the titrations which make use of conductance measurements in determining the end-point of acid-alkali reaction. These include majorly :

(a) Titration of a strong acid V_s strong base
e.g., HCl aganist NaOH.

(b) Titration of weak acid V_s strong base
e.g., CH_3COOH aganist NaOH.

(c) Titration of strong acid V_s weak base.
e.g., HCl aganist CH_3COONa.

(d) Titration of weak acid V_s weak base.
e.g., CH_3COOH aganist CH_3COONa

Theory : Electrolytic solutions obey Ohm's law just as metallic conductors do. Thus, the electric current, I carried through a given solution by the migration of ions, is proportional to the potential difference, V :

$$V = IR$$

Although water is itself a poor conductor of electricity, the presence of ionic species in solution increases the conductance considerably. The conductance depends on the type and concentration of ions present in solution, as well as the temperature and conductance monitoring device. Thus, monitoring the conductance can provide a sensitive measure that take place in the ionic composition of a solution during the course of chemical reaction occuring during conductometric titration. This titration is done using a pH sensitive dye as indicator of end point.

Advantages

1. Useful for coloured solutions where indicators cannot work satisfactorily.
2. Useful for titration of acid-alkali solutions which do not give sharp colour change with indicator.

Problems

1. Calculate the equivalent conductance and specific conductance of the solution having conductance of 0.0673 mho at 25 °C and having 0.1 N concentrations. The cell constant is 0.620 cm^{-1}.

   Solution : Data given

   Concentration = 0.1 N

   Conductance = 0.0673 mho

   Cell constant = 0.620 cm^{-1}

   Equation of equivalent conductance Λ_C.

   $$\Lambda_C = \kappa \times V$$

   $$\kappa = 0.0673 \times 0.620 = 0.0417 \text{ mho/cm}$$

   V = volume in cm^3 contains 1 gm equivalent of solute

   $$\Lambda_C = 0.0417 \times 1000/_{0.1}$$

   $$= 417 \text{ mho cm}^2/\text{Eq.}$$

2. What is osmotic pressure of a 2.0 m solution of NaCl electrolyte at 20 °C ? Correction factor = 1.9.

   Solution : Data given

   Concentration = C = 2.0 m

   Correction factor = i = 1.9

   Equation for osmotic pressure

   $$\pi = i\,RTc$$

   $$\pi = 1.9 \times 0.082 \times 293 \times 2 = 91.3 \text{ atm.}$$

3. Calculate degree of dissociation of given electrolyte if freezing point depression for 0.02 m solution is 0.0467 °C ammonium chloride.

Solution : Data given

Freezing point depression for 0.02 m solution is 0.0467 °C

Equation for degree of dissociation

$$\alpha = \frac{i-1}{\nu-1}$$

i = Van't Hoff factor

$$i = \frac{\Delta T_f}{\kappa_f \ m} = \frac{0.0467}{1.86 \times 0.02} = 1.255$$

so $$\alpha = \frac{1.255-1}{\kappa_f \ m} = 0.255.$$

4. Calculate activity or escaping tendency of water in the sucrose solution. The vapour pressure of water in solution containing 0.7 mole of sucrose in 1000 g water is 16.93 mm and vapour pressure of pure water at 20 °C is 17.54 mm.

Solution : Data given

Vapour pressure of water in sucrose solution is 16.93 mm and for pure water is 17.54 mm.

Equation for activity (ratio of the vapour pressure P_1 of the solvent in a solution to the vapour pressure of pure solvent P_1^o is approximately equal to the activity of solvent at ordinary pressure).

$$\alpha = \frac{P_1}{P_1^o}$$

$$\alpha = \frac{16.93}{17.54} = 0.9652$$

CHAPTER 11

Solubility and Distribution Phenomena

Solubility is a phenomenon which involves formation of a uniform homogenous dispersion upon interaction of two or more substances. It is dependent on many factors like temperature, nature of solute and solvent under study, pH, pressure etc.

Quantitatively the solubility is expressed in terms of concentration or amount of solute to the volume of solution.

Based on states of matter, a total of nine possible types mixtures can be formed as shown in Table 11.1.

Table 11.1 Mixtures and their examples.

Nature of solute	Nature of solvent	Example
Gas	Gas	Air
Gas	Liquid	Oxygen in water
Gas	Solid	Hydrogen in palladium
Liquid	Liquid	Ethanol in water
Liquid	Solid	Mineral oil in paraffin
Liquid	Gas	Moisture in air
Solid	Liquid	Sugar solution
Solid	Solid	Various alloys
Solid	Gas	Iodine vapour in air.

Solutions can also be classified based on the amount of solute present in the solvent are as follows.

(a) ***Super Saturated Solution :*** It is the one that contains higher amounts of dissolved solute than the solvent would take up under normal temperature and pressure condition. It is the maximum limit of solubility of a solute in a solvent.

(b) ***Saturated Solution :*** At this stage the undissolved solute is in equilibrium with dissolved solute.

(c) ***Subsaturated or Unsaturated Solution :*** It is the one in which the amount of solute present is less than that required for saturation.

The solubility of drug may be expressed in number of ways. The U.S. pharmacopoeia and National formulary list the solubility of drugs as number of mililiters of solvent in which 1 gm of solute will dissolve. Terms of approximate solubility is given in Table 11.2.

Table 11.2 Terms of approximate solubility.

Term	ml of Solvent Required for Dissolving 1 gm of Solute
Very soluble	Less than 1 ml
Freely soluble	1 to 10 ml
Soluble	10 to 30 ml
Sparingly soluble	30 to 100 ml
Slightly soluble	100 to 1000 ml
Very slightly soluble	1000 to 10,000 ml
Practically insoluble	10,000 and over.

Solvent-Solute Interactions

Water is ubiquitous in nature. It is considered as universal solvent due to its good solubilizing capacity of various compounds. Before proceeding further one needs to know about the classification of solvents based on its polarity. i.e.,

(a) Polar solvents

(b) Non-polar solvents

(c) Semipolar solvents

(a) ***Polar Solvents :*** The polarity of solvent depends up on its dipole moment. For example water has its dielectric constant value 80 and hence it falls under the category of strongly polar solvents. The solubility of compounds in solvents can be generalized under statement "*like dissolves in like*", i.e., polar solvents have strong solubilizing power for polar substances or ionic solutes. Ionic solutes include salts like sodium chloride, potassium chloride etc. The solubility of a compound also depends on ability to form hydrogen bonds. Compounds having high dipole moment tend to form hydrogen bonds to a greater extent and hence show higher solubility in polar solvents.

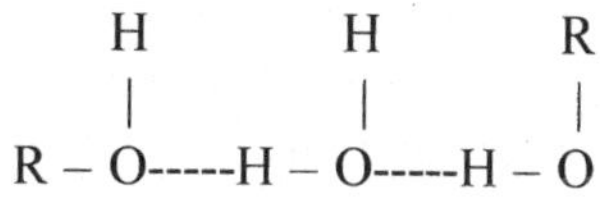

Alcohol

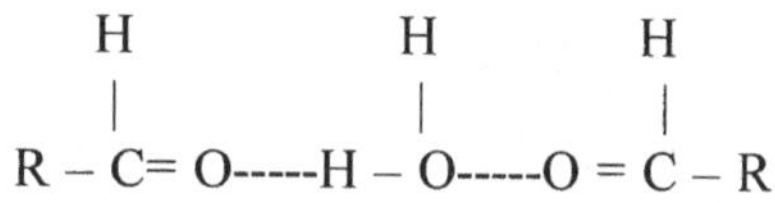

Aldehyale

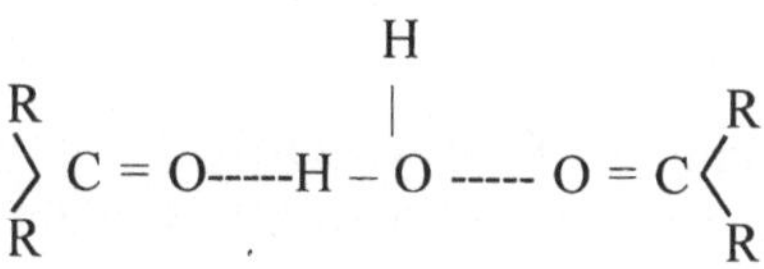

Ketone

Water dissolves phenols, alcohols, aldehydes ketones that can form hydrogen bonds with water molecules. When polar solvents like alcohol (lower alcohols) are added to water the hydrogen bonds between water molecules are replaced partly by the hydrogen bonds between alcohol and water molecules.

Apart from above mentioned factors the other parameters which play a key role in deciding the solubility include, ratio of polar to non polar groups of the molecule. The solubility is inversely proportional to the carbon chain length. E.g., The solubility of alcohols decreases with increasing carbon chain length. Branching of carbon chain increases the solubility of compound compared to its straight chain compound.

(b) ***Non-polar Solvents :*** Non-polar solvents have the capacity of dissolving non polar compounds. Generally oils, fats come under this category. They possess a very low dielectric constat value generally ranging from 0 – 10.

Due to this low dielectric constat value they fail in reducing the attraction between ions of strong and weak electrolytes.

These non-polar solvents are also called as aprotic solvents (can neither accept nor donate protons) which makes them unable to break covalent bonds or ionize weak electrolytes. Hence, non-polar solvents dissolve ionic and polar solutes only in neglible quantities.

(c) ***Semipolar Solvents :*** Ketones and alcohols have the property of inducing certain degree of polarity in non-polar solvent molecules. They are used as solvents for increasing solubility of non-polar substances in polar substances or polar substances in non-polar substances e.g., Propylene glycol has been shown to improve solubility of water in peppermint oil.

Solubility of Gases in Liquids

The solubility of gas in a liquid is the concentration of dissolved gas at equilibrium. Here, equilibrium is established between the pure gas above solution with the dissolved gas.

The common examples of gas solubilized preparations include Hydrochloric acid, Ammonia water, Beverages contain carbon dioxide dissolved under pressure.

The solubility depends primarily on pressure, temperature, presence of salts and chemical reactions that the gas sometimes undergoes with the solvent.

Effect of Pressure

The solubility of gas in a dilute solution at constant temperature, is proportional to the partial pressure of gas above solution at equilibrium. The relationship of pressure on solubility of gas is expressed by *Henry's law*.

$$C_2 = \sigma p \qquad .....(11.1)$$

where C_2 = concentration of dissolved gas in grams/liters of solvent.

p = partial pressure in millimeters of undissolved gas above the solution

σ = $1/K$,

where, K is Henry's law constant.

Effect of Temperature

With the increase in temperature solubility of most of gases decreases owing to the greater tendency of gases to expand. For the same reason gas perfumes, body sprays etc are exercised with caution in warm and hot climates. These containers should not be disposed in fire as the gas expands rapidly and results in bursting of container.

Salting Out

Introduction of electrolyte to solution that has dissolved gas results in liberation of gases from the solution. This phenomenon is called "*Salting Out*". This is due to the higher affinity of electrolyte to water molecules, which reduces the density of aqueous environment adjacent to the gas molecules.

Effect of Chemical Reaction

Henry's law is strictly applicable to gas which do not react with the solvent. The reaction between the gas and solvent alters the solubility. E.g., Hydrogen chloride is about 10,000 times more soluble in water than is oxygen.

Solubility of Liquids in Liquids

Quite often we come across the solubility of liquids in liquids in pharmaceutical solutions. These include preparation of elixirs, aromatic waters, Medicated oils etc.

As discussed earlier solutions can be classified into :

(a) ***Ideal Solutions :*** In which binary solutions obey *Raoult's law* over the whole range of compositions.

(b) ***Real Solutions :*** These are the binary solutions which show either positive or negative deviation from Raoult's law. If one compound shows positive deviation then other component also tends to show positive deviation. Positive deviations leads to decrease in solubility due to formation of dimers or polymers.

Broadly one can classify liquid-liquid systems into three categories :

(a) Complete miscibility

(b) Partial miscibility

(c) Immiscibility

(a) *Complete miscibility* represents complete solubility of two or more solvents in all proportions.

Eg : Water and Methanol, Glycerin and Alcohol

(b) *Partial miscibility* represents systems which are soluble in each other in definite proportions.

Eg : Ether and water, Nicotine and water; phenol and water

(c) *Immiscibility* represents systems that do not mix up with each other in any proportion.

Eg : Water and liquid petrolatum.

Our further discussion is concerned with partial miscible systems mainly two-component and three-component systems.

Nicotine and water is a two components system which shows both upper consolute temperature as well as lower consolute temperature. The points lying inside the curve represents systems that are immiscible. Reader is suggested to revert back to phase rule for detailed explanation.

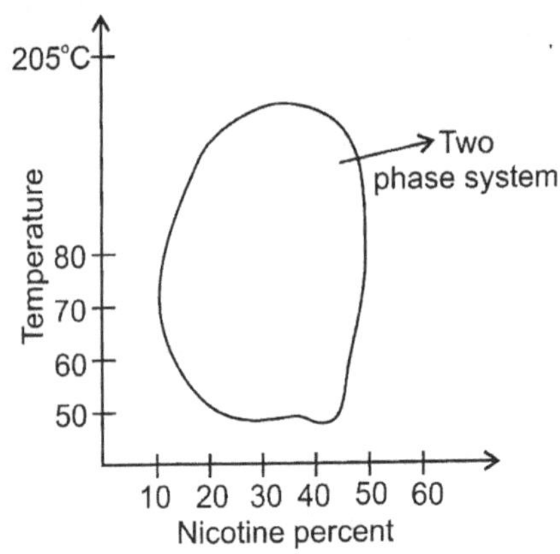

Fig. 11.1 Phase diagram for Nicotine-water system.

Ternary Systems : These systems are produced up on the addition of third component to a binary system. Affinity of the third component should be more or less same towards both binary components which reduces upper consolute temperature and elevates lower consolute temperature.

We can get a better idea of a ternary system from the Fig. 11.2. A turbid or cloudy point was observed at 67% alcohol, 27% oil, and 6% water. This indicates that alcohol which is roughly soluble in oil and water to same extent increase molal solubility of oil and water i.e., upper critical temperature of solution is lowered and lower critical temperature of solution is raised.

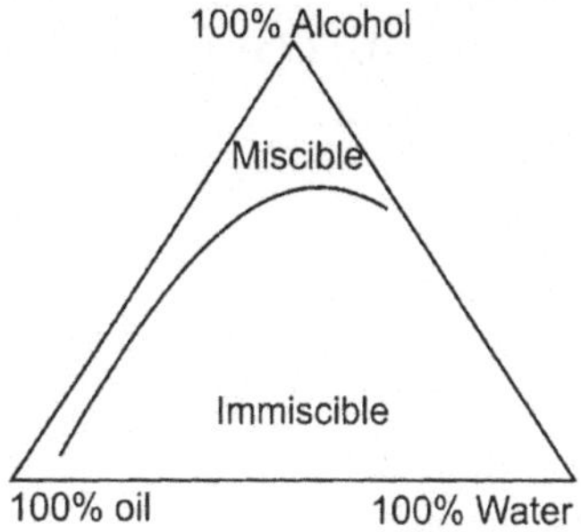

Fig. 11.2 Phase diagram of a ternary system oil, alcohol, water.

Other factors which influence solubility of liquids in liquids include :

(a) ***Dielectric Constant :*** The solubility of caffine in a mixture of dioxane and water is shown in Fig. 11.3 which depicts the solubility (mg/ml) in relation to dielectric constant ($\in$).

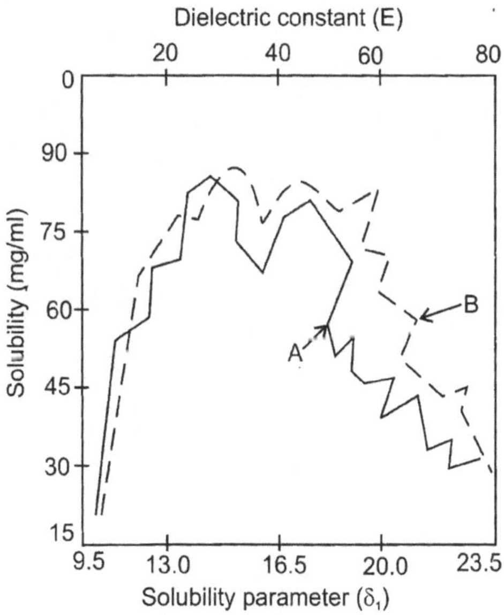

Fig. 11.3 Dielectric constant.

The dielectric properties of a mixed solvent, such as water and alcohol, can be approximated to the weighted average properties of pure components.

Hence additive in nature

$$\in_{mixture} = 0.6\,(\in_{(ethanol)}) + 0.4\,(\in_{(water)})$$
$$= 0.6\,(25) + 0.4\,(80)$$
$$= 47.$$

Molecular Connectivity

This takes into account structural features and functional groups of the molecule. It is denoted by 'X' (chi). The 'X represents first-order chi term and is obtained by summing the bonds weighted by the reciprocal square root number of each bond.

For e.g.,

Carbon atom 1 is attached to central atom which is inturn joined to other carbons by two bonds.

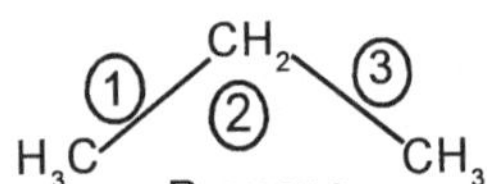

Propane

So the reciprocal square root valance is

$$\frac{1}{(1.2)^{1/2}} = 0.707.$$

The same applied to right bond also. The total value of

$$\perp_X = 0.707 + 0.707$$
$$= 1.414.$$

For isobutane,

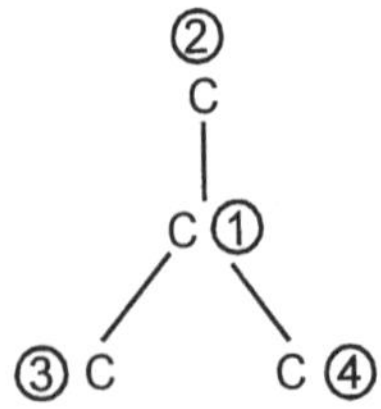

$$\perp_X = \frac{1}{(1.3)^{1/2}} + \frac{1}{(1.3)^{1/2}} + \frac{1}{(1.3)^{1/2}} = 1.732$$

Solubility of Solids in Liquids

This is yet another broader area of pharmaceutical interest. Broadly we can classify the solutions in to ideal solutions and real solutions.

For ideal solutions the behaviour can be predicted in a satisfactory manner.

Ideal Solutions : Various factors which affect the solubility of a solid include temperature, melting point, and molar heat of fusion ΔH_f (heat absorbed when solid melts). For ideal solutions heat of fusion is equal to heat of solution, which is constant independent of the temperature. The equation derived from the thermodynamics for ideal solution is

$$\log \frac{k_S, T_2}{k_S, T_1} = \frac{\Delta H(T_2 - T_1)}{2.303R\, T_1 T_2} + \text{constant}$$

where K_s, T_1 = saturation solubility at absolute temperature, T_1

K_S, T_2 = saturation solubility at absolute temperature T_2.

ΔH = heat of solution.

Effect of Temperature

As evident from the above equation the solubility of solid in a liquid depends on the temperature. If heat is absorbed in process of solution then ΔH will be positive and solubility of solute increases with increase in temperature. If a solute gives off heat during the process of solution, ΔH is negative and solubility decreases with increase in temperature. Most of the salts show positive ΔH values. Salts like calcium sulfate and calcium hydroxide show negative ΔH values. When heat is neither absorbed nor given off, the solubility is not affected by variation of temperature as is nearly the case with sodium chloride.

Solubility of Strong Electrolytes

Whenever a strong electrolyte is dissolved in a solution, we can observe the following :

(a) Rise in the temperature of system, or exothermic process.

(b) Decrease in the temperature of system or endothermic process.

(c) No change in temperature of system.

According to Lechaterlier principle, any system tends to adjust itself in a manner so as to counteract, any stress. So any change in the temperature of system will proceed in the direction, so as to nullify the change.

The effect of temperature on the solubility of some salts in water is shown in Fig. 11.4.

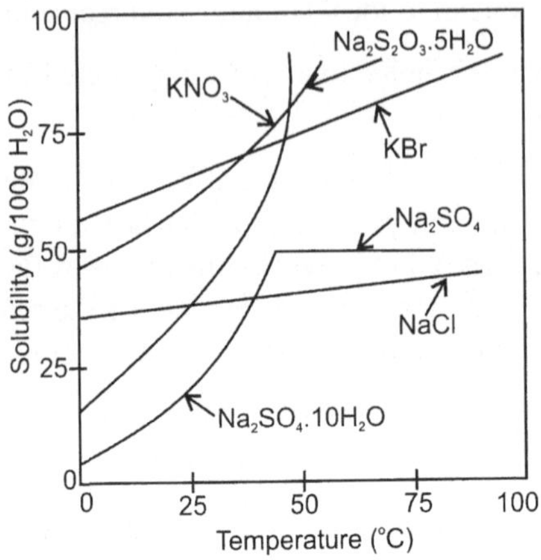

Fig. 11.4 Influence of temperature on solubility of various salts.

Solubility of Weak Electrolytes

Many drugs belong to the class influenced by the pH of the solvents. For example, a 1% solution of phenobarbital sodium is soluble at pH values greater than 8.3. If the pH is less than 8.3 the drug starts precipitating out in the form of molecular phenobarbital. Similarly alkaloidal salts such as atropine sulfate begin to precipitate as pH is elevated.

Many drugs containing carboxylic acid as a functional group are relatively insoluble in water. Upon addition of dilute sodium hydroxide, carbonate they form soluble salts. Sodium citrate is used to solubilize acetyl salicylic acid by the formation of acetyl salicylate ion.

Many compounds containing nitrogen atom are weak electrolytes that are not very soluble in water, but soluble in dilute solutions of acids. Various example, under this category include Atropine sulfate, Tetracaine hydrochloride etc.

Effect of pH on solubility of Weak Electrolytes

Take the above mentioned example of phenobarbital sodium. At pH below 8.3 phenobarbital sodium starts precipitating from solution at room temperature. The pH at which the drug precipitates from aqueous solution can be calculated in the following way :

Heat of the solution (ΔH) is the sum of heat of sublimation of the solid and heat of hydration (solvation) of the ions in the solution.

$$\Delta H_{(solution)} = \Delta H_{sublimation} + \Delta H_{hydration}$$

If $\Delta H > 0$ then absorption of heat by system

$\Delta H < 0$ then evolution of heat by system.

Solubility of Slightly Soluble Electrolyte

The solubility of slightly soluble electrolytes is described by solubility product, K_{sp}, of the compound. For example, consider silver chloride which when dissolved in excess exists in equilibrium as

$$Ag\,Cl_{solid} \rightleftharpoons Ag^{+} + Cl^{-}$$

The equilibrium expression may be written as

$$K = \frac{\left[Ag^{+}\right]\left[Cl^{-}\right]}{\left[AgCl_{Solid}\right]}$$

As the concentration of $[Ag\,Cl_{Solid}]$ is constant.

$$K_{SP} = [Ag^{+}]\,[Cl^{-}]$$

Addition of sodium chloride to above silver chloride solution results in common ion effect.

$$[Ag^{+}]\,[Cl^{-}] > K_{SP}$$

Some of the AgCl precipitates from the solution until equilibrium $[Ag^{+}]\,[Cl^{-}] = K_{SP}$ is re-established.

$$HP_{Solid} \rightleftharpoons HP_{Sol} \quad .....(11.2)$$

$$HP_{Sol} + H_2O \rightleftharpoons H_3O^{+} + P^{-} \quad .....(11.3)$$

Equilibrium constant for Eq. (11.3) is

$$K_a = \frac{\left[H_3O^{+}\right]\left[P^{-}\right]}{[HP]_{Sol}}$$

or

$$[P] = \frac{K_a\,[HP]_{Sol}}{\left[H_3O^{+}\right]}$$

And for Eq. (11.2) equilibrium constant is

$$S_o = [HP_{Sol}]$$

The total solubility of phenobarbital consists of the concentration of undissociated acid $[HP_{Sol}]$ and $[P^-]$

$$S = [HP_{Sol}] + [P^-]$$

Substituting S_o, and K_a, we get,

$$S = S_o + K_a \frac{S_o}{[H_3O^+]}$$

$$S = S_o \left(1 + \frac{K_a}{[H_3O^+]}\right)$$

or $$\frac{S - S_o}{S_o} = \frac{K_a}{[H_3O^+]}$$

Applying log on both sides

$$pH_p = pK_a + \log \frac{S - S_o}{S_o}$$

Thus we can obtain the pH below which the drug separates from the solution.

The Influence of Solvents on Solubility of Drugs

The solubility of solutes can be increased by using cosolvents. This phenomenon is called cosolvency. The solubility of phenobarbital is studied using alcohol and glycerine as cosolvents. It is observed that a mixture 40% glycerine, 22% alcohol and 38% water, could take up 1.5% w/v of phenobarbital.

Combined Effects of pH and Solvents

The addition of cosolvents like alcohol to buffered solution containing a weak electrolyte further increases the solubility of undissociated species by altering the polarity of solvent to a more favourable value.

Alcohol, being less polar than water decreases the dissociation of weak electrolyte and the solubility of drug goes down as pKa is increased. The influence of alcohol concentration on dissociation constant can be understood.

Distribution Phenomenon

When we add a solid or liquid to a system of two immiscible liquids, it will distribute itself between the two phase in a definite concentration ratio. The two immiscible liquids may be oil and water system or organic and aqueous phase system.

Let the concentration of solute in organic phase be C_{org} and aqueous phase be C_{aq} at equilibrium. The distribution co-efficient K is the ratio of concentration of solute in organic phase to concentration of solute in aqueous phase.

$$K_{o/w} = \frac{C_{org}}{C_{aq}} \text{ or } K_{w/o} = \frac{C_{aq}}{C_{org}}$$

K is also termed as partition coefficient, or distribution ratio.

Applications of Distribution Coefficient

1. Absorption and distribution of drugs in the body.
2. Drug action at non specific sites.
3. Preservation of oil-water system etc.

Effect of Ionic Dissociation and Molecular Association on K : Some solutes may exist partly or wholly as associated molecules in one phase and may exist as dissociated ions in another phase. This phenomena leads to certain deviations from the original distribution law.

If we consider the distribution of Benzoic acid in an oil/water system, we can clearly understand the above said deviation as shown in Fig. 11.5.

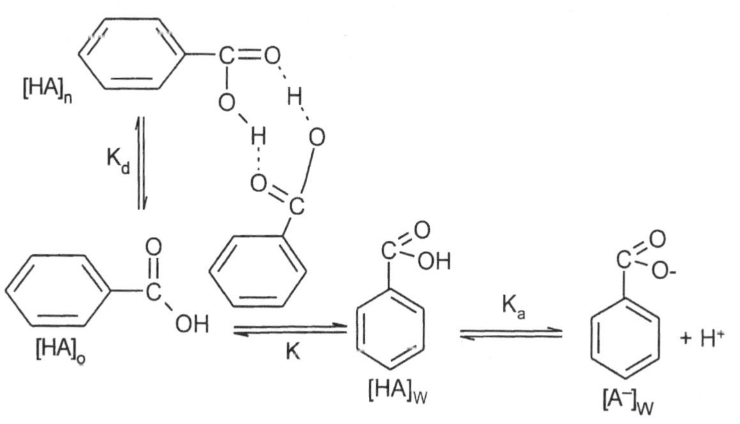

Fig. 11.5 Distribution of benzoic acid between a water and an oil.

Benzoic acid exists as a dimer in oil phase i.e., two molecules of benzoic acid associates to form a dimer of benzoic acid.

$$(HA)_n \rightleftharpoons n(HA)$$

$$\text{Associated molecules} \rightleftharpoons \text{Simple molecules}$$

And the equilibrium constant between the associated and simple molecules is denoted by

$$K_d = \frac{[HA]_o^n}{[(HA)_n]}$$

$$[HA]_o = \sqrt[n]{K_d}\ \sqrt[n]{[(HA)_n]}$$

For Benzoic acid n = 2 as it exists in dimer form so,

$$S_o = [HA]_o \cong \text{constant} \times \sqrt{C_o}$$

If we consider acidified water as aqueous phase system then benzoic acid molecules remain intact in undissociated form.

Now distribution co-efficient, $K = \dfrac{[HA]_o}{[HA]_w}$

But $[HA_o] \cong \text{constant} \times \sqrt{C_o}$

So $$K = \frac{\text{Constant} \times \sqrt{C_o}}{[HA]_w}$$

Modified distribution coefficient $K' = \dfrac{\sqrt{C_o}}{[HA]_w}$

Now consider a second case, where oil phase is peanut oil and aqueous phase having a suitable pH that can dissociate benzioc acid molecules. Unlike other oils, benzoic acid does not associate in peanut oil.

So if we consider distribution coefficient,

$$K = \frac{[HA]_o}{[HA]_w} = \frac{C_o}{C_w}$$

But $C_w = [HA]_w + [A^-]_w$

(As certain molecules exist in dissociated form)

So apparent distribution coefficient

$$K' = \frac{[HA]_o}{[HA]_w + [A^-]_w} \qquad .....(11.4)$$

The dissociation constant of benzoic acid is given by

$$K_a = \frac{[H_3O^+][A^-]_w}{[HA]_w} \qquad .....(11.5)$$

Eq. (11.4) and Eq. (11.5) can be combined to give

$$\frac{K_a + [H_3O^+]}{C_w} = \frac{K_a}{C} + \frac{K+1}{C}[H_3O^+]$$

A plot of $\frac{K_a + [H_3O^+]}{C_w}$ on y-axis and $[H_3O^+]$ on x-axis yields a straight line with slope equal to $\frac{K+1}{C}$ and intercept $= \frac{K_a}{C}$

The oil/water distribution co-efficient is an indication of lipophilic or hydrophobic charactor of drug molecule. For the purpose of study of drug, passage through lipodial membrane, good correlation is observed by using octanol / water system.

Problems

1. How many grams of oxygen can be dissolved in 500 ml of aqueous solution when the total pressure above the mixture is 760 mm.Hg. The partial pressure of oxygen in the solution is 0.263 atm.

   Solution : Data given

   Partial pressure = 0.263 atm

   Henry's law constant $= \sigma = 5.33 \times 10^{-5}$

   Equation

$$\sigma = \frac{C_2\,(\text{g/liter})}{p\,(\text{mm.Hg})}$$

$$5.33 \times 10^{-5} = \frac{C_2\,(\text{g/liter})}{(0.263 \times 760)\,\text{mm}}$$

$$C_2 = 0.0107 \text{ g/liter}$$

$$= 0.00535 \text{ g/500 ml}$$

2. Compute the internal pressure of water if the molar heat of vaporization of water 25 °C is 12,500 cal and V is 20.03 cm^3; gas constant R is 1.987 cal/mole.deg.

   Solution : Data given

   Molar heat of vaporization $= \Delta H_V$

   R = gas constant = 1.987 cal/mole.deg

   Temperature = 298 °K

   and molar volume = 20.03 cm^3

   Equation for internal pressure

$$P_i = \frac{\Delta H_V - RT}{V}$$

$$= \frac{12{,}500 - (1.987 \times 298)}{20.03}$$

$$= 594.50 \text{ cal/cm}^3$$

3. What is the solubility of given substance at 20 °C in an ideal solution? The melting point of given substance is 80 °C and the molar heat of fusion is 4500 cal/mole.

   Solution : Data given

   Melting point = 80 °C = 353 °K

   Molar heat of fusion = 4500 cal/mole

   Equation for ideal solubility

$$\log X_2^i = \frac{\Delta H_f}{2.303R}\left(\frac{T_o - T}{T\,T_o}\right)$$

$$\log X_2^i = \frac{4500}{2.303 \times 1.987}\frac{(353-293)}{293 \times 353}$$

$$X_2^i = 0.27.$$

4. A solid material is to be comminuted so as to increase its solubility by 10% i.e., S/S_0 is 1.10. What is final radius of particles in cm, assuming that the surface tension of solid is 110 dynes/cm and volume per mole is 70 cm^3. Temperature is 27 °C.

   Solution : Data given

   γ = surface tension = 110 dynes/cm

   T = 300 K

   Volume per mole = 70 cm^3

   Equation

$$\log {}^{S}\!/_{S_o} = \frac{2\gamma V}{2.303\,RTr}$$

$$r = \frac{2 \times 110 \times 70}{2.303 \times 8.314 \times 10^7 \times 300 \times 0.0414}$$

$$= 6.4 \times 10^{-6} \text{ cm}$$

$$= 0.064\ \mu\text{m}.$$

CHAPTER 12

The Solid State

Solids are the substances which possess rigid structure and have the tendency to maintain definite shape and volume. Unlike liquids they have high values of Young's modulus and shear modulus of elasticity. The branch of physics that deals with the behavior of solids is called solid-state physics and the branch of chemistry which deals with the synthesis and identification of novel solid materials is called as solid-state chemistry. The atoms, molecules and ions are held together by strong chemical forces. Solids can be classified into two types based on the arrangement constituent units :

(a) ***Crystalline Solids :*** These are characterised by definite geometric shape. The atoms, molecules or ions have regular, repeating crystal arrangement.

Examples include various salts like sodium chloride, potassium chloride etc.

(b) ***Amorphous Solids :*** These solids lack ordered crystalline lattice structure. The constituent units are arranged randomly in a disordered structure.

Examples include plastic, rubber, glass etc.

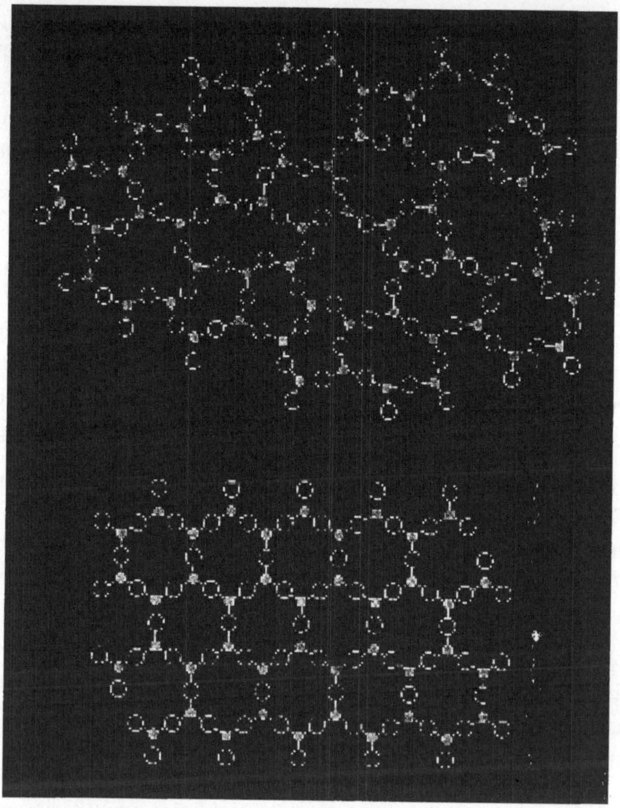

Schematic representation of a random-network glassy form (top) and ordered crystalline lattice (bottom) of identical chemical composition. *Courtesy: Logger9*

Depending upon the nature of forces acting the solids can be divided into four types :

(i) ***Covalent Solids :*** In these solids the constituent units are attached by covalent linkages. The electrostatic glue between the particular ions is piled up into distinct bonds resulting in covalent linkages. Depending on arrangement, these can be divided into isotropic and anisotropic substances.

(I) ***Isotropic Substances :*** These systems show uniform velocity of light in all directions. Amorphous substance exhibit this property. Other parameters like refractive index, thermal and electrical conductivities are also uniform in all directions.
Eg : Water, glass

(II) ***Anisotropic Substances :*** The velocity of light is not uniform in all directions. When a ray enters anisotropic substance it splits up into two separate components which travel with different velocities. The other physical properties which are mentioned in isotropic substance also vary in anisotropic substances.

Eg : Silver iodide.

(ii) ***Ionic Solids :*** In these substances the unit constituents are ions (positive and negative). These ions are held together by electrostatic forces maintaining overall electroneutrality. Ionic solids have high melting and boiling points because of very strong forces between the ions throughout the crystal and have poor electrical conductivity as the electrons are tightly bound to each ion (positive or negative).

(iii) ***Metallic Solids :*** These are good conductors of heat and electricity. The elements in the periodic table that have cubic closed-packed or hexagonal closed-packed unit cells come under this category of solids. Their coordination number is 12. They also possess other properties like malleability, *ductility* and shining luster.

(iv) ***Molecular Solids :*** These are held together by weak Van der Waal's forces. Rare gases fall under this category of solids. At very low temperatures these exist as solids. They are characterized by low melting and boiling points.

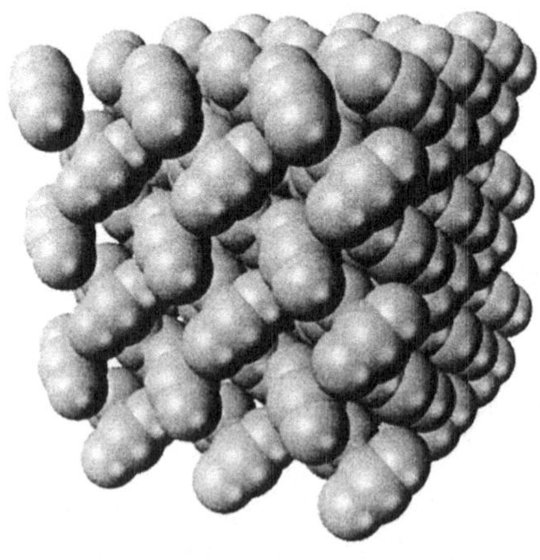

Crystal structure of solid carbon dioxide, molecular solid containing discrete CO_2 molecules, *Courtesy: Ben Mills*

Bragg's equation : In 1913 W.L. Bragg made a successful attempt in determining the interatomic distance in a crystal lattice using X-rays. The study of crystal structure with the help of X-rays is called X-ray crystallography.

He showed that :

(i) X-rays obey laws of reflection

(ii) The extra distance travelled by the second ray [P] is an integral number of wavelength

So $n\lambda = 2d \sin\theta$ (Bragg's equation)

For a given set of lattice planes d and λ are fixed.

d - distance between

λ - wavelength of x-rays

θ - Angle at which the X-rays strike the crystal

n - order of reflection.

Methods of Crystal Analysis

When a beam of X-rays is allowed to pass through crystal lattice, a large number of images of different intensities are formed. A crystal lattice is considered to be made up of regular planes which are separated by equal distance. So, if the diffracted waves are in the same phase, they reinforce each other and a series of bright spots are produced on a photographic plate placed in their path as shown in Fig. 12.1.

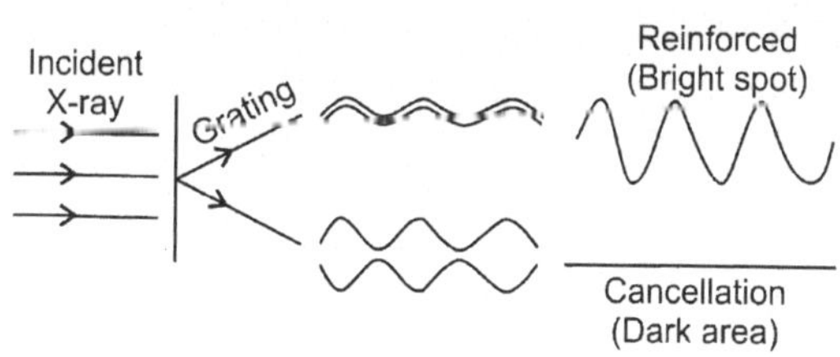

Fig. 12.1 Diffraction pattern produced by the crystals.

X-ray crytallography is the study of crystal structure with help of X-rays.

Procedure

In this method a beam of X-rays of known wavelength is made to fall on the crystal mounted on a graduated turn table as shown in Fig. 12.2.

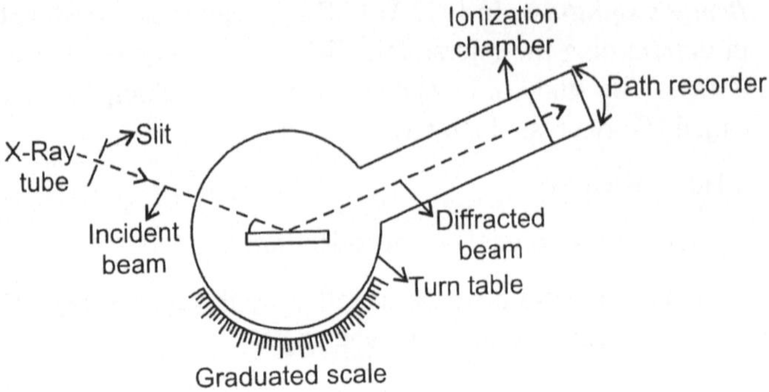

Fig. 12.2 Rotating Crystal Method.

The diffracted rays are allowed to pass through ionization chamber of the recorder. The reading obtained on the electrometer is proportional to the intensity of X-rays. This method is also known as Rotating Crystal Method as the recorder along with the crystal is rotated for the angles of maximum intensity. Using the values of θ, λ and n, one can calculate "d" value.

Powder Method

In this method a powdered sample containing many small crystals arranged in all orientations is placed in a capillary tube, which is attached to camera contaning a film strip. The sample is rotated by means of a motor. The X-rays pass through the gaps between the ends of the film. The mechanism of powder method is given in Fig. 12.3.

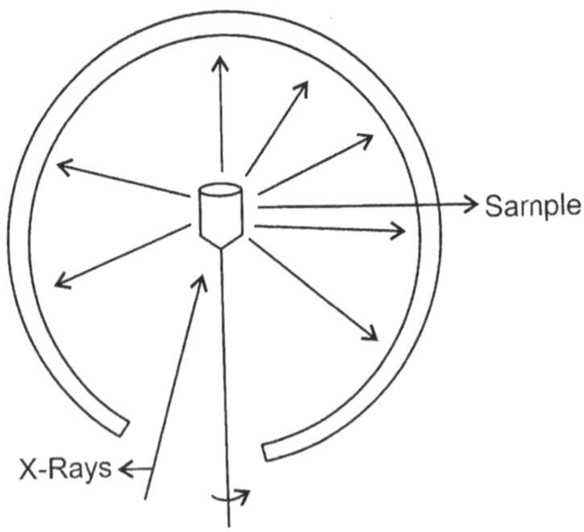

Fig. 12.3 Powder method.

The reflected X-rays make an angle of 2θ with the incident X-ray. From the geometry of camera, θ can be calculated for different crystal planes.

Bragg's Method

W. L. Bragg in 1913, used X-rays for the purpose of studying the internal structure of crystals. The reflection of X-rays from different planes is shown in Fig. 12.4.

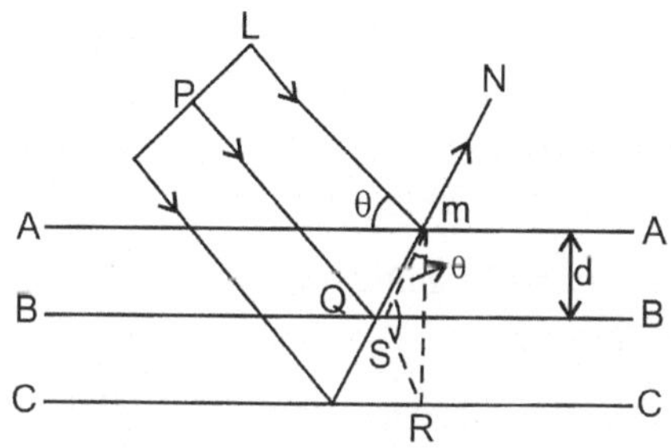

Fig. 12.4 Reflection of X-rays from different of planes of crystals.

Polymorphism

Many substances exist in more than one form in crystalline state; this phenomenon is known as polymorphism. This phenomenon of polymorphism occurs in various elements, organic, inorganic substances.

Allotropy is synonymous to polymorphism. Elements like carbon, sulfur and phosphorus etc show allotropy.

A substance existing in two different forms it is called diamorphic, if there are three different forms it is trimorphic and so on.

Isopolymorphism : If each of the two forms of a polymorphic substance is isomorphous with a form of another polymorphic substance the phenomenon is known as isopolymorphism. e.g., Arsenic and antimony trioxides are isodiamorphous.

Polymorphs generally have different melting points, X-ray diffractions and solubilities.

Theobroma oil or Coca butter is a polymorphous natural fat. It exists in four polymorphic forms. Unstable gamma form has melting point at 18 °C.

Alpha form melts at 22 °C.

Beta prime form melts at 28 °C.

Stable Beta form melts at 34.5 °C.

This study helps in preparation of Coca butter suppositories.

Polymorphs study also proved to be useful in the case of slightly soluble drugs and hence its therapeutic activity. e.g., chloramphenicol in its ester form as chloramphenicol palmitate is found to have significant activity.

Cortisone acetate has been found to exist in atleast five different forms. But only one form is found to stable in suspension form. Other polymorphic forms of cortisone acetate were found to be unstable in presence of water and accompanied by appreciable caking of crystals.

Tamoxifen citrate, an antiestrongenic and antineoplastic drug exist in two forms (form A and form B).

Form B is found to be more stable due to formation of hydrogen bonding. Form A is metastable and immediately rearranges spontaneously into form B in ethanolic suspension.

Problems

1. The diffraction of crystal with X-radiation of wavelength 2.29 Å gives a first order reflection at $27^{o}\ 8^{1}$. Calculate distance between the diffracted planes.

   Solution : Data given

   $$n = 1$$

   $$\lambda = 2.29\ \text{Å}$$

   $$\theta = 27^{o}\ 8^{1}$$

   Equation : Bragg's Equation

   $$n\lambda = 2d \sin\theta$$

   $$1 \times 2.29\ \text{Å} = 2.d \sin 27^{o}\ 8^{1}$$

   $$d = 2.51\ \text{Å}$$

CHAPTER 13

Micromeritics

Micromeritics is science of small particles and the study of particle size distribution. Micromeritics is the study of a number of characteristics, including particle size and distribution, shape, angle of repose, porosity, true volume, bulk volume, apparent density, and bulkiness.

The unit of particle size used most frequently is micrometer, μm or micron, μ and is equal to 10^{-6} m or 10^{-3} mm. Sometime millimicron unit is used and is equal to 10^{-9}m. The millimicron is commonly referred to as the nanometer, nm.

The Applications of Micromeritics

The knowledge of particle technology is essential in the formulation and manufacturing of dosage forms such as powders, tablets, suspensions, emulsions, aerosols etc. The particle size or surface area and other properties can be related to physical, chemical and pharmacological properties of a drug. Clinically, the particle size of a drug can affect its release from dosage forms. Higher the dissolution, faster the absorption, and hense quicker and greater the drug action. The physical stability and pharmacological response of many dosage form depends on the particle size. Smaller the size of particles, better the physical stability of dosage form, example – suspension, emulsion.

Particle size is important in extraction process. Flow properties of grannules and powders are important in manufacture of tablets and capsules. Rate of dissolution depends upon particle size. The Whitney-Noyes equation shows that rate of dissolution is proportional to the area.

Particle size and size Distribution : When a powder sample contains of uniform size, it is said to be monodisperse. In collection of particles of more than one size, it is said to be polydisperse. The pharmaceutical powders are almost always be polydisperse and hence it is necessary to charcterise particle size and their distribution. For characterisation two properties are important i.e., (a) the shape and surface area of the individual particles, and (b) the size range and number or weight of particles present and hense, the total surface area.

The size of a sphere can compleatly be expressed in terms of its diameter. When particle is asymmetrical the diameter which is related to an equivalent spherical diameter, which relates the size of the particles to the diameter of a sphere having the same surface area, volume or diameter.

The size of particles may be expressed as :

(i) ***Surface diameter, d_s :*** Is the diameter of a sphere having the same surface area as that of the asymmetric particle.

(ii) ***Volume diameter, d_v :*** Is the diameter of of a sphere having same volume as that of the asymmetric particle.

(iii) ***Projected diameter, d_p :*** Is the diameter of sphere having the same observed area as the particle when viewed normal to its most stable plane.

(iv) ***Stokes' diameter, d_{st} :*** Is the diameter of an equivalent sphere undergoing sedimentation at the same rate as the asymmetric particle.

(v) ***Sieve diameter, d_{sieve} :*** Is the diameter of a sphere that will just pass through the same square or sieve aperture as the particle.

(vi) ***Volume-surface diameter; d_{vs} :*** Is the diameter of a sphere that has the same volume to surface area ratio as the asymmetric particle.

Averge Particle Size : An average or mean diameter is usually used for comparison of particle size of two different batches for same material. The data obtained from one batch is compared with data obtained from second batch to determine the batch to batch variation by same method : Example – the data obtained from microscopic method; Counted more than 200 particles using a calibrated ocular on a microscope. Given following data, calculate the average diameter of the particles.

Size of counted particles (mm)	Middle value 'mm'	No. of ' particles 'N	ND
40 – 60	50	15	750
60 – 80	70	25	1750
80 – 100	90	95	8550
100 –120	110	140	15400
120 – 140	130	80	10400

$\Sigma_n = 355$ $\Sigma_{nd} = 36850$

$$d_{av} = \frac{\Sigma_{nd}}{\Sigma_n} = \frac{36850}{355} = 103.8 \ \mu m$$

Similarly data obtained from second batch the average particle size can be calculated and compared and one can find out batch to batch variation.

Particle Size Distribution : When the number, or we ight of particles lying within a certain size range is plotted against the size range or mean particle size, a frequency distribution curve can be obtained, as shown in Fig. 13.1. An alternative method for representation of particle size distribution is to plot either the cumulative percentage over or under a particular size versus particle size, as given in Fig.13.2. A frequency distribution plot as shown in Fig.13.3 can be plotted for both number distribution and weight distribution.

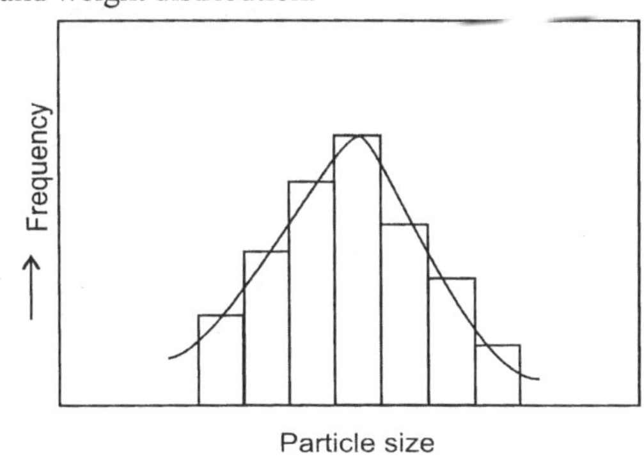

Fig. 13.1 A size-frequency distribution as a bar graph or histogram (Normal distribution curve).

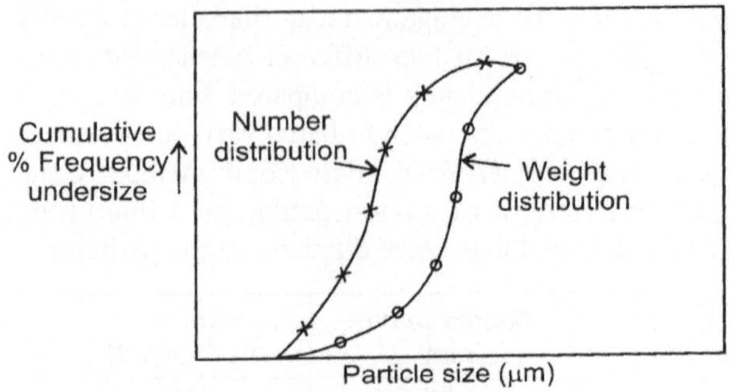

Fig. 13.2 Cummulative frequency plot.

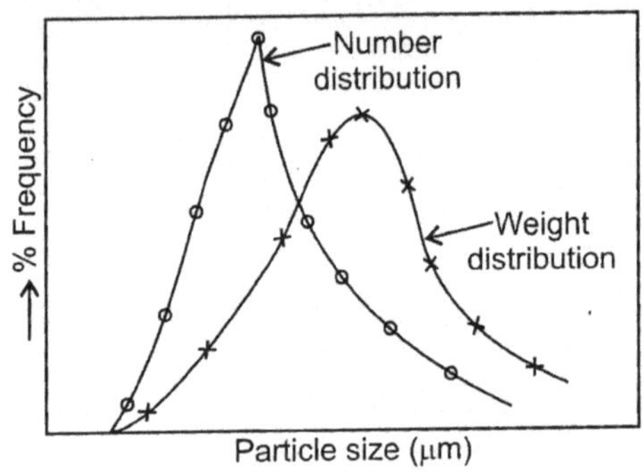

Fig. 13.3 Frequency distribution plot.

The normal distribution, as shown in Fig. 13.1, is uncommon in pharmaceutical powders. The maximum pharmaceutical powders have an unsymmetric, or skewed, distribution depicted in Fig.13.4.

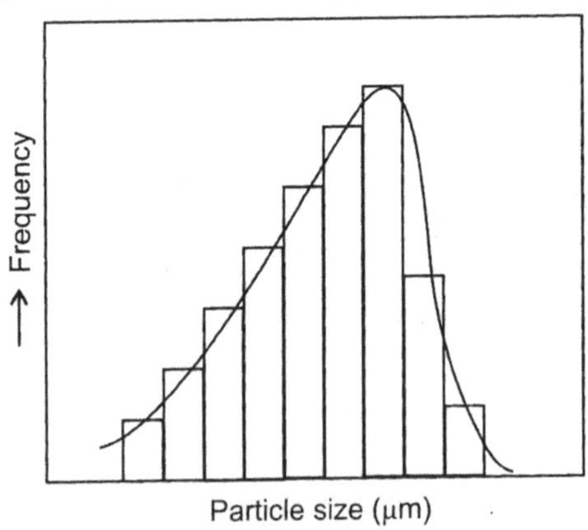

Fig. 13.4 Skewed distribution curve.

Sometime log-normal distribution curve can be used for represent particle size distribution-depicted Fig.13.5.

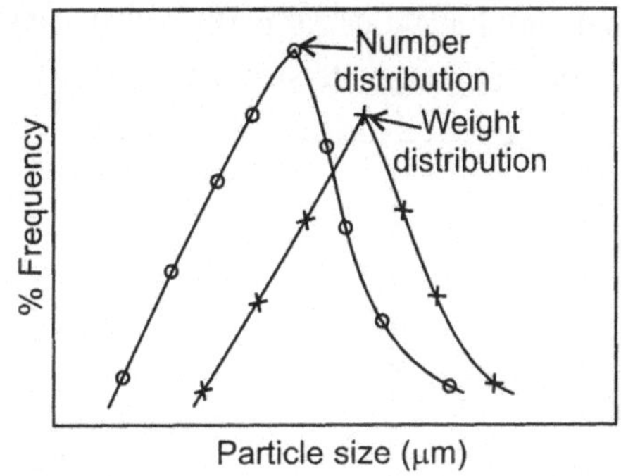

FIg. 13.5 Log-normal distribution curve.

Particle Number : The particle number is important in dose of drugs specially for potent drugs or drugs having low dose. Knowledge of particle number is important in preparation of tablets and capsules. The number of particles per unit weight, N, is expressed in terms of volume-number mean diameter, d_{vn}. Assuming that the particles are spheres, the volume of a single particle is $\frac{\pi\, d_{vn}^3}{6}$ and the mass (volume × density) is $\frac{\pi\, d_{vn}^3\, \rho}{6}$ gram per particle. The number of particles per gram may be obtained from following relationship,

$$\frac{\left(\pi d_{vn}^3\, \rho\right)/6g}{\perp \text{ particle}} = \frac{1\text{ g}}{N}$$

So $$N = \frac{6}{\pi\, d_{vn}^3\, \rho}$$

Particle Size Determination

A number of techniques can be used to determine particle size and size distributions. The particle size provides information concerning any characteristic dimension. The methods used for particle size distribution may be direct or indirect method. None of the measurement are truly direct methods. Microscope allows to view the actual particles. Selection of a particular method largely depends upon the desired application.

Following are the most commonly used methods for determination of particles size of particular size range given in Table 13.1.

Table 13.1 Commonly used methods for particle size determination and their approximate size ranges.

Name of method	Approximate size ranges
Electron microscope	10 Å to 1 μm
Optical microscope	1 μm to 1000 μm
Sedimentation	1 μm to 1 mm
Coulter counter	1 μm to 1 mm
Air permeability	1 μm to 100 μm
Sieving	10 μm to 1cm

(a) **Optical Microscopy :** The optical microscopy can be used to measure the particles size in the range of 0.2 μm to about 100 μm. In this method the size is expressed as d_p, projected diameter. By this method the number distribution data can be obtained and it can be converted to weight distribution. The resolving power of optical microscope is less as compared to ultramicroscope or electron microscope. In this method, an emulsion or suspension, diluted or undiluted, is mounted on a slide or ruled cell. Eye-piece of the microscope is fitted with a micrometer, called ocular micrometer. The eyepiece or ocular micrometer is calibrated using a stage micrometer. The slide or ruled cell is placed on a mechanical stage. The size of particle is determined with the help of ocular micrometer. The field can be projected onto a screen where particles are measured more accuratly and photograph can be taken. The optical microscopy method can be used to determine the particle size analysis in suspensions, in aerosols or in emulsion (droplet size). The figure of optical microscope is given in Fig. 13.6. In order to get statistically valid results the counting of particles should be in the range of 500 to 1000 particles for every sample.

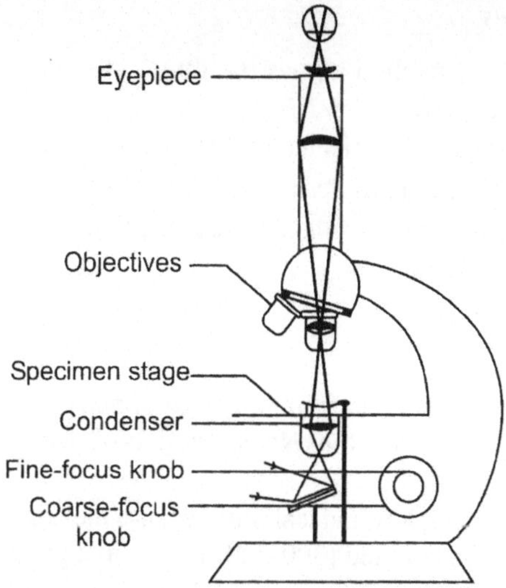

Fig. 13.6 The student microscope.

From the obtained data the size frequency distribution curves, cumulative frequency curves are plotted.

Other popular measurements includes – Feret diameter, the Martin diameter and Projected area diameter. For the measurement purpose of these diameters, the following Fig. 13.7 can be considered.

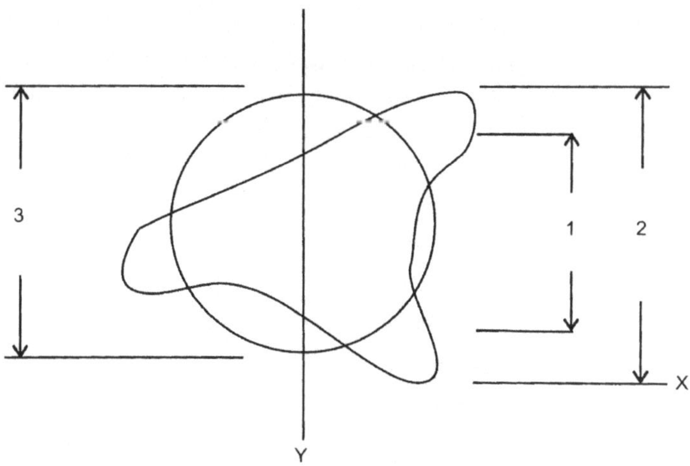

Fig. 13.7 A general diagram to express the particle diameter by microscopy. Key-1- projected diameter; 2-The Martin diameter; 3-Feret diameter.

Advantages

1. Microscopy method allows the direct observation (shape and size) of particles
2. The field can be projected and a photograph can be taken.
3. Aggregation of particles can be easily detected.
4. Provides accurate results and reproduciability.
5. Simple and economic.
6. Easy to handle.

Disadvantages

1. Diameter is obtanied from only two dimensions of the particle i.e., length and breadth. No estimation of depth (thickness) of particle.
2. The method is slow and tealious, because the number of particles that must be counted (300-500) to obtain a good estimation of the distribution.
3. Time consuming method.

(b) ***Sieving method :*** Mechanical sieving is generally used for the particles having size range between 50μm to 1500μm. It consist of a series of standard sieves calibrated by the N.B.S. [National Bureau of Standards]. Sieves are produced by photoetching and electroforming techniques. This method directly gives weight distribution. Sieves are generally used for grinding coarser particles. This method is useful in the development of some dosage forms like tablets and capsules.

Sieves for pharmaceutical testing are constructed from wire cloth with square meshes. Standard sieves of different mesh numbers are available commercially. The sieves are arranged in a nest of about five with the coarsest at top as shown in Fig. 13.8.

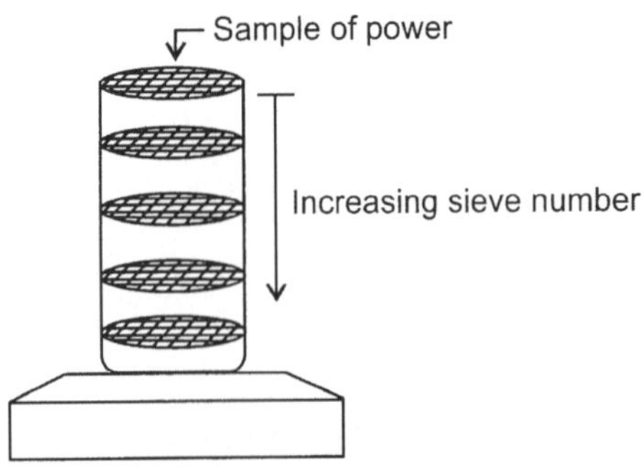

Fig. 13.8 Arrangement of sieves.

According to the method of pharmacopoeia (USP/IP) for testing powder fineness the following procedure is used. Arrange set of at least five sieves in descending order of aperture size as shown in Fig. 13.8. Place the weighed quantity usually 50gm of sample on top sieve. Start mechanical shaker and shaken for a certain period of time (usually 15 to 20 min.). Collect the powder retained on each sieve and record the weight. Data obtained will be analyzed for normal, log-normal, cumulative percent frequency distribution.

Sieving errors can be arise from many variables including sieve loading, duration and intensity of agitation. Care must be excersized to get reproducible results.

Advantages

1. It is simple for handling.
2. It is inexpensive and rapid.
3. Provides reproducible results.
4. Specially useful for weight distribution.
5. It can be used for very small particles having particle diameter upto 5μm.

Disadvantages

1. It cannot used for very small particles is below 5μm.
2. The powder sample should be dried every time, otherwise it may clog with particles, resulting improper sieving.
3. During shaking, attrition of particles may cause reduction of particle size. This may leads to errors in estimation.
4. Time consuming method.
5. Approximate results can be obtained.

(c) ***Sedimentation Method :*** The sedimentation method can be used for formulation and evaluation of suspensions, emulsions and determination of molecular weight of polymers. The particle size in the subsieve range may be obtained by gravity sedimentation and is expressed as stokes' diameter, d_{st}, in Stokes' law.

$$V = \frac{h}{t} = \frac{d_{st}^2 \left(\rho_s - \rho_o\right)g}{18\eta_o} \qquad \text{..... (13.1)}$$

$$d_{st} = \sqrt{\frac{18\eta_o h}{(\rho_s - \rho_o)gt}} \quad \text{....(13.2)}$$

Where, V = rate of settling

h = distance of fall in time, t

η_o = viscosity of medium

ρ_s = density of particles

ρ_o = density of the dispersion medium

g = aceleration due to gravity

d_{st} = mean diameter of particles

Physical stability of a suspension depends on the rate of settling of the particles in the dosage forms.

The equation 13.2 holds exactly for spheres falling freely at a constant rate without hindrance. The law is applicable to irregularly shaped particles of various sizes. The particles should not be aggregated or clumped together in the suspension. The clumps may fall rapidly than the individual particles. To avoid the aggregation the deflocculating agent may be in corporated.

The suspension should be diluted (1-2%) . The flow should be laminar, i.e., the rate of sedimentation of particles must not be too rapid to create turbulance. Whether the flow is turbulent or laminar is inicated by the dimensionless Reynolds number, R_e, which is defined as.

$$R_e = \frac{V_d \rho_o}{\eta_o} \quad \text{.....(13.3)}$$

If Reynolds number is greater than 0.2, the flow is turbulent and Stokes'law cannot be used.

Rearranging Eq. 13.1 and 13.3 gives

$$V = \frac{R_e \eta}{d\rho_o} = \frac{d^2(\rho_s - \rho_o)g}{18\eta} \quad \text{.....(13.4)}$$

and so

$$d^3 = \frac{18 R_e \eta^2}{(\rho_s - \rho_o)\rho_o g} \quad \text{.....(13.5)}$$

Equation 13.5 allows calculation of the maximum particle diameter.

Many methods based on sedimentation are used for determination of particle diameter. The methods may include pipette method, the balance method, the hydrometer method etc. Pipette method is mostly used because of its certain merits like ease of analysis, accuracy and economy etc.

The Andreasen apparatus is shown in Fig. 13.9

The apparatus usually consist of 550ml vessel containing a 10ml pipette sealed into a ground glass stopper. When the pipette is in place in the cylinder, its lower tip is 20cm below the surface of the suspension.

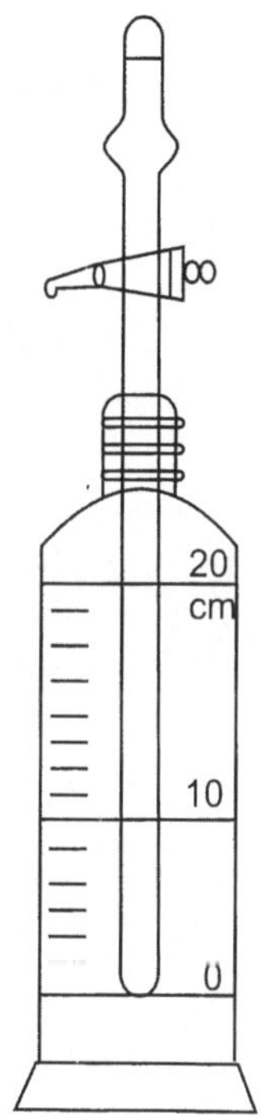

Fig. 13.9 Andreasen apparatus for determining particle size by the gravity sedimentation method.

The procedure is as follows :

1 or 2% suspension of powder in a suitable medium firstly prepared and to that add suitable deflocculating agent. Transfer this mixture (suspension) into the Andreasen vessel. Place the stopper and shake the vessel to distribute the particles uniformly throughout the suspension and the apparatus is place in a constant temperature bath. Remove the stopper and attach two-way stopcock. At various time intervals, 10ml samples are withdrawn and discharged by means of the two way stopcock. The samples are evaporated and weighed or analyzed by any method, correcting for the deflocculating agent that has been added. The weight or the amount of particles obtained in each time interval is referred to as weight undersize. The weights are converted into cumulative weight undersize.

(d) **Particle Volume Measurement :** The popular instrument to measure the volume of particles is the coulter counter, Fig. 3.10 This method gives number distribution. Here the particle volume is measured and is converted into particle diameter, and size is expressed as volume diameter d_v. The method is useful in the study of particle growth in suspension and solutions, useful in dissolution studies and to study the effect of antibacterial agents on the growth oof microorganisms. This method gives a quick and accurate results.

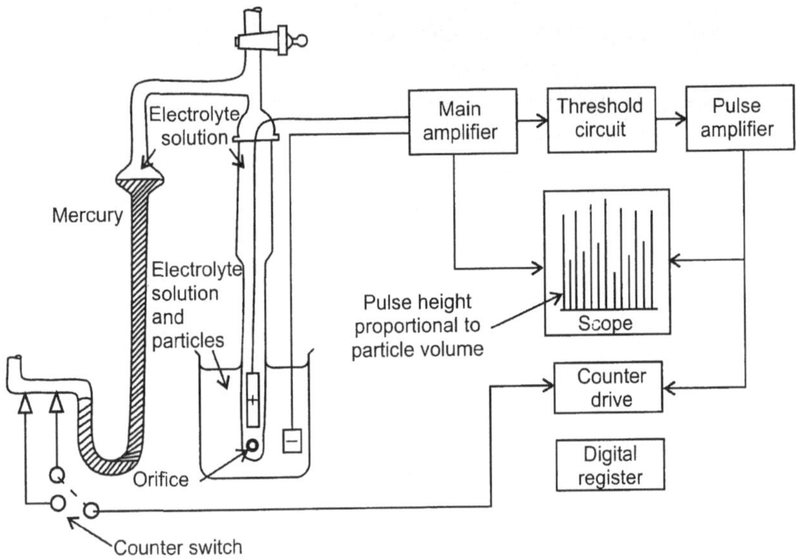

Fig. 13.10 Coulter counter apparatus

The working principle of coulter counter (Fig. 13.10) is that when a particle suspended in a liquid containing electrolyte (sodium chloride) passed through a small orifice, and maintains contact with the external medium. Generally, a known volume of a dilute suspension is pumped through the orifice. The suspension is sufficiently diluted so that only one particle can pass at a time through an orifice. A constant voltage is applied across the two electrodes. Here the current produces. When a suspended particle travels through the orifice, it displaces its own volume of electrolyte. The resistance, between two electrodes increases. The net result is a change in the electrical resistance, which is related to the particle volume, causes a voltage pulse. The voltage pulse are amplified and fed to a pulse height analyzer calibrated in terms of particle size.

The pulses are electronically counted for a given threshold value. By adjusting the threshold setting the number of particles of each size range is obtained. Thus the particle size distribution can be obtained.

The instrument is capable of counting particles at the rate of approximately 4000 per second. The data may be converted from a volume distribution to a weight distribution.

Advantages

1. It gives very fast results [approximately 4000 particles per second]
2. Short period of time is required for size distribution analysis.
3. It provides accurate results.
4. It can be used to measure particulate contamination in parenteral solutions.
5. Submicron particle sizing instrument, the coulter Model N_4 has been developed for analyzing particles in the range of 0.003 to 0.3 μm.
6. It is used in the study of the clustering process and the packing of the mineral components of renal stones.
7. It is also useful in quality control of large volume parenteral [LVP] solutions.

Disadvantages

1. It is not suitable for polar and highly water soluble materials due to solvation.
2. It is expensive method.

(e) ***Surface Area Method :*** Surface area of a powder can be determine from particle size data. The shape and surface area of a particle plays an important role in flow and packaging properties of a powder. Specific surface is defiined as the surface area per unit weight (S_w) or unit volume (S_v) of the material.

A sphere has minimum surface area per unit volume. The more asymmetric a particle, the greater the surface area per unit volume. The surface area or volume of a sphere can be written as –

$$\text{Surface area} = \pi d^2 \text{ and} \qquad .....(13.6)$$

$$\text{Volume} = \frac{\pi d^3}{6} \qquad .....(13.7)$$

where, d is diameter of the particle.

Specific Surface

$$S_v = \frac{\text{Surface area of particles}}{\text{Volume of particles}}$$

$$= \frac{\text{number of particles} \times \text{Surface area of each particle}}{\text{number of particles} \times \text{Volume of each particle}}$$

$$= \frac{\eta \alpha_s d^2}{\eta \alpha_v d^3} = \frac{\alpha_3}{\alpha_v d} \qquad .....(13.8)$$

$$S_w = \frac{\text{Surface area}}{\text{Weight}} = \frac{\text{Surface area}}{\text{Density} \times \text{Volume}}$$

$$S_w = \frac{S_v}{\rho} = \frac{\eta \alpha_s d_{vs}^2}{\eta \alpha_v d_{vs}^3 \times \rho}$$

$$= \frac{\alpha_s}{\alpha_v \, d_{vs} \, \rho} \qquad .....(13.9)$$

When the particles are spherical, equation (13.9) simplifies to

$$S_w = \frac{6}{\rho d_{vs}} \qquad .....(13.10)$$

Since $\frac{\alpha_s}{\alpha_v} = 6.0$ for a sphere.

Methods for Determining Surface Area

Two methods are commonly used for determination of surface area are :

(i) Adsorption Method

(ii) Air permeability Method

(i) ***Adsorption Method :*** The amount of a gas or liquid solute that is adsorbed onto the sample of powder to form a monolayer is a direct function of the surface area of the sample.

This principle is used to estimate the specific surface and is also used to estimate surface diameter, d_s. At low pressure the adsorbed layer is monomolecular and becomes multimolecular at high pressures. The completion of the monolayer of nitrogen on a powder is shown in Fig. 13.11.

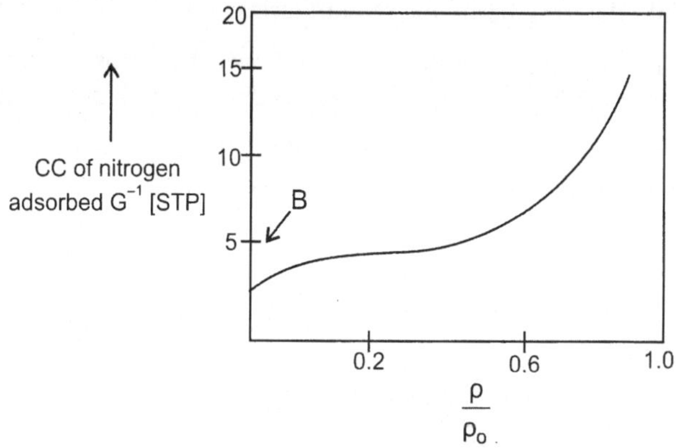

Fig. 13.11 Isotherm showing completion of monolayer.

The volume of nitrogen gas V_m in Cm^3 that 1 gram of the powder can adsorb when the monolayer is complete. In the Fig. 13.10, the point B represent the volume of adsorbed gas corresponding to the completion of a monomolecular film. The Quantasorb instrument manufactured by Quantachrome corporation can be used for determination of surface area and pore structure of powders.

(ii) ***Air permeability Method :*** This method can be used in powder manufacturing in controlling batch to batch variations. The resistance to the flow of a fluid, such as air, through a plug of compacted powder is the surface area of the powder. The resistance to flow is greater if surface area per gram of powder, S_w, is greater.

Powder is packed in the sample tube in between porous plugs. A surface-surface contacts between particles or a plug of powder may be regarded as a series of capillaries whose diameter is related to the average particle size. According to poiseuille's equation.

$$V = \frac{\pi d^4 \Delta pt}{128\ln} \quad .....(13.11)$$

Where, V = volume of air flowing through a capillary.

d = internal diameter

l = length

t = time in second

Δp = pressure difference

η = viscosity of the fluid in poise.

The flow rate through the plug or bed is affected by

(i) the degree of compression of the particles

(ii) the irregularity of the capillaries.

The more compact the plug, the lower the porosity [ratio of the total space between the particles to the total volume of the plug].

From the Poiseuille equation, the Kozeny-Carman equation is derived and is used to estimate surface area.

$$v = \frac{A}{\eta Sw^2} \cdot \frac{\Delta pt}{Kl} \cdot \frac{\epsilon^3}{(1-\epsilon)^2}$$

Where,

A = cross–sectional area of the plug.

K = constant.

ϵ = porosity.

A fisher subsieve sizer is commercially available. This method is official in I.P. The arrangement or operation is illutrated in Fig. 13.12.

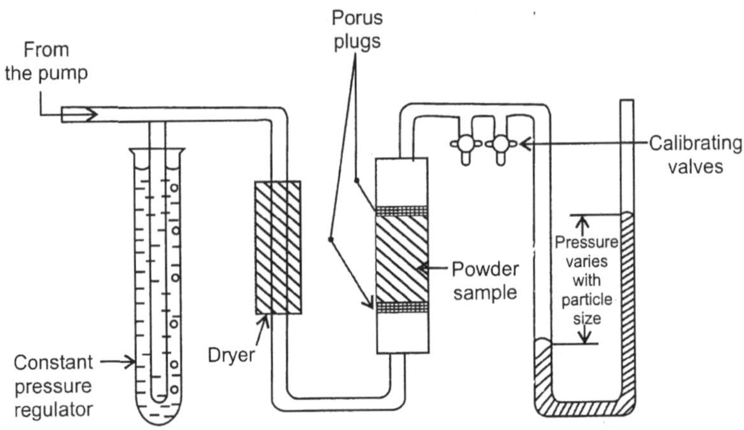

Fig. 13.12 The fisher subsieve sizer.

If consist of a sample tube and one end connected to an air pump through a constant pressure regulator. The other end attached to calibrated manometer. The air is allowed to pass through constant pressure regulator. Air is passed through the dryer to remove any moisture. Then the air (dried) is allowed to pass through sample tube and the flow of air is measured by the manometer. The pressure is measured on the manometer which varies with particle size and average diameter of the particles can be determined.

Advantages

(i) Simple instrumentation and high speed, it is widly used pharmaceutically for specific surface determinations.

(ii) Bephenium hydroxynaphthoate, official in the B.P.C., 1973 is standardized by air permeability method.

(iii) Activity of some drugs is related to the specific surface. Ex : Anthelmintic drugs in suspension dosage form, must possess a surface area of not less than 7000 cm^2/g. As the specific surface of the material is reduced, the activity of the drug also falls.

(iv) Air permeability method, officially in U.S. pharmacopoeia used for determining the spedific surface area of griseofulvin.

(v) This method is also used for measuring the fineness of portland cement.

Derived Properties of Powders

The size distribution and surface area of powders are two fundamental properties of any collection of particles. Derived properties are based on fundamental properties.

Porosity : The volume of space between particles may vary depending on the size, shape and density of the particles. Suppose a powder is placed in a graduated cylinder and total volume noted. The volume occupied known as bulk volume, V_b . The bulk volume of powder consists of the true volume of solid particles plus the volume of the spaces between particles, if the powder is nonporous, that is, has no internal pores or capillary spaces. The volume of the spaces, known as the void volume, V, i.e.

$$V = V_b - V_p \qquad .....(13.13)$$

Where, V_p = true volume

$$\text{The porosity or voids } \in = \frac{V_b - V_p}{V_b} = 1 - \frac{V_p}{V_b} \qquad .....(13.14)$$

Porosity is generally expressed in percent $\in \times 100$

Packing arrangements : There are two ideal packing arrangements for the powder beds of uniform sized spheres as shown in Fig. 13.13

(i) closest or rhombohedral and

(ii) loosest or cubic packing

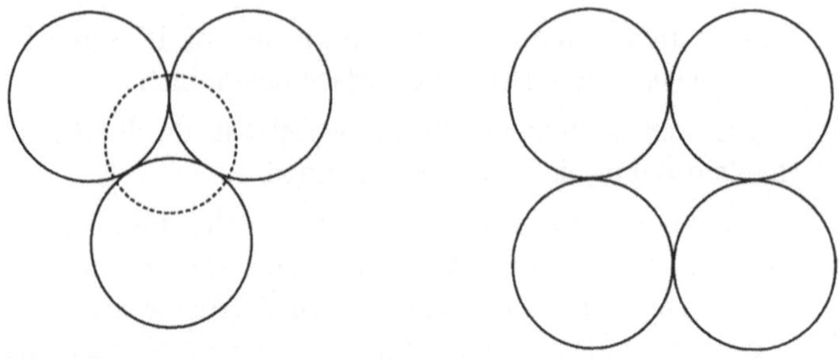

Fig. 13.13 Packing arrangements (a) closest and (b) loosest.

The particles in real powder are neither spherical in shape nor uniform in size. The powder may therefore have any arrangement between two ideal packings.

Densities of particles : Systems of particulate solids are most complex physical systems encountered in pharmacy. Basically density is defined as weight per unit volume. Three types of densities.

(i) Bulk density (ii) Granule density (iii) True density.

(i) Bulk density, ρ_b, is defined as the mass of a powder divided by the bulk volume. On the basis of bulk volume, powders may be classified as, "light" and "heavy". Light powders have high bulk volume. The bulk density of a powder depends mainly on particle size distribution, particle shape and the tendancy of particles to adhere to one another.

A sample of about 50gm, which has previously been passed through standard No.20 sieve, and is introduced into a 100-ml graduated cylinder. The cylinder is dropped at 2- seconds intervals into a hard wood surface three times from a height of 1 inch. This method is also called three-tap method. Sometimes 500 tap method is used where the cylinder dropped 500 times on hard wood surface. The final bulk volume is determined and bulk density is calaculated.

The determination of bulk density is used to check the uniformity of bulk in given sample. It is important in capsule manufacturing.

(ii) Granule density, ρ_g, is determined by liquid displacement method. Mercury is generally used since it fills the void spaces but fails to penetrate into the internal pores of the particles.

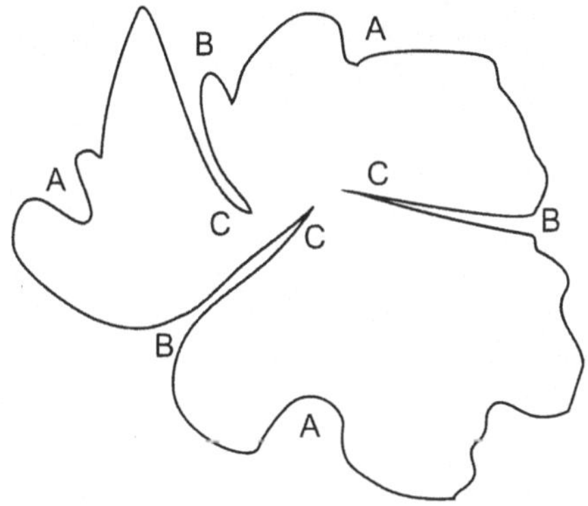

Fig. 13.14 Pores and crevices of a granule.

As shown in Fig. 13.14 water or mercury surrounds such a particle and rests only in the surface irregularities such as regions A & B. The volume of particles together with their intraparticle spaces gives the granule volume. From the knowledge of weight the granule density can be calculated.

(iii) True density, ρ, is the density of the actual solid material. The volume occupied by voids (inter-particle spaces) and intra-particle pores are excluded or not included in the measurement. The most common method used is helium densitometer, as suggested by Franklin, as shown in Fig. 13.14, where water or mercury can not penetrate to the regions C, however, helium can penetrate regions C.

The known quantity of helium is introduced in the empty apparatus and volume of the empty apparatus (dead space) is determined. A exactly weighed amount of powder is then introduced into the sample tube. The adsorbed gases are removed from the powder by an out-gassing procedure; and helium is again introduced. The pressure is determined by mercury manometer. The difference between the volume of helium filling the empty apparatus and the volume of helium in the presence of the power sample yields the volume occupied by the powder. From the knowledge of weight of the powder, true density can be determined.

The different types of densities or volumes are illustrated in the Fig. 13.15.

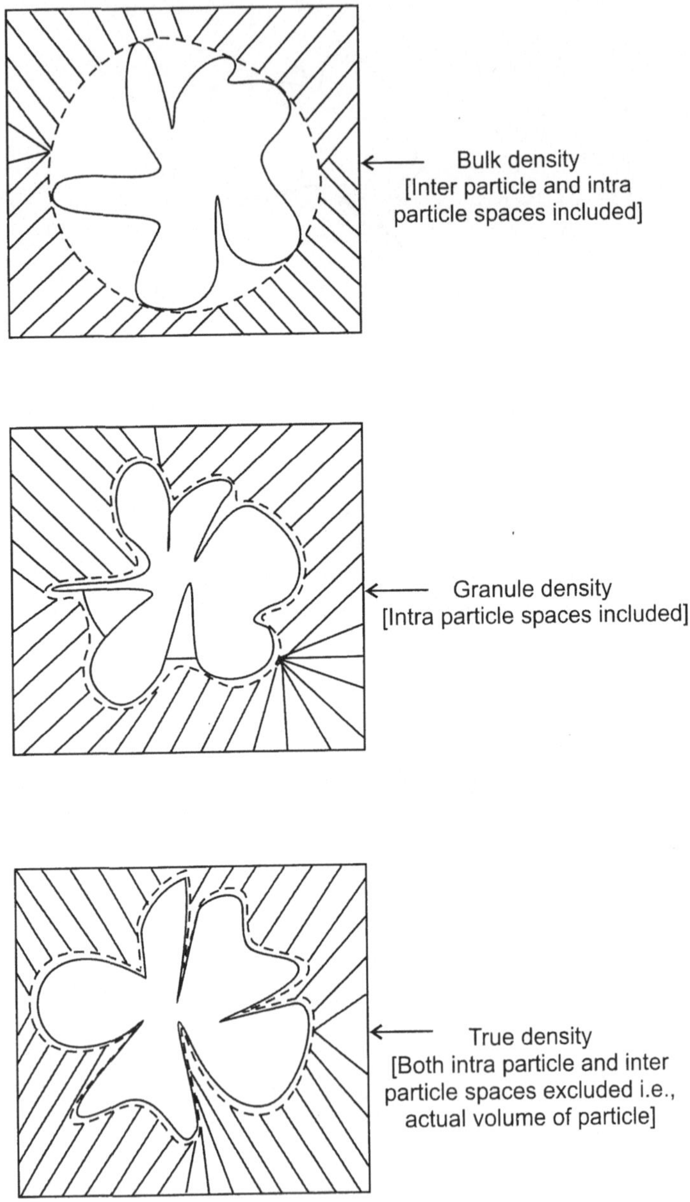

Fig. 13.15 Comparison of bulk density, granule density and true density.

As shown in Fig. 13.15, different densities, the interparticle, intraparticle and toal porosity can be computed.

The intraparticle porosity of granule may be determined from the knowledgte of true and granule density.

$$\in_{intraparticle} = \frac{V_g - V_p}{V_g} = 1 - \frac{V_p}{V_g}$$

$$= 1 - \frac{\text{weight/true density}}{\text{weight/granule density}} \quad .....(13.15)$$

$$\in_{intraparticle} = 1 - \frac{\text{granule density}}{\text{true density}}$$

$$= 1 - \frac{\rho_g}{\rho} \quad .....(13.16)$$

Where, V_p is the true volume and V_g - granule volume. Similarly interparticle or interspace or void porosity of a powder can be computed.

$$\in_{interspace} = \frac{V_b - V_g}{V_b} = 1 - \frac{V_g}{V_b}$$

$$= 1 - \frac{\text{weight/granule density}}{\text{weight/bulk density}} \quad .....(13.17)$$

$$\in_{interspace} = 1 - \frac{\text{bulk density}}{\text{granule density}}$$

$$= 1 - \frac{\rho_b}{\rho_g} \quad .....(13.18)$$

where, V_b is bulk volume.

The total porosity is defined as

$$\in_{total} = \frac{V_b - V_p}{V_b} = 1 - \frac{V_p}{V_b} \quad .....(13.19)$$

where, V_p – volume of solid itself.

$$\in_{total} = 1 - \frac{\text{weight/true density}}{\text{weight/bulk density}}$$

$$= 1 - \frac{\text{bulk density}}{\text{true density}}$$

$$\in_{total} = 1 - \frac{\rho_b}{\rho} \quad .....(13.20)$$

Flow Properties : The flow properties of powder plays an important role in the manufacturing of tablet or capsules. Weight variation of tablets is common problem in tablet manufacturing and is mainly due to poor or irregular flow of powder from the hopper to the die. Flow properties depenpds on particle size, shape, porosity and density, and surface texture.

Powder may be free-flowing or cohesive. If the particle size is less than 10 μm, the powder flow is restricted because the cohesive forces between particles are of the same magnitude as gravitational forces. The presence of moisture, excess amount of small particles and surface roughness leads to poor flow due to friction and cohesiveness. Smooth surface of particles improves the flow. Particles having high density and low internal porosity shows good flow properties.

Free-flowing powders are characterized by "dustibility". [opposite of stickiness]. Lycopodium shows greatest degree of dustibility; if it is arbitrarily assigned a dustibility of 100% ; talcum powder has value of 57%, potato starch 27% ; charcoal 23% & caromel 0.7%.

The flow rate of a tablet granulation increased with an increase in the quantity of fines added and the combination of lubricant. Glidants are frequently added to granular powders to improve flow characteristics. Ex : Magnesium Stearate, starch, talc.

The flow characteristics are measured by angle of repose; ϕ. This is the maximum angle possible between the surface of a pile of powder and the horizontal plane.

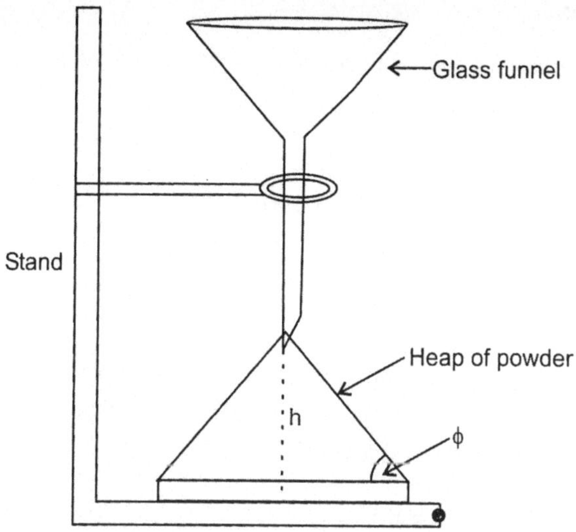

Fig. 13.16 Angle of repose measurement.

As shown in Fig 13.16 the angle of repose is related to the coefficient of interparticle friction μ.

$$\tan \phi = \frac{h}{r} = \mu$$

Where, h = height of pile, r = radius of the base of the pile, ϕ angle of repose.

The rougher and more irregular the surface of the particles, the higher will be the angle of repose. The relationship between angle of repose (ϕ) and powder flow is given in Table 13.2.

Table 13.2 Relationship between angle of repose and powder flow.

Flow	Angle of repose ϕ, (degrees)
Excellent	< 25
Good	25 – 30
Poor	30 – 40*
Very poor	> 40

* Addition of glidant, flow porperties may be improved.

The flow properties of powders is also important factor involving in mixing different materials to form a powder blend.

Problems

1. If the surface area of a particle is 4×10^{-4} cm^2. What is its equivalent surface diameter?

   Solution : Data given

   Surface area = $4\pi r^2 = 4 \times 10^{-4}$

   $r = 0.564 \times 10^{-2}$ cm.

   $d_s = 1.128 \times 10^{-2}$ cm.

2. The mean volume number diameter of the given sample is 2.41×10^{-4} cm. What is the number of particles per gm when the density of the powder is 4.0 g/cm^3?

   Solution : Data given

   Density = 4.0 g/cm^3.

   $$\text{Volume number diameter} = N = \frac{6}{\pi d_{vn}^{3} \rho}$$

   $$= \frac{6}{3.14 \times \left(2.41 \times 10^{-4}\right)^3 \times 3.0} = 3.41 \times 10^{10}$$

3. What are the specific surfaces, S_w and S_v of a zink oxide powder having density 1.5 g/cm^3 and average particle diameter, d_{vs} is 1.25 μm?

   Solution : Data given :

   Density = ρ = 1.5 g/cm^3 ; d_{vs} = 1.25 μm.

   $= 1.25 \times 10^{-4}$ cm.

   Equation for specific surface,

   $$S_w = \frac{6}{\rho d_{vs}} = \frac{6}{1.5 \times 1.25 \times 10^{-4}}$$

   $$= 3.18 \times 10^3 \text{ cm}^2/\text{g}$$

Equation for specific surface,

$$S_v = \frac{6}{d_{vs}} = \frac{6}{1.25 \times 10^{-4}}$$

$$= 4.8 \times 10^4 cm^2/cm^3$$

4. A zinc stearate powder having density 2.3 g/cm^3 is suspended in water. The viscosity of water at 20° is 0.01 poise and density 1.0 g/cm^3. What is the size of largest particle that will settle in suspension?

Solution : Data given

Density = ρ_s = 2.3 gm/cm^3

Density (water) = ρ_o = 1 gm/cm^3

Reynolds number = R_e = 0.2

Viscosity of water = 0.01 poise

Acceleration due to gravity = g = 981.

Equation for particle size

$$d^3 = \frac{18R_e\eta^2}{(\rho_S - \rho_o)\rho.g}$$

$$= \frac{(18)(0.2)(0.01)^2}{(2.3-1.0)1.0 \times 981}$$

$$= 2.82 \times 10^{-3} \text{ cm}$$

$$= 28.2 \text{ µm}.$$

5. Calculate the intraparticle porosity if the granule density, ρ_g of given powder is 1.360 and the true density, ρ is 2.010.

Solution : Data given

Granule density, ρ_g = 1.360.

True density ρ = 2010.

Equation for intraparticle porosity =

$$\in_{\text{intraparticle}} = 1 - \frac{1.360}{2.010}$$

$$= 0.3238$$

$$= 33\%$$

6. What is the bulk density and the total porosity of the tablet if the weight of tablet is 0.4320 g, bulk volume is 0.08762 cm^3, and true density is 3.010 g/cm^3?

Solution : Data given

Weight of Tablet = 0.4320 g

Bulk volume = 0.08762 cm^3 and

True density = 3.010 g/cm^3.

Equation for Bulk density = $\rho_b = \frac{\text{weight}}{\text{volume}}$

$$= \frac{0.4320}{0.08762} = 4.930 \text{ g/cm}^3.$$

$$\in_{\text{total}} = 1 - \frac{\rho_b}{\rho} = 1 - \frac{\text{Bulk density}}{\text{True density}}$$

$$= 1 - \frac{4.930}{3.010}$$

$$= 0.06762 = 6.762\%$$

7. Compute the angle of repose of the given granules, if a pile of granules has the base of 9.2 cm diameter and height of 3.6 cm.

Solution : Data given

Diameter = d = 9.2 cm = r = $\frac{9.2}{2}$ = 4.6 cm.

Height = h = 3.6 cm

Equation for angle of repose

$$\tan \phi = \frac{h}{r}$$

$$\phi = \tan^{-1} \frac{h}{r}$$

$$= \tan^{-1}\left(\frac{3.6}{4.6}\right) = \tan^{-1} 0.782$$

$$\phi = 38.05^{\circ}$$

CHAPTER 14

Interfacial Phenomena

All the liquids have a tendency to assume a shape having the minimal surface area exposed. For a drop of a liquid, that shape is the sphere. The boundary that forms between two phases [e.g. solid and liquid] is called interface. Surface tension is property of liquids arises from the intermolecular forces of attraction. Interfacial phenomena is important property in the formulation of various dispersions include –

Suspensions [solid in liquid]

Emulsions [liquid in liquid]

Foams [vapour in liquid].

Interfacial phenomena is significant in pharmacy and medicine that affects absorption of drugs onto solid in dosage forms, penetration of molecules through biologic membrane, stability of emulsion, formulation of suspensions.

The interfaces can be classified into six classes as given in Table 14.1.

Table 14.1 Classification of Interfaces.

Phase	Interfacial Tension	Examples
Gas-gas	–	No interface possible
Gas-liquid	γ_{LV}	Body of water exposed to atmosphere
Gas-solid	γ_{SV}	Table top
Liquid-liquid	γ_{LL}	Emulsion
Liquid-solid	γ_{LS}	Suspension
Solid-solid	γ_{SS}	Powder particles in contact

The combinations given in Table 14.1 can be divided into two groups, namely liquid interfaces and solid interfaces and can be illustrated as shown in Fig. 14.1.

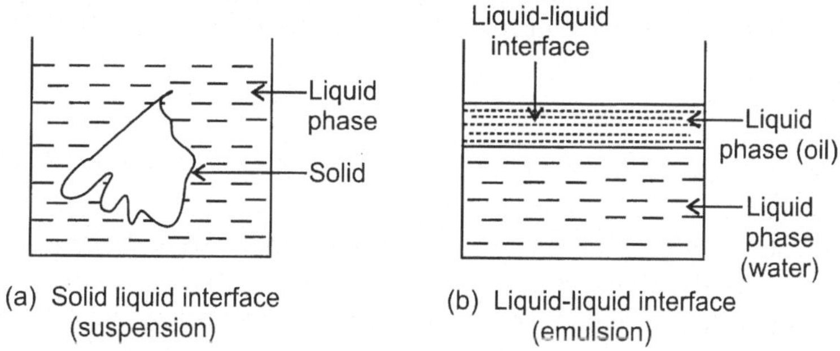

Fig. 14.1 Representation of different types of surfaces and interfaces.

The term surface is generally used to denote interface, in which one of the phases is gas.i.e., either a gas-solid or a gas-liquid interface. Ex: table top forms a gas-solid interface and the rain drop constitutes a gas-liquid interface. This phenomena can be illustrated as shown in Fig. 14.2.

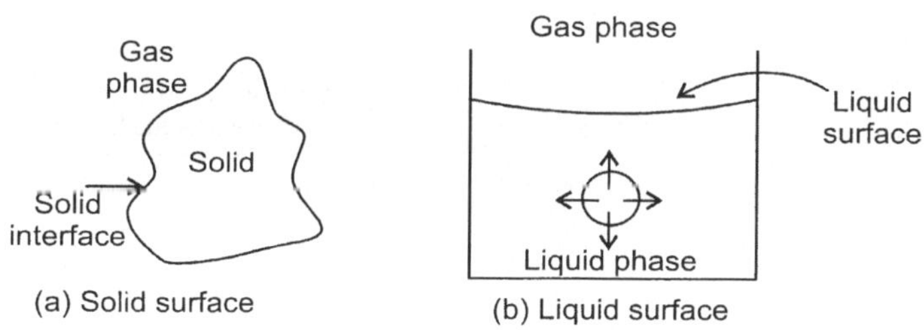

Fig. 14.2 Representation of different types of surfaces and interfaces.

If two or more drops of the same liquid come into contact with one another, the tendancy for them is to join or to coalesce, making one larger drop. This larger drop will have a smaller surface area than the total surface area of the individual drops. This tendancy of liquids may be measured quantitatively, and when the surrounding of the liquid is air, it is referred to as the liquid's surface tension.

The surface tension (γ) is defined as : the force in dynes along the surface of a liquid at right angle to any line 1 cm in length.

Units of Surface Tension

The unit of surface tension in CGS system is dynes per centimeter (dyne cm^{-1}). In SI system, the unit is Newton per metre (Nm^{-1}). The relation of these units :

$$1 \text{ dyne cm}^{-1} = 1 \text{ m Nm}^{-1}$$

In the liquid state, the cohesive forces (intermolecular attractions between like molecules) between adjacent molecules are well developed. A molecule in the interior of a liquid is attracted equally in all directions by the molecules around it as shown in Fig 14.3. A molecule in the surface of a liquid is attracted with other liquid molecules that are situated below and adjacent to them.

A change in temperature causes change in surface tension of a liquid. Generally surface tension decreases with increase in temperature.

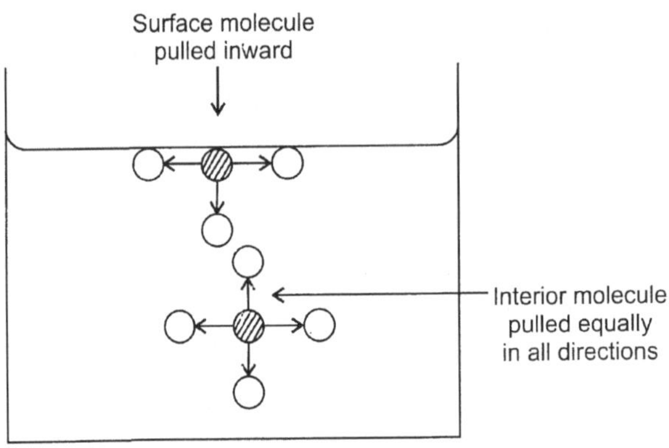

Fig. 14.3 Surface tension due to net inward pull on the surface molecules.

Interfacial tension is the force per unit length existing at interface between two immiscible liquid phases, unit is dyne/cm. In two liquids which are completely miscible no interface is observed and hence do not possess interfacial tension. Ex : water and ethanol

When benzene and water are mixed together, there is formation of boundary and shows interfacial tension. Interfacial tensions are less than surface tensions. Some example of surface tension and interfacial tension are given in Table. 14.2

Table 14.2 Surface tension and interfacial tension (20°).

Substance	Surface Tension (dyne/cm)	Substance	Interfacial tension Against water (dyne/cm)
Water	72.8	Mercury	375
Mercury	476	n-Hexane	51.1
Glycerin	63.4	Benzene	35.0
Oleic acid	32.5	Chloroform	32.8
Benzene	28.9	Oleic acid	15.6
Chloroform	27.1	Olive oil	22.9
Olive oil	35.8	Ethyl ether	10.7

The surface tension phenomena may be illustrated by means of a three sided wire frame across which a movable bar is place as shown in Fig. 14.4. A soap film is formed over the area ABCD and can be streached by force F, to the movable bar, length L. When mass is removed, the film will contract. The surface tension, γ is the force that must be applied to break the film.

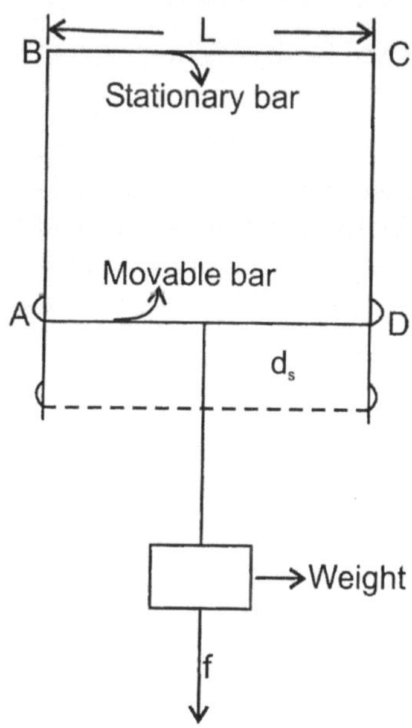

Fig. 14.4 Apparatus used to demonstrate the surface tension.

The soap film has two liquid-gas interfaces (above and below the plane of the paper), the total length of contact is infact equal to twice the length of the bar. So

$$\gamma = \frac{f_b}{2L} \quad .....(14.1)$$

where, f_b = force required to break the film

L = length of the movable bar.

Surface Free Energy

As shown in Fig. 14.4, the mass is added to extend the surface by a distance d_s, the work d_W [force × distance] can be written as

$$d_w = f \times d_s = \gamma \times 2L \times d_s$$

$$d_w = \gamma \times dA$$

where, $dA = 2L \times d_s$, and for a finite change

$$W = \gamma \Delta A \quad .....(14.2)$$

in which W is the work done or surface free energy. Unit is ergs.

Measurement of Surface and Interfacial Tensions

Methods commonly employed for the determination of surface tension are :

(a) ***Capillary Rise Method :*** When a capillary tube of radius 'r' is vertically inserted into a liquid, the liquid rises to a height 'h' and forms a concave meniscus Fig. 14.5(a) and Fig. 14.5(b). This is because of the adhesive forces between liquid molecules and glass are stronger than cohesive forces between liquid molecules. The liquid is said to wet the capillary wall, spreading over it, and rising in the tube. The rise in the tube continue until the upward movement is just balanced by the downward force of gravity due to the weight of the liquid.

The upward vertical component of the force resulting from surface tension on the circumferece is given by

$$a = \gamma \cos\theta$$

The total upward force around the inside circumference of the tube is

$$2 \pi r \gamma \cos \theta \quad .....(14.3)$$

where, θ = contact angle between surface of liquid and the capillary wall.

$2\pi r$ = inside circumference of the capillary.

For water θ is insignificant as shown in Fig. 14.5(b). The contact angle is very small for the liquids used in pharmacy similar to water, Cosθ approaches 1 i.e., Cos θ = 1 and equation 14.3 can be changed as

$$a = 2\pi r \gamma \qquad .....(14.4)$$

This is also called upward component

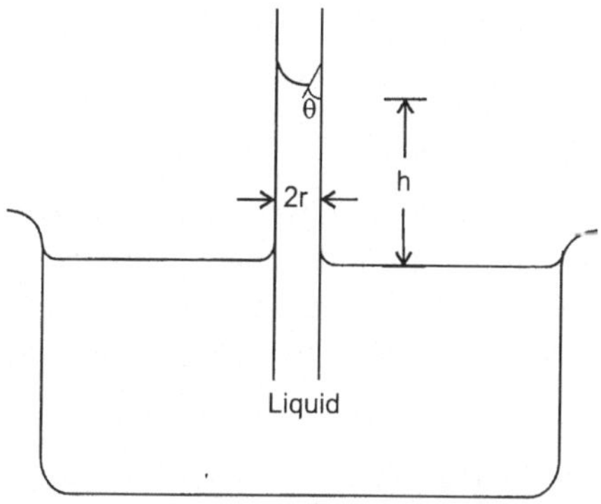

Fig. 14.5(a) Measuring surface tension by means of the capillary rise principle.

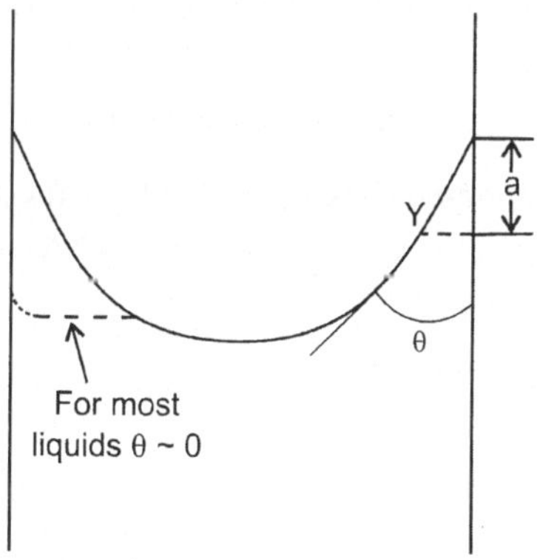

Fig. 14.5(b) Force components and contact angle at the meniscus of a liquid.

The counteracting force is gravity (mass × acceleration).

b = mass × acceleration

= (volume × density) × acceleration

= cross sectional area × height × density × acceleration

$$b = \pi r^2 \times h \times \rho \times g \qquad \text{..... (14.5)}$$

This is also called downward component.

At equilibrium a = b

$$2 \pi r \gamma = \pi r^2 h \rho g$$

$$\gamma = \frac{1}{2} r h \rho g \qquad \text{.....(14.6)}$$

The equation (14.6) is used to calculate the surface tensions of liquids. This method is most accurate and simple.

(b) ***Drop Formation Method***

A drop of liquid is allowed to form at the lower end of a capillary tube as shown in Fig. 14.6 Stalagmometer.The drop is supported by the upward force of surface tension and weight of the drop (mg) pulls it downward. The drop breaks when the two forces are balanced.

At the point of breaking,

$$mg = 2 \pi r \gamma$$

where, m = mass of drop

g = acceleration due to gravity

r = outer radius of the tube.

The stalagmometer (Drop pipette) is the apparatus used for determination of surface tension and one of the two methods are used as given below.

(i) ***Drop – Weight Method :*** In a weighing bottle about 20 drops of liquid are received from stalagmometer and weighed. Thus weight of one drop is found. Repeat the procedure for second liquid (reference, usually water) and weight of one drop determined as before. Using following equation one can calculate the surface tension of unknown liquid.

$$\frac{\gamma_1}{\gamma_2} = \frac{m_1}{m_2} \qquad \text{.....(14.7)}$$

where, γ_1 = surface tension of unknown liquid

γ_2 = surface tension of known (water) liquid

m_1 = weight of one drop of unknown liquid

m_2 = weight of one drop of known liquid.

(ii) ***Drop–number Method :*** The number of drops is counted as the meniscus travels from mark X to mark Y for the experimental liquid and repeat the procedure for reference liquid (Fig. 14.6). The densities of experimental and reference

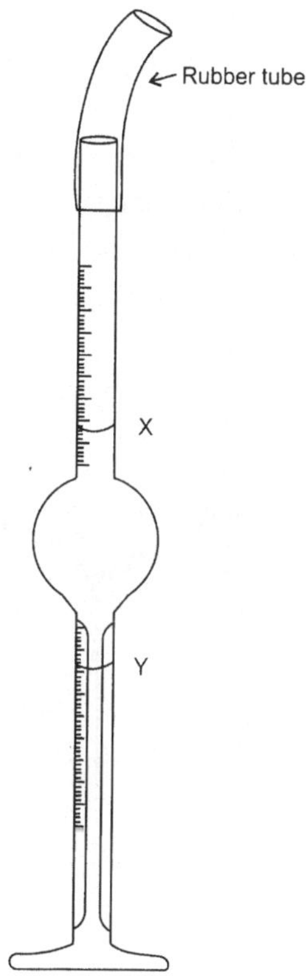

Fig. 14.6 Stalagmometer.

liquid are determined with a pyknometer. The surface tension can be calculated using formula.

$$\frac{\gamma_1}{\gamma_2} = \frac{n_2 d_1}{n_1 d_2} \quad .....(14.8)$$

where, γ_1 and γ_2 are surface tension of unknown and reference liquid respectively.

n_1 and n_2 are number of drops of experimental liquid and reference liquid respectively. d_1 and d_2 are densities of experimental and reference liquid respectively.

(c) Ring–detachment Method

Thė DuNouy tensiometer, as shown in Fig. 14.7 is commonly used for measuring surface and interfacial tensions. The force necessary to detach a platinum-iridium ring immersed at the surface or interface is proportional to the surface or interfacial tension; is the principle of this instrument. The main parts are shown in Fig. 14.8. One end of the torsion wire is fixed while the other attached to a knob having a pointer; which moves on a fixed scale. The force required to detach the ring is recorded in dynes on a calibrated dial.

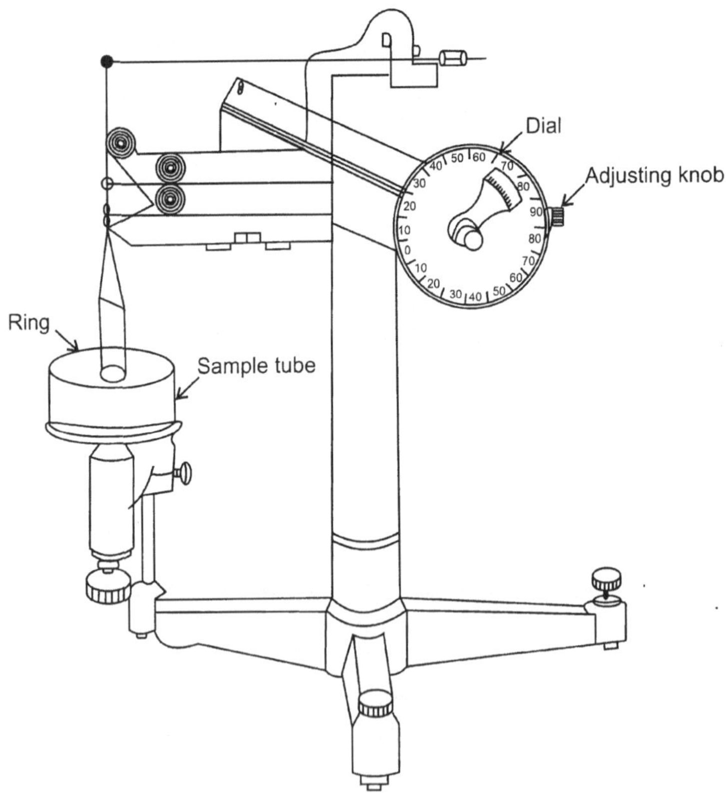

Fig. 14.7 Cenco DuNouy Tensiometer.

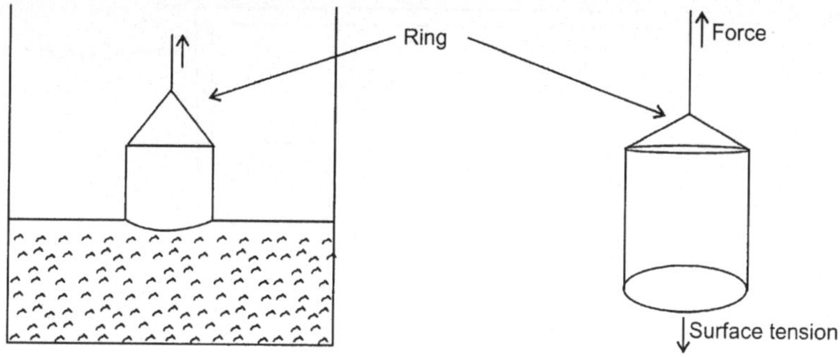

Fig. 14.8 DuNouy ring tensiometer : The representation of the tensiometer ring pulling a column of water above the surface.

The surface tension can be computed from following formula

$$\gamma = \frac{\text{dial reading (dynes)}}{2 \times \text{ring circumference}} \times \text{correction factor B} \quad .....(14.9)$$

In equation (14.9), the correction factor is essential because certain variables must be consider to avoid errors like radius of ring, radius of wire used to form the ring and volume of the liquid raised out of the surface.

(d) ***Maximum Bubble pressure Method***

In this method the maximum pressure required to break a bubble at the end of the capillary and at the moment of breaking it is determined. As shown in Fig. 14.9, air pressure is applied slowly through a tube dipping in experimental liquid. A bubble is formed and slowly grows and then breaks. The pressure at which the air bubble breaks is determined on manometer and surface tension calculated using following formula.

$$P = hdg + \frac{2\gamma}{r} \quad .....(14.11)$$

Where, p = maximum pressure

γ = surface tension

r = radius of capillary

d = density of the liquid

h = depth of liquid.

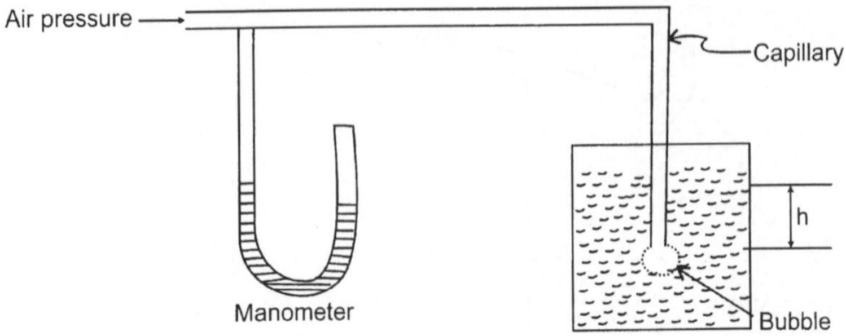

Fig. 14.9 Apparatus for Maximum bubble pressure method.

Spreading Coefficient

When a drop of liquid (oleic acid) is placed on the surface of water, it will spread as a film if force of adhesion is greater than cohesive forces. This phenomena is important in absorption of medicament from dosage form eg. from cream or lotion. For the stabilization of emulsion spreading coefficient phenomena is useful.

The work of adhesion, which is the energy required to break the attraction between the unlike molecules.

Now consider the hypothetical cylinder (cross-section area, $1 cm^2$) of the sublayer liquid S overlaid with a similar section of the spreading liquid L, as shown in Fig. 14.10.

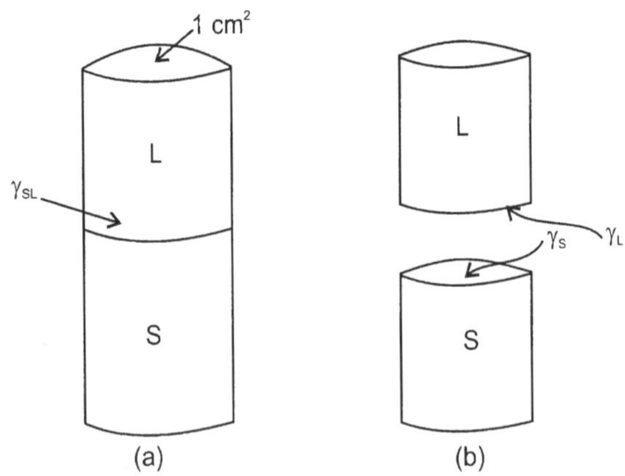

Fig. 14.10 Representation of the work of adhesion involved in separating a substrate and an overlying liquid.

The work of adhesion = $W_a = \gamma_L + \gamma_S - \gamma_{LS}$ .....(14.12)

Where,

γ_S and γ_L are newly created surface tension and γ_{LS} interfacial tension that has been destroyed in the process.

The work of cohesion, required to separate the molecules of the spreading liquid so that it can flow over the sublayer, as shown in Fig. 14.11. Here is no interfacial tension. Now consider a hypothetical cylinder is divided two new surfaces are created. Fig. 14.11.

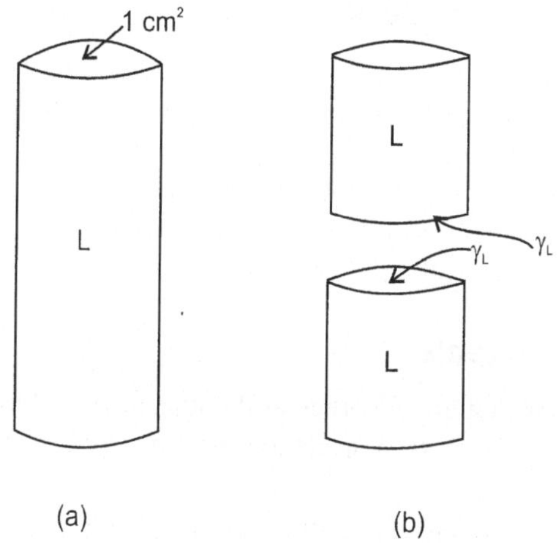

Fig. 14.11 Representation of the work of cohesion involved in separating like molecules in a liquid.

The work of cohesion = $W_c = 2\gamma_L$ .....(14.13)

The work of adhesion is greater than the work of cohesion. The spreading coefficient, S, is obtained from Eqs. (14.12) and (14.13).

$$S = W_a - W_c = (\gamma_L + \gamma_S - \gamma_{LS}) - 2\gamma_L \quad .....(14.14)$$

$$S = \gamma_s - (\gamma_L + \gamma_{LS}) \quad .....(14.15)$$

If, S, is positive, it indicates spreading and if negative indicates no spreading. For the organic liquids spread on water, initial spreading coefficient may be positive or negative, but the final spreading coefficient always negative. Some examples of substances and their spreading coefficient are given in Table 14.3.

Table 14.3 Initial spreading coefficients, S, at 20°.

Substance	S (dynes/cm)
Ethyl alcohol	50.4
Propionic acid	45.8
Ethyl ether	45.5
Chloroform	13
Benzene	8.9
Hexane	3.4

Adsorption at Liquid Interfaces

Adsorption to solid surfaces from solution may occur if the dissolved molecules and the solid surface have chemical groups capable of interacting. When the added molecules move on their own accord to the interface, called positive adsorption. Example - surface active agents. Certain molecules prefer to remain in the bulk of solution, called negative adsorption. Example - electrolytes (sodium chloride) are added to water.

Surface-Active Agents

Molecules and ions that are adsorbed at the interface are termed surface - active agents or surfactants. Surfactants or amphiphiles have a certain affinity for both polar and non polar solvents. Amphiphile may be hydrophilic (water - loving); lipophilic (oil - loving) or well balanced between these two extremes. Ex: straight - chain alcohols, amines and acids. Three types of surfactants

(a) Anionic Surfactant
(b) Cationic Surfactant
(c) Amphoteric Surfactants

(a) ***Anionic Surfactants :*** Mostly anionic surfactants are those containing carboxylate, sulfonate and sulfate ions. Carboxylate ions are known as soaps and generally are prepared by the saponification of natural acid glycerides in alkaline solution.

(b) ***Cationic Surfactants :*** It includes long chain cations such as amine salts and quaternary amonium salts. Mostly used as antimicrobial preservatives.

(c) ***Amphoteric Surfactants :*** Those surfactants containing carboxylate or phosphate groups as the anion, and amino or quaternary amonium groups as the cation.

When a surfactant is dissolved in water at low concentration, a fraction of it will be adsorbed at the air-water interface, and remainder will reside in the bulk in the form of monomers. As the concentration is increased 50 or more monomers come together to form colloidal aggregates termed micelles. The concentration at which aggregation occurs is called critical micelle concentration or CMC. Surfactants are added in pharmaceutical preparations for various purposes such as solubilizing agents, wetting agents, foaming agents, suspending or emulsifying agents etc.

Hydrophilic – Lipophilic Balance : [HLB]

Generally, each emulsifying agent has a hydrophilic portion and a lipophilic portion may be categorized on the basis of their chemical makeup as to their hydrophil – lipophil balance or HLB. By this method each surfactant or emulsifying agent is assigned as HLB value or number indicating the substance's polarity. Although the numbers have been assigned up to about 40, the usual range is between 1 and 20.

Griffin, devised an arbitrary scale of values to serve as a measure of hydrophilic - lipophilic balance as shown in Fig. 14.12.

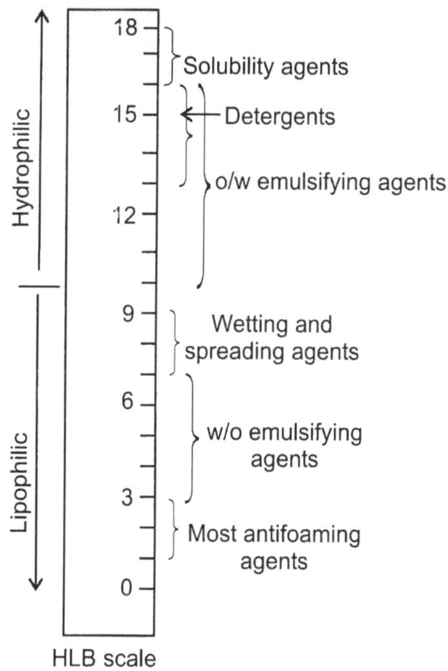

Fig. 14.12 A scale showing surfactant function on the basis of the HLB values.

Wetting agents are surfactants with HLB values of 7 to 9. These agents aid in attaining intimate contact between solid particles and liquids.

Emulsifying agents are surfactants with HLB value of 3 to 6 and 8 to 18 and these agents reduce interfacial tension between oil and water. Detergents having HLB of 13 to 16 and reduce surface tension and aid in wetting the surface and the dirt. Solubilizing agents have HLB of 15 to 20. The HLB of surfactant can be estimated by the formula.

$$HLB = 20\left(1 - \frac{S}{A}\right) \qquad ..... (14.16)$$

in which S is the saponification number of the ester and A is the acid number of fatty acid. Ex : HLB of poly oxyethylene sorbiton monolaurate (Tween 20), for which S = 45.5 and A = 276,

$$\text{So the HLB} = 20\left(1 - \frac{45.5}{276}\right) = 16.7$$

The oil phase of an oil-in-water (o/w) emulsion requires a specific HLB, called the required hydrophile - lipophile balance, RHLB.

Some commonly used amphiphilic agents HLB value are given Table 14.4.

Table 14.4 Some amphiphilic agents and their HLB value.

Substance	HLB
Sodium lauryl sulphate	40
Potassium oleate	20
Oleic acid	1
Sorbitan tristearate	2.1
Glyceryl monostearate	3.8
Gelatin (pharmagel B)	9.8
Sodium oleate	18
Tween 20	16.7
Tween 80	15

Types of Monolayer at Liquid Surfaces

Adsorbed materials are divided into two groups : those that forms "soluble" monolayers and those that form "insoluble" films. Ex: Amyl alcohol may be said to form a soluble monolayer on water. Cetyl alcohol would form an insoluble film on the water. The addition of amphiphiles to a liquid leads to a reduction in surface tension and these molecules adsorbed as a monolayer, this phenomena first expressed quantitatively by Gibbs in 1878 as follows :

$$\Gamma = -\frac{c}{RT}\frac{d\gamma}{dc} \qquad \text{..... (14.17)}$$

where, Γ is the surface excess or concentration,

c is concentration of amphiphile in the liquid bulk

R is gas constant; T is absolute temperature

$\frac{d\gamma}{dc}$ is the change in surface tension of solution

Langmuir, and others have made quantitative studies of the properties of films that are spread over a surface of the substrate liquid (water). The film can be compressed against a horizontal float. The force exerted on float is measured by an apparatus called film balance. The compressive force per unit area on the float is known as surface or film pressure, π; it is difference in surface tension between the pure substrate, γ_0 and that with a film spread on it, γ i.e.

$$\pi = (\gamma_0 - \gamma) \qquad \text{.....(14.18)}$$

This phenamenon is useful in pharmacy especially in stabilization of emulsions, wetting and detergency etc.

Adsorption at Solid Interfaces

When a solid surface exposed to a gas or a liquid, molecules from the gas/ solution accumulate at the surface. The phenomenon of concentration of molecules of a gas or liquid at a solid surface is called adsorption. Ex: Adsorption of a dye by charcoal; Adsorption of a gas by charcoal.

Absorption indicates penetration of molecules into the body of the solid. Ex: Water absorbed by a sponge is distributed throughout the sponge uniformly. Sorption is general term used to indicate both the adsorption and absorption.

Adsorption may be classified into two classes i.e., physical adsorption (physisorption) and chemical adsorption (chemisorption). Physisorption is reversible, nonspecific and mainly due to weak Van Der Waals forces and commonly observed at low temperature. Chemisorption is irreversible, more specific and forms strong chemical bonds and generally occurs at high temperature.

Adsorption is applicable in the removal of objectionable odors from rooms and foods, the operation of gas masks, and the measurement of the dimensions of particles in a powder. The principles of solid – liquid is used in decolorizing solutions, chromatography, detergency and wetting.

The Solid–Gas Interface

The adsorption of gas by solid depends on chemical nature of the adsorbent (the material used to adsorb the gas) and adsorbate (the substance being adsorbed); the surface area of the adsorbent, the temperature and the partial pressure etc. The removal of adsorbate from adsorbent is known as desorption.

To study the adsorption of gas (vapours) onto solid surface, one must measure the amount of gas adsorbed per unit area or unit mass of solid; at different pressures of gas. The plots of volume adsorbed versus pressure at constant temperature are known as adsorption isotherms. If adsorption process is monomolecular, the adsorption isotherm should appear similar to those shown in Fig. 14.13

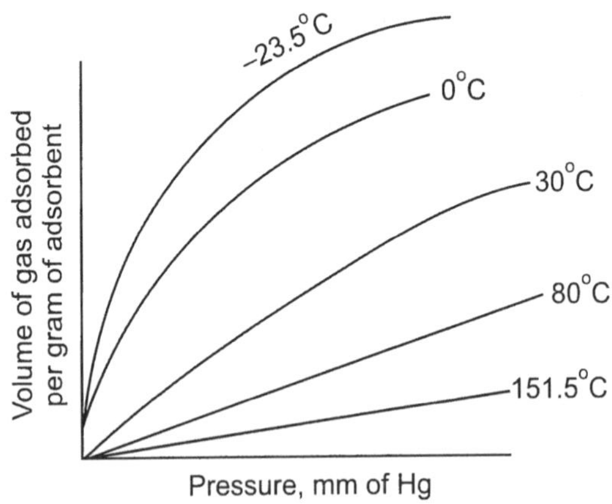

Fig. 14.13 Adsorption isotherms for ammonia on charcoal.

If adsorption process is multimolecular where vapour molecules essentially condense upon themselves as the liquefaction pressure of the vapour is approached. Fig. 14.14 illustrates the multilayered physisorption.

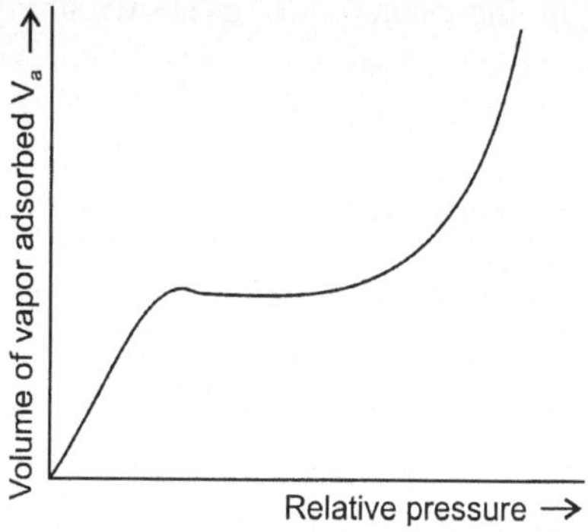

Fig. 14.14 A plot of multilayer physical adsorption of a vapour on a solid surface.

The relationship between the equilibrium pressure of a gas and its amount adsorbed on the solid at any constant temperature is called adsorption isotherm as shown in Fig. 14.15.

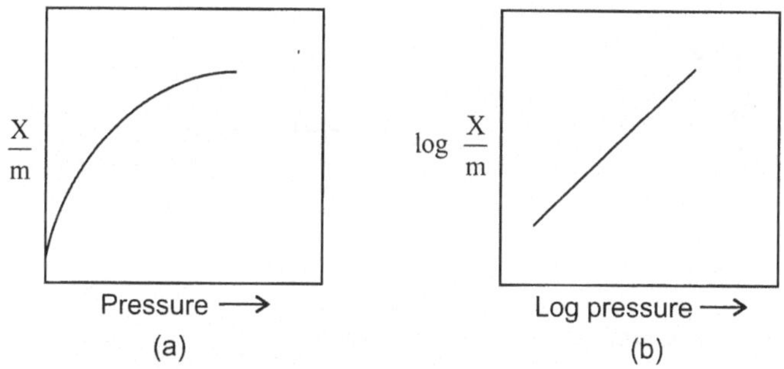

Fig. 14.15 Adsorption isotherms for a gas on a solid.

Freundlich Adsorption Isotherm

Freundlich proposed an empirical relation as

$$y = \frac{x}{m} = kp^{\frac{1}{n}} \qquad .....(14.19)$$

in which y is the mass of gas x adsorbed per unit mass m of adsorbent, and k and n are constants. Equation (14.19) can be written in the logarithmic form,

$$\log \frac{x}{m} = \log k + \frac{1}{n} \log p \qquad .....(14.20)$$

which yield a straight line when plotted as shown in Fig. 14.15(b). The constant, log k, is the intercept on the ordinate and 1/n is slope. Freundlich isotherm is not applicable at high pressures.

Langmuir Adsorption Isotherm

Langmuir (1916) derived a simple adsorption isotherm based on some assumptions. These assumptions are :

1. The molecules or gas atoms are adsorbed on active sites of the solid to form a layer one molecule thick (monolayer).
2. The adsorbed layer is uniform all over the adsorbent.
3. There is no interaction between the adjacent adsorbed molecules.

Derivation : Langmuir considered the fraction of centers occupied by gas molecules at pressure p is represented by θ, and the fraction of sites not occupied is $1 - \theta$. This can be illustrated in Fig. 14.16.

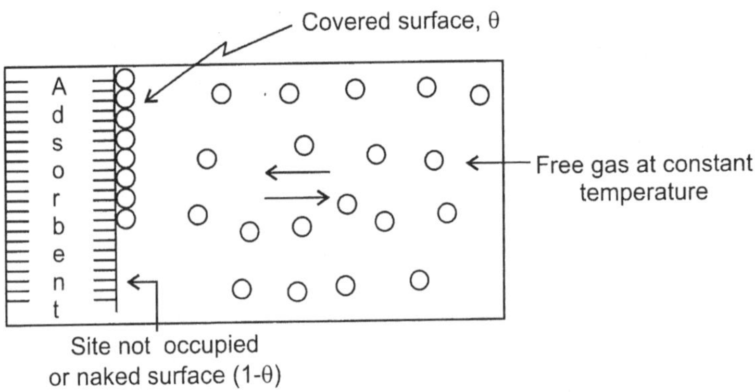

Fig. 14.16 Representation of adsorption of gas molecules on the fraction of adsorbent surface.

The rate r_1 of adsorption or condensation of gas molecules on the surface is proportional to the unoccupied spots $1 - \theta$ and to the pressure p. i.e.

$$r_1 = k_1 (1 - \theta)p \quad .....(14.21)$$

where k_1 is rate constant for adsorption process.

The rate r_2 of evaporation of molecules bound on the surface is proportional to the fraction of surface occupied, θ or.

$$r_2 = k_2\theta \quad .....(14.22)$$

and at equilibrium $r_1 = r_2$ or

$$k_1(1-\theta)p = k_2\theta \qquad .....(14.23)$$

By rearrangement we obtain

$$\theta = \frac{k_1 p}{k_2 + k_1 p} = \frac{(k_1/k_2)}{1+(k_1/k_2)p} \qquad .....(14.24)$$

After replacing k_1/k_2 by b and θ by γ/γ_m in which γ is mass of gas adsorbed per gram of adsorbent at pressure p and at constant temperature and y_m is mass of gas that 1 gram of the adsorbent can take up when the monolayer is complete. So equation (14.24) will becomes

$$y = \frac{y_m bp}{1+bp} \qquad .....(14.25)$$

Equation (14.25) represents the Langmuir isotherm.

Inverting and multiplying by 'p' the equation (14.25) gives,

$$\frac{p}{y} = \frac{1}{by_m} + \frac{p}{y_m} \qquad ..... (14.26)$$

A plot of p/γ against p gives a straight line and y_m and b can be obtained from the slope and intercept.

As shown in Fig (14.14) curve is sigmoidal in shape and occur due to physical adsorption to form monolayer and when pressure increases there is formation of multilayer. This isotherm is also called Type II isotherm and described by an expression derived by Brunauer, Emmett and Teller i.e., BET equation and may be written as.

$$\frac{p}{y(p_0 - p)} = \frac{1}{y_m b} + \frac{b-1}{y_m b}\frac{p}{p_0} \qquad .....(14.27)$$

Where, p = pressure of the adsorbate, (mm Hg)

y = mass of vapor per gram

p_0 = vapor pressure at saturation

y_m = amount of vapor adsorbed per unit mass of adsorbent, when the surface is covered with monomolecular layer.

b = constant, proportional to the difference between the heat of adsorption of the gas in the first layer and the latent heat of condensation of subsequent layers.

Adsorption Isotherms : There are five different types of adsorption isotherms as shown in Fig. 14.17.

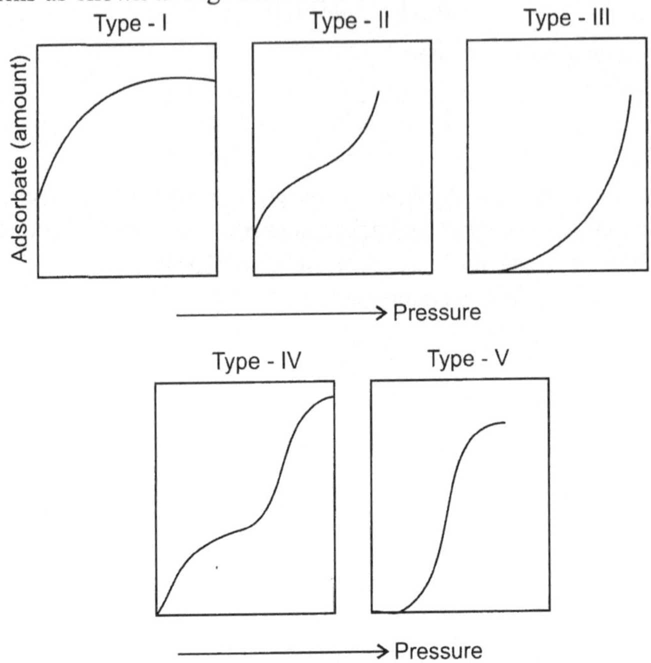

Fig. 14.17 Various types of adsorption isotherms.

Type I : This represent increase in adsorption with increasing pressure. Ex: Freundlich and Langmuir adsorption isotherm. [Adsorption of nitrogen gas at 78 °k on charcoal].

Type II : This is sigmodial in shape and occur when gas undergo physical adsorption onto nonporous solids to form a monolayer. When the pressure is increased multilayer is formed. Type - II is described by BET equation as explained earlier.

Type III : It is not commonly observed. The heat of adsorption of gas in the first layer is less than the latent heat of condensation of successive layers.

Type IV : This represents the adsorption of gas on porous solids. It shows capillary condensation. Ex. Adsorption of benzene on silica gel.

Type V : This is uncommon and shows capillary condensation. Ex. water vapour on charcoal at 100 °C.

The Solid – Liquid Interface : From the solution the solute molecules may be adsorbed on solid. Drugs such as dyes, alkaloids, fatty acids, inorganic acids and bases may be adsorbed from solution onto solids such as alumina or charcoal. The adsorption of strychnine, atropine and quinine from aqueous solutions by different clays was expressed by Langmuir equation in the following form.

$$\frac{c}{y} = \frac{1}{by_m} + \frac{c}{y_m} \qquad \text{..... (14.28)}$$

where, c is equilibrium concentration (mg/100ml)

y is amount of alkaloidal base x in milligrams adsorbed per gram m of clay. The adsorption of strychnine from aqueous solution onto three different clays such as activated attapulgite, halloysite and kaolin have been studied, and shown in Fig. 14.18.

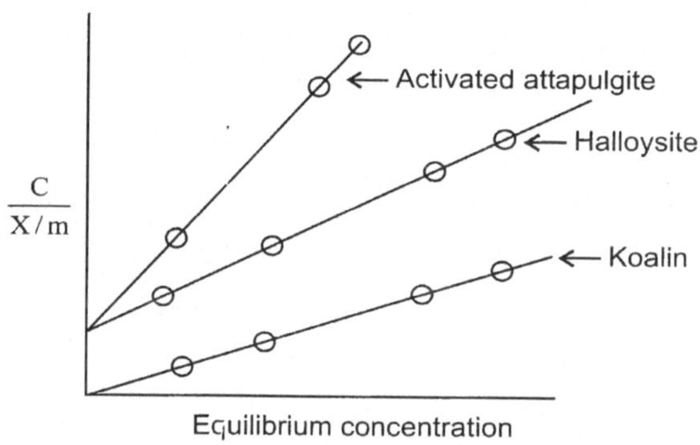

Fig. 14.18 Adsorption of strychnine on various clays.

The smaller the slope, the better the absorption. From the Fig. 14.18 one can conclued that attapulgite is superior than halloysite and kaolin.

Applications of Activated Charcoal

Activated charcoal is used as an antidote in poisoning by sulfonyl ureas such as tolbutamide acetohexamide and other drugs. In large overdosage, paracetamol my cause liver damage, renal failure and death due to hepatotoxicity. Activated charcoal enhance the diffusion of drugs from tissues of GI tract into GI contents so facilitating the elimination of drugs. This process called gastrointestinal dialysis. Charcoal is used to purify water, used in HPLC as analytical tool, etc.

Wetting : When talc or charcoal sprinkled onto the surface of water, it float on the surface. For immersion of the solid, the liquid must displace air and spread over the surface of the solid. When liquids cannot spread over a solid surface, S, spreading coefficient, is negative, i.e., solid is not wetted.

Wetting is an adsorption process in which an intimate contact of the solids with liquid phase is achieved. Wetting phenomenon is useful in pharmacy and medicine include the displacement of air from the surface of charcoal sulfer and other powders, the displacement of dirt and debris by the use of detergents in washing of wounds, application of lotions, sprays to the skin etc.

Surfactants are used as wetting agents because, they can lower interfacial tension, lowering of contact angle between solids and liquids, and can displace air from surface.

The important property of wetting agent is to lower the contact angle between surface and the wetting liquid. The contact angle may be defined as an angle between the liquid droplet and surface over which it spreads.

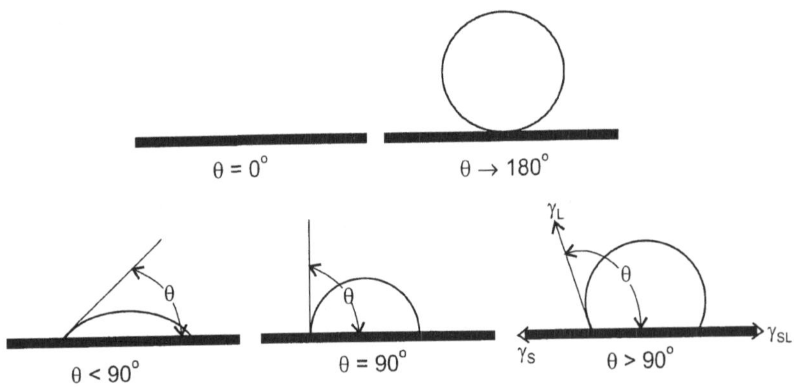

Fig. 14.19 Contact angles from 0° to 180°.

As shown in Fig. 14.19. the contact angles may have values between 0° and 180°, When $\theta = 0$, signifies complete wetting and when $\theta > 90°$ at which wetting is insignificant.

At equilibrium, the surface and interfacial tensions can be written as

$$\gamma_s = \gamma_{SL} + \gamma_L \cos\theta \qquad .....(14.29)$$

Equation (14.29) known as Young's equation and can be written as

$$S = \gamma_L (\text{Cos } \theta - 1) \qquad .....(14.30)$$

and combining Eq. (14.29) in Eq. (14.12) of spreading coefficient we can write

$$W_a = W_{SL} = \gamma_L (1 + \text{Cos } \theta) \qquad .....(14.31)$$

Detergents : Detergents are surfactants used for removal of dirt from glass, febric, skin etc., Detergency is complex process and involved number of steps of its actions include -

* initial wetting of the dirt and surface.
* solubilization of dirt particles.
* removing the insoluble dirt.
* suspending particles in the detergent solution.
* removing of oil soluble material
* foaming washing away the particles.

The HLB for the detergency is about 13 to 16.

Electric Properties of Interfaces

The colloidal dispersions or suspensions consists of suspended particles possess either a positive or negative charge. The similarly charged particles prevent aggregation and settling due to mutual force of repulsion between similarly charged particles. This gives the stability to the colloidal dispersion or sol. This can be illustrated by Fig. 14.20.

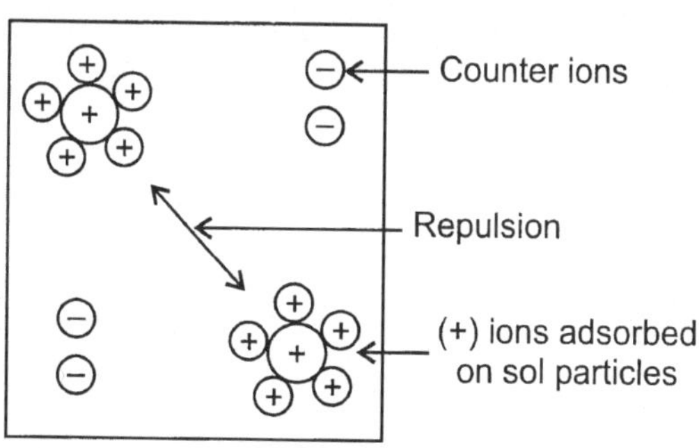

Fig. 14.20 Representation of the mutual forces of repulsion between similarly charged particles prevent aggregation.

The surface of colloidal particle acquires a positive charge by selective adsorption of positive ions around it. This layer attracts counter ions from medium which form second layer of negative charge as seen in Fig. 14.21, this is called Helmholtz Double layer.

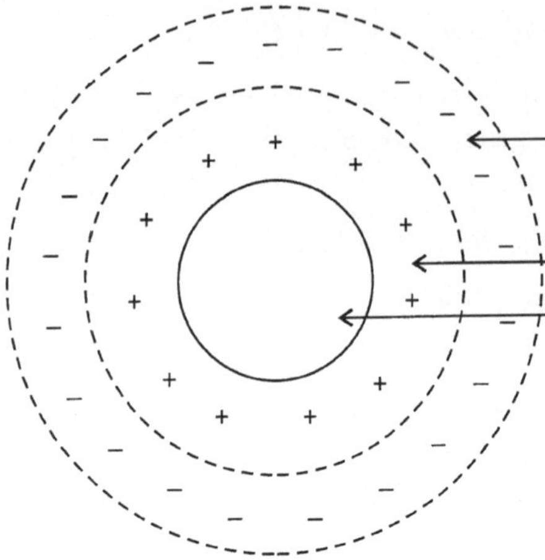

Fig. 14.21 Helmholtz Double layer.

The study of electrical properties is useful in stabilization of colloidal dispersions, suspensions and stabilization of emulsions.The concept of electrical double layer at interface can be studied with the help of Fig. 14.22.

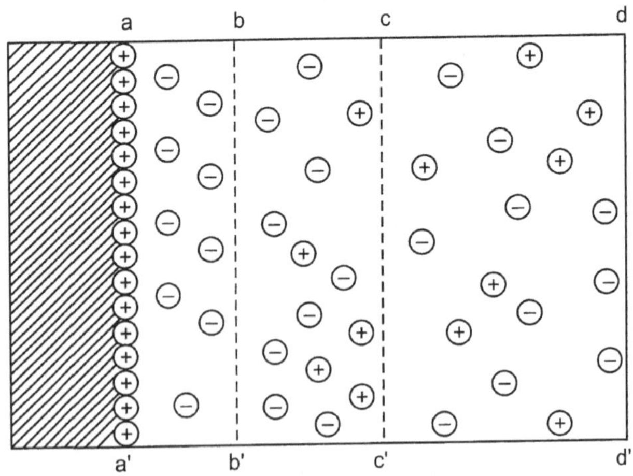

Fig. 14.22 Electrical Double Layer.

Suppose a solid surface is in contact with a polar solution containing ions (an aqueous solution of an electrolyte). Further consider some of the cations are adsorbed onto the surface, impart a positive charge. In the remaining solution cations plus total number of anions are present.The anions are attracted to positively charged surface by electric forces and complete initial adsorption. At a particular distance from the surface, the concentration of anions and cations are equal i.e., electric neutrality.

As shown in Fig. 14.23, where aa' is the surface of the solid. The adsorbed ions gave the positive charged surface are referred as potential determining ions. Immediately adjacent to this surface layer is a region of tightly bound solvent molecules, together with some negative ions. This layer extends upto bb'. Anions are generally termed as counter ions or gegenions. The boundary bb' is termed as shear plane. In the region bb' and cc', there is an excess of negative ions. The potential at bb' is still positive. Beyond cc', the ions are equally distributed and electric neutrality is obtained.

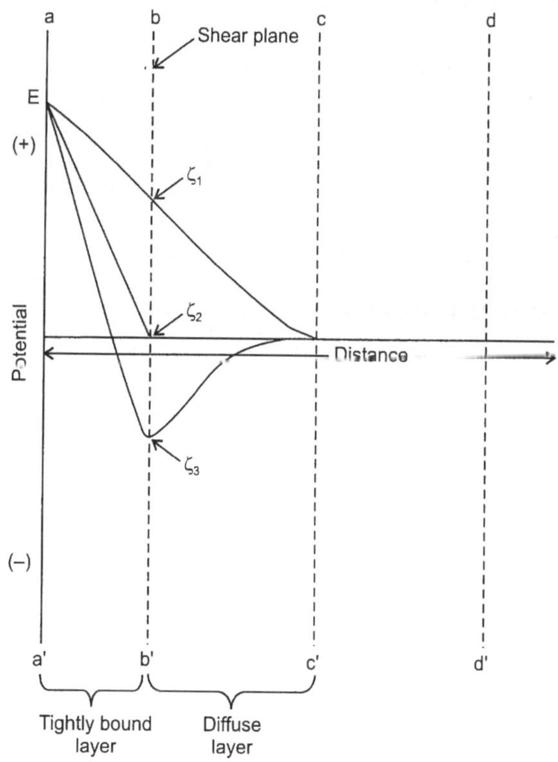

Fig. 14.23 Electrokinetic potential at solid-liquid boundaries.

The potential charges are represented in Fig. 14.23 and can be expressed by different ways.

Nernst and Zeta Potentials

The potential at the solid surface aa', due to the potential determining ions is Nernst potential, E and is defined as the difference in potential between the actual surface and the electroneutral region of the solution. This is also called electrothermodynamic potential. The potential located at the shear plane bb' is known as the electrokinetic or Zeta potential, ζ; and is defined as the difference in potential between the surface of tightly bound layer and electroneutral region of the solution.

Zeta potential plays an important role in the stabilization of systems containing dispersed particles. An optimum Zeta Potential is essential for the maximum stability. If the Zeta Potential is falls below a particular value, the attractive forces exceed than repulsive forces and it may cause aggregation of particles. This phenomenon is known as flocculation observed in colloids or suspension. Zeta potential decreases rapidly when concentration of electrolytes is increased.

Problems

1. What is the surface tension of sodium lauryl sulphate solution if the length of the bar L, is 7 cm and the mass required to break a soap film is 0.80 gm ?

   Solution : Data given

   Length of bar $= L = 7$ cm

   Mass required to break soap film $= 0.8$ gm.

   Acceleration due to gravity $= 981$ cm/sec^2

   Equation for surface tension $= \gamma = fb/2L$.

   fb = mass × acceleration due to gravity

$$\gamma = \frac{0.8 \times 981}{2 \times 7} = 56.05 \text{ dynes/cm.}$$

2. Ethanol rises 1.22 cm in a capillary rise apparatus of 25 °C. The radius of capillary tube was found to be 0.057 cm. The density of ethanol is 0.781 g/cm^3. Compute the surface tension of ethanol.

Solution : Data given

Height = h = 1.22 cm; Radius = r = 0.057 cm.

Density = ρ = 0.781 g/cm^3.

Acceleration due to gravity = g = 981 cm/sec^2.

Equation for surface tension = γ = 1/2 rρhg

$$= \frac{0.057 \times 0.781 \times 1.22 \times 981}{2}$$

$$= 26.63 \text{ dyne/cm.}$$

3. Calculate the surface tension of the soap solution from the following data obtained by the use of DuNouy tensiometer. The ring circumference of tensiometer was found to have 10.47 cm and the correction factor was 0.880. The dial reading was found to have 886.

Solution : Data given

Ring circumference = 10.47 cm

Equation for surface tension = γ

$$= \frac{\text{dial reading in dynes}}{2\times \text{ ring circumference}} \times \text{ correction factor}$$

$$= \frac{886}{2 \times 10.47} \times 0.880$$

$$= 37.23 \text{ dynes/cm.}$$

4. From the surface pressure method following data was obtained. The surface tension of soap is 2.3 dyne/cm; radius of bubble expands to 8.4 cm. Calculate pressure difference across the surface film of the soap bubble.

Solution : Data given

Surface tension = γ = 2.3 dyne/cm

radius = r = 8.4 cm

Equation for pressure difference

$\Delta p = \frac{2\gamma}{r}$ called young Laplace equation.

$$\Delta p = \frac{2 \times 2.3}{8.4} = 0.54 \text{ dynes/cm}^2$$

5. Calculate the HLB of polysorbate (Tween 20). The Saponification number of Tween 20 is 45.5 and acid number is 276.

   Solution : Data given

   Saponification number = S = 45.5

   Acid number = A = 276

   $$\text{Equation for HLB} = 20\left[1-\frac{S}{A}\right] = 20\left[1-\frac{45.5}{276}\right]$$

   $$= 16.7.$$

CHAPTER 15

Units and Measures

Compounding of prescriptions is a rapidly growing component of pharmacy practice. Pharmacists are creative and should have the ability to formulate patient-specific preparations for providing pharmaceutical care. Most compounded prescriptions require a number of calculations as part of preparation, packing and dispensing. One of the greatest potentials for error in prescription compounding is in the area of pharmaceutical calculations and conversions. There is no excuse for ignorance in this area and an individual unprepared to do necessary calculations should not be involved in pharmaceutical compounding. The idea in including this topic is to make the students well aware of the conversions that often puzzle them in calculations.

The International System of Units (SI) comprises three categories of units, namely basic units, derived units and supplementary units. The basic units are given in Table 15.1. The derived units are obtained by combining the basic units according to certain algebraic relationships between the corresponding quantities. Some of these derived units have special names and symbols, which are shown in Table 15.2.

Table 15.1 Basic units for various quantities.

Quantity	Name of basic SI Unit	Symbol
Length	metre	m
Mass	kilogram	kg
Tme	second	s
Eletric current	ampere	A
Thermodynamic temperature	kelvin	K
Amount of substance	mole	mol
Luminous intensity	candela	cd

Table 15.2 Derived units for various quantities.

Quantity	Name of derived SI unit	Symbol	Expression in basic SI units	Equivalence with other units
Absrobed dose of ionising radiation	gray	Gy	m^2s^{-2}	1 Gy = 1 joule per kg
Energy, work, qauntity of heat	joule	J	$kg\,m^2\,s^{-2}$	1 J = 10^7 ergs
Electrical potential, potential"	volt	V	$kg\,m^2A^{-1}\,s^{-3}$	
Electric resistance	ohm	Ω	$kg\,m^2A^{-1}\,s^{-3}$	
Force	newton	N	$kg\,ms^{-2}$	1 N = 10^5 dynes
Frequency	hertz	Hz	s^{-1}	1 Hz = 1 cycle per second
Power	watt	W	$kg\,m^2\,s^{-3}$	
Pressure	pascal	Pa	$kg\,m^{-1}\,s^{-2}$	1 kPa = 7.5 mm Hg = 7.5 torr
Radioactivity	becquerel	Bq	s^{-1}	1 Bq = 2.703 × 10^{-11} curies

Further we will discuss on some of the conversions of most commonly used physical quantities in pharmacy so as to make these calculations handy.

Length

The S I unit of length is the metre. To change any of the other units of length into their equivalent values in metres use the operation and conversion factor given below in Table 15.3. All the values are given to an appropriate degree of accuracy.

Table 15.2 .1 Derived units for various quantities.

Derived units for various quantities			
Quantity of electricity, electric charge	coulomb	C	s A
Capacitance	farad	F=C/V	$s^4 A^2/m^2 kg$
Surface tension	newton per metre	N/m	kg/s^2
Moment of force	metre newton	N m	$m^2 kg/s^2$
Heat capacity, entropy	joule per kelvin	J/K	$m^2 kg/s^2 K$
Conductance	siemens	S = A/V	$s^3 A^2/m^2 kg$
Magnetic flux	weber	Wb = V s	$m^2 kg/s^2 A$
Specific heat capacity, specific entropy	joule per kilogram kelvin	J/kg K	$m^2/s^2 K$
Specific energy	joule per kilogram	J/kg	m^2/s^2

Area

The S I unit of area is square metre. To change any of these other units of area into their equivalent values in square metres use the operation and conversion factor given below in Table 15.4. All the values are given to an appropriate degree of accuracy.

Table 15.3 Conversion table for length,

angstroms	divide by 10^{10}
astronomical units	x 149 598 550 000
barleycorns	x 0.008 467
centimetres	x 0.01
chains (surveyors')	x 20.1168
cubits	x (0.45 to 0.5)
ells (UK)	x 0.875 *(but many variations)*
ems (pica)	x 0.004 233 3
fathoms	x 1.8288
feet (UK and US)	x 0.3048
feet (US survey)	x 0.304 800 609 6
furlongs	x 201.168
hands	x 0.1016
inches	x 0.0254
kilometres	x 1000
light years	x 9 460 500 000 000 000
metres [m]	x 1
microns(micrometres)	x 0.000 001
miles (UK and US)	x 1609.344
miles (nautical)	x 1852
parsecs	x 30 856 770 000 000 000
yards	x 0.9144

Table 15.4 Conversion table for area.

acres	x 4046.856 422 4
ares	x 100
hectares	x 10 000
square centimetres	x 0.000 1
square feet (UK and US)	x 0.092 903 04
square feet (US survey)	x 0.092 903 411 613
square inches	x 0.000 645 16
square kilometres	x 1 000 000
square metres	1
square miles	x 2 589 988.110 336
square millimetres	x 0.000 001
square yards	x 0.836 127 36

Volume or Capacity

The SI unit of volume is the cubic metre. However, this seems to be much less used than the litre (1000 litres = 1 cubic metre). To change any of these other units of volume into their equivalent values in litres use the operation and conversion factor given. All the values are given to an appropriate degree of accuracy. There can be some ambiguity about the size of the litre. When the metric system was introduced in the 1790's the litre was intended to match up with the volume occupied by 1 kilogram of pure water at a specified pressure and temperature. As the ability to measure things got better (by 100 years later) they found that there was a mismatch between the kilogram and the litre. As a result of this they had to redefine the litre (in 1901) as being 1.000028 cubic decimetres. Here the litre is taken as being a cubic decimeter. The conversion chart is given below in Table 15.5.

Table 15.5 Conversion table for volume.

cubic centimeters	x 0.001
cubic decimeters	x1
cubic decameters	x 1 000 000
cubic feet	x 28.316 846 592
cubic inches	x 0.016 387 064
cubic meters	x 1000
cubic millimeters	x 0.000 001
cubic yards	x 764.554 857 984
decilitres	x 0.1
fluid ounces (UK)	x 0.028 413 062 5

fluid ounces (US)	x 0.029 573 529 562 5
gallons (UK)	x 4.546 09
gallons, dry (US)	x 4.404 883 770 86
gallons, liquid (US)	x 3.785 411 784
litres [l or L]	x1
litres (1901 - 1964)	x 1.000 028
millilitres	x 0.001
pints (UK)	x 0.568 261 25
pints, dry (US)	x 0.550 610 471 357 5
pints, liquid (US)	x 0.473 176 473
quarts (UK)	x 1.136 522 5
quarts, dry (US)	x 1.101 220 942 715
quarts, liquid (US)	x 0.946 352 946

Mass or Weight

The SI unit of mass is the kilogram. To change any of these other units of mass into their equivalent values in kilograms use the operation and conversion factor given below in Table 15.6. All the values are given to an appropriate degree of accuracy.

Table 15.6 Conversion table for mass.

grains	x 0.000 064 798 91
grams	x 0.001
hundredweights, long	x 50.802 345 44
hundredweights, short	x 45.359 237
kilograms [kg]	x 1
ounces, avoirdupois	x 0.028 349 523 125
ounces, troy	x 0.031 103 476 8
pounds	x 0.453 592 37
slugs (or g-pounds)	x 14.593 903
tons (UK or long)	x 1016.046 908 8
tons (US or short)	x 907.184 74
tonnes	x 1000

Temperature

There have been five main temperature scales, each one being named after the person who invented it.

G D FAHRENHEIT (1686-1736) a German physicist, in about 1714 proposed the first practical scale. He called the freezing point of water 32 degrees (so as to avoid negative temperatures) and the boiling point 212 degrees.

R A F de REAUMUR (1673-1757) A French entomologist, proposed a similar scale in 1730, but set the freezing point at 0 degrees and the boiling point at 80 degrees. This was used quite a bit but is now obsolete. Anders CELSIUS (1701-1744) a Swedish astronomer, proposed the 100-degree scale (from 0 to 100) in 1742. This was widely adopted as the centigrade scale. But since grades and centigrades were also measures of angle, in 1947 it officially became the Celsius scale. Also, the S I system of units gives preference to naming units after people where possible. William Thomson, 1st Lord KELVIN (1824-1907) a Scottish mathematician and physicist, worked with J P Joule - about 1862 - to produce an absolute scale of temperature based on laws of heat rather than the freezing/boiling-points of water. This work produced the idea of 'absolute zero', a temperature below which it was not possible to go. Its value is -273.15 degrees on the Celsius scale. William J M RANKINE (1820-1872) a Scottish engineer and scientist, promoted the Kelvin scale in its Fahrenheit form, when the equivalent value of absolute zero is -459.67 degrees Fahrenheit. Nowadays, while scientists use the KELVIN scale, the CELSIUS scale is the preferred scale in our everyday lives. However, the Fahrenheit scale is still widely used and there frequently is a need to be able to change from one to the other. The formula for interconversion of temperature is given below in Table 15.7.

Table 15.7 Conversion table for temperature.

To change temperature given in Fahrenheit (*F*) to Celsius (*C*) Start with (*F*); subtract 32; multiply by 5; divide by 9; the answer is (*C*)
To change temperature given in Celsius (*C*) to Fahrenheit (*F*) Start with (*C*); multiply by 9; divide by 5; add on 32; the answer is (*F*)

Deg C = (Deg F – 32) × 5/9

Deg F = (Deg C × 9/5) + 32

Density

Density is the shortened term generally used in place of the more accurate description *volumetric density.* It is a measure of mass per unit volume. The S I compatible unit of density is kilograms/cubic metre. However, this a rather large unit for most purposes (iron is over 7000, wood is about 600 and even cork is over 200). A much more useful size of unit is kilograms/litre (for which the previous values then become 7, 0.6 and 0.2 respectively). This unit also has the great advantage of being numerically unchanged for grams/cubic centimeter and tones/cubic metre (or megagrams/cubic metre). To change any of these other units of density into their equivalent values in kilograms/litre use the operation and conversion factor given. All the values are given to an appropriate degree of accuracy in Table 15.8.

Table 15.8 Conversion table for density.

grains/gallon(UK)	divide by 70 157
grains/gallon(US)	divide by 58 418
grams/cubic centimetre	1
grams/litre	divide by 1000
grams/millilitre	1
kilograms/cubic metre	divide by 1000
megagrams/cubic metre	1
milligrams/milliliter	divide by 1000
milligrams/litre	divide by 1 000 000
kilograms/litre	1
ounces/cubic inch	x 1.729 994 044
ounces/gallon(UK)	x 0.006 236 023
ounces/gallon(US)	x 0.007 489 152
pounds/cubic inch	x 27.679 905
pounds/cubic foot	x 0.016 018 463
pounds/gallon(UK)	x 0.099 776 373
pounds/gallon(US)	x 0.119 826 427

Force

The S I unit of force is the Newton. To change any of these other units of force into their equivalent values in newtons use the operation and conversion factor given below in Table 15.9. All the values are given to an appropriate degree of accuracy.

Table 15.9 Conversion table for force.

dynes	divide by 100 000
kilograms force	x 9.806 65
kilonewtons [kN]	x 1000
kips	x 4448.222
meganewtons [MN]	x 1 000 000
newtons [N]	1
pounds force	x 4.448 222
poundals	x 0.138 255
sthenes (=kN)	x 1000
tonnes force	x 9806.65
tons(UK) force	x 9964.016
tons(US) force	x 8896.443

Pressure or Stress

The S I unit of pressure is the Pascal. The units of pressure are defined in the same way as those for stress - force/unit area. To change any of these other units of pressure (or stress) into their equivalent values in Pascal use the operation and conversion factor given below in Table 15.10. All the values are given to an appropriate degree of accuracy. Measures based on water assume a density of 1 kg/litre - a value that is rarely matched in the real world, though the error is small.

Table 15.10 Conversion table for pressure.

atmospheres	x 101 325
bars	x 100 000
centimetres of mercury	x 1333.22
centimetres of water	x 98.066 5
feet of water	x 2989.066 92
hectopascals [hPa]	x 100
inches of water	x 249.088 91
inches of mercury	x 3386.388
kg-force/sq.centimetre	x 98 066.5
kg-force/sq.metre	x 9.806 65
kilonewton/sq.metre	x 1000
kilopascal [kPa]	x 1000
kips/sq.inch	x 6 894 760
meganewtons/sq.metre	x 1 000 000

metres of water	x 9806.65
millibars	x 100
pascals [Pa]	1
millimetres of mercury	x 133.322
millimetres of water	x 9.806 65
newtons/sq.centimetre	x 10 000
newtons/sq.metre	1
newtons/sq.millimetre	x 1 000 000
pounds-force/sq.foot	x 47.880
pounds-force/sq.inch	x 6894.757

Speed

The S I compatible unit of speed is metres/second. To change any of these other units of speed into their equivalent values in metres/second use the operation and conversion factor given below in Table 15.11. All the values are given to an appropriate degree of accuracy.

Table 15.11 Conversion table for speed.

centimetres/minute	divide by 6000
centimetres/second	divide by 100
feet/hour	divide by 11 811
feet/minute	x 0.005 08
feet/second	x 0.3048
inches/minute	divide by 2362.2
inches/second	x 0.0254
kilometres/hour	divide by 3.6
kilometres/second	x 1000
knots	x 0.514 444
Mach number	x 331.5
metres/hour	divide by 3600
metres/minute	divide by 60
metres/second [m/s]	1
miles/hour	x 0.447 04
miles/minute	x 26.8224
miles/second	x 1609.344
yards/hour	divide by 3937
yards/minute	x 0.015 24
yards/second	x 0.9144

The SI unit of work of energy or quantity of heat is Joule (symbol J), named after James Prescott Joule. It is defined as "the amount of work done by a force of one newton moving an object through a distance of one meter". To convert the other units of energy into their equivalents values in Joules conversion factor is given below in Table.

Units	Symbol	Conversion factor
Watt-second	W*s	multiply with 1
Newton meter	N*m	multiply with 1
Ergs	erg	multiply with 1×10^{7}
Electron volts	eV	multiply with 6.24×10^{18}
British thermal unit	BTU	multiply with 9.48×10^{-4}
Foe	foe	multiply with 1×10^{-44}
Kilowatt hour	kW.h	multiply with 2.77×10^{-7}
Foot-pound force	ft·lb	multiply with 0.7376
Calories	cal	multiply with 0.2390

Problem 1: Covert 50 lb to kg

$$50 \text{ lb} \times 0.453\_= 22.65 \text{ kg}$$

Problem 2:

Solve the following problems:

1. How many cc in ½ tsp?
2. Convert 20 gtt to cc.
3. How many qt in 4 fl oz?
4. Convert 1.5 inches to cm.
5. Convert 0.05 g to ìg.
6. Convert 0.0025 L to cc.
7. Convert 0.25 g to gr.
8. Convert 1/40 gr to mg.
9. How many tsp in 2 Tbs?
10. Convert 88 lb to kg.

Answer:

1. 2.5 cc
2. 1.3 cc
3. 0.125 qt
4. 3.81 cm
5. 50,000 ìg
6. 2.5 cc
7. 4.17 gr
8. 1.5 mg
9. 6 tsp
10. 40 kg

Problem 3:

1. 1 g to mg
2. 5 mg to μg
3. 0.0025 L to ml
4. 10 gr to mg
5. 68 lb to kg
6. 15 cc to tsp
7. 500 cc to L
8. 36.8° C to ° F
9. 15 ml to Tbs
10. 1 fl oz to ml
11. 2 gr to g
12. 25 cc to ml
13. 1 tsp to cc
14. 10 km to ft
15. 180 lb to kg
16. 0.0005 mg to μg
17. 500 ìg to kg
18. 98.6° F to Celsius
19. 25 gr to mg
20. 1 hr to min

21. 20 kg to lb
22. 1 pt to fl oz
23. 1 pt to ml

Hints:

1. 1 g = 1000 mg
2. 1 mg = 1000 ìg
3. 1000 ml = 1 L
4. 60 mg = 1 gr
5. 2.2 lb = 1 kg
6. 5 cc = 1 tsp
7. 1000 ml = 1 L, 1 cc = 1 ml
8. 98.2° F
9. 5 ml = 1 tsp, 3 tsp = 1 Tbs
10. 1 fl oz = 30 ml
11. 1 gr = 60 mg, 1000 mg = 1 g
12. 1 cc = 1 ml
13. 5 cc = 1 tsp
14. 2.54 cm = 1 in, 12 in = 1 ft
15. 2.2 lb = 1 kg
16. 1000 ìg = 1mg
17. 1,000, 000 ìg = 1 kg
18. 37°C
19. 60 mg = 1 gr
20. 60 min = 1 hr
21. 2.2 lb = 1 kg
22. 16 fl oz = 1 pt
23. 1 pt = 16 fl oz, 30 cc = 1 fl oz

CHAPTER 16

Buffers and Buffered Isotonic Systems

A buffer system is a solution consisting of a mixture of a weak acid and its conjugate base or a weak base and its conjugate acid which has the capacity to resist changes in pH. Addition of a small amount of acid or base to an aqueous/water solution results in change of pH. However, addition of a buffer system to these solutions helps in resisting pH changes. Buffer systems have been widely used in various pharmaceutical dosage forms (especially aqueous solutions) for achieving stability and optimum physiological effect of drugs.

Examples of Weak Acid Buffer Systems:

- Acetic acid and Sodium acetate
- Boric acid and Sodium borate
- Citric acid and Sodium citrate
- Phosphoric acid and Potassium phosphate

Theory

As mentioned above buffer systems contain a mixture of a weak acid and its conjugate base or a weak base and its conjugate acid. For a system containing a weak acid (HA), and its conjugate base (A^-), there exists an equilibrium which is between

$$HA + H_2O \rightleftharpoons H_3O^+ + A^-$$

According to Le Chatelier's principle when H^+ ions are added to the solution the equilibrium moves to the left and when OH^- ions are added the equilibrium moves to the right. Thus, a part of the reagent added to the system is consumed in shifting the equilibrium and the pH will be slightly affected if the solution is not buffered.

The acid dissociation constant for a weak acid, HA, is defined as

$$K_a = \frac{[H^+][A^-]}{[HA]}$$

Applying logarithm on both sides we obtain Henderson-Hasselbalch equation,

$$pH = pK_a + \log_{10}\frac{[A^-]}{[HA]}.$$

In this equation [HA] is the concentration of acid and $[A^-]$ is the concentration of conjugate base. At $[HA] = [A^-]$ we obtain half-neutralization point where, pH = pK_a. The calculated pH may not be always equal to the measured pH. The same considerations also apply to a mixture of a weak base, B and its conjugate acid BH^+.

$$B + H_2O\ BH^+ + OH^-$$

The pK_a value to be used is that of the acid conjugate to the base.

In general a buffer solution may be made up of more than one weak acid and its conjugate base.

The resistance to changes in pH makes buffer solutions very useful in chemical and pharmaceutical manufacturing processes. An ideal buffer system for a particular pH requires pK_a equal to that pH, since such a solution has maximum buffer capacity.

Applications of Buffer Systems

- Blood plasma contains buffer system [carbonic acid (H_2CO_3) and bicarbonate (HCO_3)] which maintains the pH between 7.35-7.45.
- Buffer solutions are necessary to keep the correct pH for enzymes in many organisms to work.
- Ionized form of a drug is more water soluble than the unionized form. So, buffers are used to maintain the drug in ionized form for aqueous solutions.

- Unionized form of a drug is more lipid soluble than the ionized form. So buffer systems are used to maintain the drug in unionized forms to increase the absorption.
- Aqueous solutions containing ester drugs are maintained at low pH (3-5) so as prevent the hydrolytic reactions.
- Control of gelling in pectin-based products.
- Flavor intensity changes with change in pH.
- Changes in sourness, sweet/sour balance with pH.
- Decrease variation in color shade of natural colors.
- In ophthalmic products high or low pH can causes tissue irritation. So pH is maintained in between 5.5-7.5.

Buffer Capacity

It is defined as the resistance to pH change. The equation for buffer capacity is:

$$\text{Buffer capacity} = \frac{dn}{d(pH)}$$

where, dn= an infinitesimal amount of base added

d(pH)= an infinitesimal change in pH

Buffer capacity is also defined as the number of equivalents of a strong base (ΔB) required for increasing pH (ΔpH) by one unit in 1 L of solution. Greater the buffer capacity smaller is the change in pH from addition of a given amount of strong acid or base. Buffer capacity is dependent on the total concentration of the buffer system and on the HA/A- ratio.

Buffer capacity is highest when pH = pKa and can be increased by following ways:

- increasing the concentration of the buffer system components (e.g. doubling the total molar concentration of the buffer system will double the buffer capacity at a given pH).
- using equimolar concentrations of the acid (HA) and its conjugate base (A-). Buffer capacity is maximal when pH = pKa ([HA] = [A-]).

  Maximum buffer capacity (β) = $0.576 \times C$

  where, C is the total buffer concentration

Buffer capacity of a solution containing strong acid (β) = 2.303 × $[H_3O^+]$

Buffer capacity of a solution containing strong base (β) = 2.303 × $[OH^-]$

Buffer capacity of a solution containing strong acid (β) = 2.303 × $([H_3O^+] + [OH^-])$

Isotonic Solution

These are the solutions that have the same osmotic pressure as the body fluids and hence said to be isotonic with the body fluid. Isotonic solutions does not cause contraction or swelling of the tissues and produce no discomfort following ocular, nasal, or intravenous administration.

Example: isotonic sodium chloride (0.9% w/v solution)

Experiment

1. When blood (defibrinated) is added to 0.9g NaCl/100 mL (0.9%), cells retain their normal size.
2. When blood (defibrinated) is added to 2.0% NaCl solution (hypertonic), cells shrink and wrinkle (crenate) because the water molecules come out of the cells through the membrane until the concentration of salt on both sides of the membrane are identical.
3. When blood (defibrinated) is added to 0.2% NaCl solution (hypotonic), cells swell and burst.

Calculating Isotonicity

1. ***Hemolytic method:*** As mentioned above the interaction of red blood cells can be observed in suspended solutions.
2. ***Colligative properties:*** Based on the colligative properties of the drug solutions.

$$\Delta T_f = i\, K_f\, m$$

$$\Delta T_f = L_{iso}\, c$$

c = molar concentration

L_{iso} = applicable value at isotonicity

L_{iso} = value for 0.9% solution of NaCl

$c = 154$ M

$\Delta T_f = 0.52$

$L_{iso} = \Delta T_f/c = 0.52/0.154 = 3.4$

Methods of Adjusting Tonicity

- ***Class I:*** Substances such as sodium chloride and dextrose are added to drug solution to lower the freezing point of solution to -0.52 ^{0}C and thus make the solution isotonic with body fluids. This is also known as cryoscopic method.
- ***Class II:*** Water is added to the drug solution in sufficient amount to make it isotonic with body fluids.

Class I

A. Cryoscopic Method

Quantity of each substance required for the preparation of an isotonic solution can be calculated from the freezing point depression values. Any solution which is isotonic with blood has a T_f of 0.52 ^{0}C. So, the freezing point of the drug solution should be adjusted to this value to make it isotonic. For example the freezing point depression of 1% w/v NaCl solution of sodium chloride is 0.576 ^{0}C. Therefore, the concentration of sodium chloride required to make isotonic saline solution is then

$$(0.52 \ / \ 0.576) \times 1.0 = 0.9\% \text{ w/v}$$

However, it is not possible to adjust tonicity by altering the drug concentration and an "adjusting" substance must be added to achieve tonicity. The weight (in grams) of adjusting substance can be calculated. Taken that the drug concentration in 100 mL solution is k grams, then:

ΔT_f (for drug solution) = k (ΔT_f of 1% drug solution) = a

If w are the grams of the adjusting substance to be added to 100 mL of drug solution to make it isotonic:

ΔT_f (for adjusting solution) = w ΔT_f (1% adjusting substance) = wb

Equation for the preparation of isotonic solution:

$$a + (wb) = 0.52$$

or

$$w = (0.52 - a) / b$$

B. Sodium Chloride Equivalent Method (E):

It is the use of sodium chloride (NaCl) equivalents as an adjusting agent so as to make the solution isotonic. The sodium chloride equivalent for any drug substance is the amount of sodium chloride that has the same colligative properties (or) osmotic effect as 1 gram of the drug.

$$E = 17 \times (L_{iso} / MW)$$

L_{iso}: It is a factor which depends on ionic state of the salt.

Electrolytes	L_{iso} values
Non electrolytes	1.9
Weak electrolytes	2.0
Divalent electrolytes	2.0
Uniunivalent electrolytes	3.4
Unibivalent electrolytes	4.3
Diunivalent electrolytes	4.8
Unitrivalent electrolytes	5.2
Triunivalent electrolytes	6.0

Class II methods

A. White-Vincent Method

Using this method we can calculate the volume (V) in ml of water that needs to be added to specified amount of drug to prepare an isotonic buffered solution

$$V = w * E * 111.1$$

w = wt. of drug (gm)

E = sodium chloride equivalent value

B. Sprowls Method

This is much simplified form White-Vincent method. In this method the V values of drugs are calculated using a constant or arbitrarily fixed value for the weight of drug (0.3 gm).

Problems

1. A buffer solution was made by dissolving 10.0 grams of sodium acetate in 200.0 mL of 1.00 M acetic acid. Estimate the pH of the acetic acid/sodium acetate buffer solution (assumption: change in volume when the sodium acetate is not significant). The K_a for acetic acid is 1.7×10^{-5}.

   Solution:

   The equation can be written as

   $$CH_3COOH\,(aq) + H_2O(l) \rightarrow H_3O^+(aq) + CH_3COO^-(aq)$$

   $$[H_3O^+] = K_a \frac{[CH_3COOH]}{[CH_3COO^-]}$$

   Number of moles of acid:

   (1.00 M CH_3COOH) * (200.0 mL) * (1 L/1000 mL) = 0.200 mol CH_3COOH

   Number of moles of conjugate base:

   (10.0 g $NaCH_3COO$) * (1 mol/82.03 g) = 0.122 mol $NaCH_3COO$

   Substituting the values in the above equation:

   $$[H_3O^+] = (1.7 \times 10^{-5})\,(0.200/0.122) = 2.79 \times 10^{-5}$$

   or

   pH = 4.56

2. Calculate the ratio of $NH_4Cl : NH_3$ that is required to make a buffer solution with a pH of 9.00. The Ka for ammonium ion is 5.6×10^{-10}.

   Solution:

   $$NH_4^+(aq) + H_2O(l) \rightarrow H_3O^+(aq) + NH_3(aq)$$

   $$K_a = \frac{[H_3O^+]\,[NH_3]}{[NH_4^+]}$$

   $$[H_3O^+] = K_a \frac{[NH_4^+]}{[NH_3]}$$

   $$[H_3O^+] = \text{Antilog}\,(-9) = 1 \times 10^{-9}\ M$$

$1 \times 10^{-9} = 5.6 \times 10^{-10}(NH_4^+/NH_3)$

Therefore, the ratio of $(NH_4^+/NH_3) = 1.786/1$

3. What is the pH of a solution that is 0.13 M HCOOH and 0.24 M $KHCO_2$? The K_a of the acid, HCOOH, is 1.8×10^{-4}.

Solution:

$$KHCO_2 \rightarrow K^+ + HCO_2^-$$

$$[K^+] = [HCO_2^-] = 0.24\ M$$

And the weak acid reacts as

$$HCOOH + H_2O \rightleftharpoons H_3O^+ + HCO_2^-$$

In the equilibrium, HCOOH is the acid and HCO_2^- is its conjugate base.

The $pK_a = -\log K_a = -\log (1.8 \times 10^{-4}) = 3.74$

So using the Henderson–Hasselbalch equation,

$$pH = pK_a + \log([base]/[acid])$$

$$pH = 3.74 + \log (0.24/0.13)$$

$$pH = 3.74 + 0.27$$

$$pH = 4.01$$

4. What is the maximum buffer capacity of acetate buffer containing a total concentration of 0.020 moles/liter?

Solution:

$$\beta = 0.576 \times C$$

$$= 0.012$$

5. What is the freezing point depression of a 1% solution of sodium propionate (MW = 96)? $CH_3CH_2C00^-Na^+$ is a univalent electrolyte

Solution:

$$L_{iso} = 3.4;\ c = 1/(96 \times 100/1000) = 0.104\ M$$

$$\Delta T_f = L_{iso}\ c = 3.4 \times 0.104 = 0.35\ ^0C$$

6. Calculate the approximate E value for a new amphetamine hydrochloride derivative (MW=187).

This drug is uni-univalent salt, therefore, $L_{iso} = 3.4$

$$E = 17\ (3.4/187) = 0.31$$

7. How much sodium chloride is required to render 100ml of a 1% solution of apomorphine hydrochloride isotonic with blood serum? E value is 0.14. (Use White-Vincent Method)

Solution:

Weight of drug = 1g

Volume of solution = 100ml

Sodium Chloride Equivalent E = 0.14

$$V = w \times E \times 111.1 = 0.14 \times 111.1$$

$$= 15.55 \text{ ml}$$

So for preparing an isotonic solution 1g of apomorphone hydrochloride should be dissolved in 15.5 ml of water and remaining volume should be made up to 100ml using 0.9% sodium chloride solution.

8. How much sodium chloride is required to render 100ml of a 1% solution of apomorphine hydrochloride isotonic with blood serum? V value is 4.7. (Use Sprowls Method).

Solution:

This is the volume of water required for 0.3g of drug for isotonicity.

So for 1 gm of drug= $(4.7 \times 1)/0.3 = 15.66$

Dissolve 1g of drug in 15.6 ml of water and make up the solution to 100ml with 0.9% sodium chloride solution.

CHAPTER 17

Ionic Equilibria

Acids and Bases

Chemical substances can be broadly classified as acids, bases and salts. Acids and bases generally display opposite characteristics. Acids are sour in taste and change color of the litmus paper red. They have the property to react with some metals to produce hydrogen gas. Bases are bitter in taste and turn litmus paper blue. When aqueous solutions of an acid and a base are mixed, a neutralization reaction occurs. This reaction is fairly rapid and generally produces water and a salt. As simple reaction of sulfuric acid (H_2SO_4) with sodium hydroxide (NaOH) yields water (H_2O) and sodium sulfate (Na_2SO_4).

Reaction: $$H_2SO_4 + 2NaOH \rightleftarrows 2H_2O + Na_2SO_4$$

Early Theories: In 1884 the Swedish chemist Svante Arrhenius proposed the definition of acids and bases.

Arrhenius definition for acids

An acid is a substance which, upon being dissolved in water, increases the concentration of hydrogen ions (H^+)

For example hydrochloric acid (Strong Acid)

$HCl_{(g)}$ in water gives: $H^+_{(aq)} + Cl^-_{(aq)}$

Arrhenius Definition for Bases

A base is a substance which, upon being dissolved in water, increases the concentration of hydroxyl ions (OH^-).

For example sodium hydroxide (caustic soda, Strong base)

$NaOH_{(s)}$ in water gives: $OH^-_{(aq)} + Na^+_{(aq)}$

Ammonia (Weak base)

$NH_{3(aq)}$ in water gives: $OH^-_{(aq)} + NH_4^+{}_{(aq)}$

When acids and bases are combined a neutralization reaction takes place resulting in:

$$H^+ + OH^- \rightleftarrows H_2O$$

However, this theory was criticized because acids are restricted to H^+ containing species and bases to OH^- containing species. Moreover, this theory is applicable to aqueous solutions, whereas many acid-base reactions are known to take place in the absence of water.

Bronsted-Lowry Theory

In the year 1923, a Danish chemist Johannes Bronsted and Thomas Lowry proposed this theory independently. This theory states that an acid is a proton (hydrogen ion, H^+) donor and a base a proton acceptor. Though acids contain hydrogen ions, Bronsted-Lowry theory does not require an aqueous medium.

For example, liquid ammonia (NH_3), which acts as a base in aqueous solution, can act as an acid in the absence of water by transferring a H^+ to a base and forming the amide anion (negative ion) NH_2^-:

$$NH_3 + \text{base} \rightleftarrows NH_2^- + \text{base} = H^+$$

The Bronsted-Lowry definition of acids and bases also explains why a strong acid displaces a weak acid from its compounds (and likewise for strong and weak bases). In terms of a general chemical equation, the reaction of Acid (1) with Base (2), results in transfer of a proton from Acid (1) to Base (2). After losing the proton, Acid (1) becomes its conjugate base, Base (1). After gaining a proton, Base (2) becomes its conjugate acid, Acid (2). The equilibrium shifts towards the direction that produces the weaker acid-base pair.

$$\text{Acid (1)} + \text{Base (2)} \rightleftarrows \text{Acid (2)} + \text{Base (1)}$$

For example, hydrochloric acid, HCl, (strong acid) in water readily transfers a proton to water to form a hydronium ion.

$$HCl + H_2O \rightleftarrows H3O^+ + Cl^-$$

Equilibrium shifts to towards right hand side because the conjugate base of HCl, Cl^-, is a weak base, and H_3O^+, the conjugate acid of H_2O, is a weak acid.

In contrast, hydrogen fluoride, HF, (weak acid) in water does not readily transfer a proton to water.

$$HF + H_2O \rightleftarrows H_3O^+ + F^-$$

In this reaction, equilibrium shifts to left hand side because H_2O is a weaker base than F^-, and because HF is a weaker acid (in water) than H_3O^+. The Bronsted-Lowry theory also explains why water can be amphoteric, that is, why it can serve as either an acid or a base. Water serves as a base in the presence of an acid that is stronger than water (such as HCl), in other words, an acid that has a greater tendency to dissociate than does water.

$$NH_3 + H_2O \rightleftarrows NH_4^+ + OH^-$$

Water can also serve as an acid in the presence of a base that is stronger than water (such as ammonia.

Lewis Acid-Base Theory

Gilbert N. Lewis's (1923) theory is based on chemical bonding. According to his theory, Lewis acid (A) is a molecule or ion that can accept a pair of electrons and Lewis base (B) is a molecule or ion that can donate a pair of electrons. The combination of Lewis acid and Lewis base is known as adduct (AB).

$$A + :B \rightarrow A - B$$

In a simple reaction of hydrochloric acid and sodium hydroxide:

$$HCl\ (aq) + NaOH\ (aq) \rightarrow H_2O\ (l) + NaCl\ (aq),$$

Lewis base or OH^- ion donates an electron pair to the H^+ ion (Lewis acid) forming a covalent bond and thus producing water (H_2O).

Both Lewis acid base theory and Bronsted-Lowry acid-base theory were published in the same year. The two theories are distinct but complementary to each other. A Lewis base can also be called as Bronsted-Lowry base, while a Lewis acid need not be a Bronsted-Lowry acid.

Some examples of reactions of Lewis acids (shown on the left):

- $H^+ + :NH_3 \rightarrow NH_4^+$
- $BF_3 + F^- \rightarrow BF_4^{\check{s}}$
- $AlF_3 + 3F^- \rightarrow AlF_6^{3-}$
- $SiF_4 + 2F^- \rightarrow SiF_6^{2-}$
- $SF_4 + F^- \rightarrow SF_5^-$

Some examples of Lewis base:

- compounds of N, P, As, and Bi in oxidation state 3.
- compounds of O, S, Se and Te in oxidation state 2, including water, ethers, ketones, sulphoxides.

Differences between acids and bases

Acids	Bases
Acids release hydrogen or H^+ ions into water (aqueous) solution	Bases release hydroxide or OH^- ions into water solution
Neutralize bases in a neutralization reaction	Bases neutralize acids in a neutralization reaction
Corrode most of active metals	Denature protein
Turns blue litmus to red	Turns red litmus to blue
Taste sour	Bases taste bitter
Examples of some strong acids: HNO_3 - nitric acid HCl - hydrochloric acid H_2SO_4 - sulfuric acid $HClO_4$ - perchloric acid HBr - hydrobromic acid HI - hydroiodic acid	Examples of some strong bases: LiOH - lithium hydroxide NaOH - sodium hydroxide KOH - potassium hydroxide RbOH - rubidium hydroxide CsOH - cesium hydroxide $Mg(OH)_2$ - magnesium hydroxide $Ca(OH)_2$ - calcium hydroxide $Sr(OH)_2$ - strontium hydroxide $Ba(OH)_2$ - barium hydroxide

Salts

Salt is a combination of an anion ("- ve" ion) and a cation ("+ve" ion). The neutralization of sodium hydroxide with hydrochloric acid produces water and the salt, sodium chloride. When salt is dissolved in water solution, it usually dissociates into anions and cations that make up the salt. The pH of solution depends on the type of anion and cation. Salts made of the anion of a strong acid and the cation of a strong base will be neutral salts. When neutral salts are dissolved in water pH of solution becomes approximately seven. Salt containing anion of a strong acid and cation of a *weak* base will be acidic salts (i.e. salt solution in water will have a pH < 7).

E.g. ammonium chloride

Salts made of anion of a *weak* acid and a strong base will be an alkali salt. (i.e. salt solution in water will have a pH > 7).

E.g. sodium bicarbonate

However, it is difficult to estimate the pH of a salt solution when the salt consists of anion of a weak acid and the cation of a weak base.

Ionization of Weak Acids

When a weak acid (HA) is dissolved in water it gets slightly ionized.

i.e., exists in equilibrium with its ions

$$HA(aq) \square H^+ (aq) + A^- (aq)$$

Equilibrium constant for the above reaction is given by the law of mass action:

$$K_a = \frac{[H^+][A]}{[HA]}$$

or

$$\log K_a = \log[H^+] + \log([A^-]/[HA])$$

Substituting, $pK_a = \log_{10} K_a$, and $pH = \log_{10} [H^+]$, the equation can be written as

$$pKa = pH + \log([A^-]/[HA])$$

This equation is called as Henderson-Hasselbalch equation and it serves as a basis for the determination of the ionization constant, K_a. One can determine the concentrations of A^- and HA in a solution using this equation.

Similarly for weak bases,

$$B + H_2O \rightleftharpoons BH^+ (aq) + OH^- (aq)$$

Equilibrium constant for the above reaction is given by the law of mass action:

$$K_b = \frac{[BH^+][OH^-]}{[B]}$$

$$pK_b = p[OH^-] + \log([BH^+]/[B])$$

Conjugate Acid-Base Pairs

A pair of compounds or ions that differ by one proton (H^+) is called a conjugate acid-base pair. For example in the above equation of base hydrolysis, BH^+ and B form a conjugate acid-base pair. More common example is water and hydroxide ion. The acid equilibrium constant and the base equilibrium constant for a conjugate acid and a conjugate base can be related as:

$$K_a K_b = K_w$$

If K_a of a weak acid (HA) is known then K_b for its conjugate base (A-) can be calculated.

The pH values of the five solutions will be measured, and a best-fit line will be obtained using linear regression.

Also, $pH + pOH = pK_w$ and $pK_a + pK_b = pK_w$

Ionization of Water

Two water molecules react with each other to produce a hydronium ion (H_3O^+) and a hydroxide ion (OH^-). This is known as ionization of water.

$$2H_2O\ (l) \rightleftharpoons H_3O^+ (aq) + OH^- (aq)$$

Equilibrium constant (K_{eq}) for the above reaction can be written as

$$K_{eq} = \frac{([H_3\ O^+][OH^-])}{[H_2O]^2}$$

Also, Dissociation constant = $K_w = [H_3O^+] \times [OH^-] = [H_2O]^2 \times K_{eq}$

The K_w for pure water at 25°C is 1×10^{-14}

But at 25 ^{0}C the amount of $[H_3O^+]$ ions equals to $[OH^-]$ ions.

So, $[H_3O^+] = [OH^-] \sim 1 \times 10^{-7}$

pH SCALE

The concept of pH was first introduced by S.P.L. Sorensen in the year 1909. This scale represents acid and base concentrations in small numbers. pH represents the hydronium ion concentration and pOH represents the hydroxide ion concentration. They are related by the equations below.

$$pH = -\log[H_3O^+]$$

$$pOH = -\log[OH^-]$$

$$pH + pOH = 14$$

At pH 7.0, a solution is neutral

- At lower pH (1-6), a solution is acidic
- At higher pH (8-14), a solution is basic

pH in various part of body:

- Gastric acid pH: 0.7
- Lysosomes pH: 4.5
- Granules of chromaffin cells pH: 5.5
- Urine pH: 6.0
- Cytosol pH: 7.2
- Cerebrospinal fluid (CSF) pH: 7.3
- Blood pH: 7.34 – 7.45
- Mitochondrial matrix pH: 7.5
- Pancreas secretions pH: 8.1

Calculation of pH

The general way of calculating pH is using Proton Balance Equation (PBE).

For a system containing hydrochloric acid in water is:

$$[H_3O^+] = [OH^-] + [Cl^-]$$

Steps involved:

(a) Start with the species added to water.

(b) On the left hand side (LHS) of the equation, place all ionic species which are formed when protons are consumed.

(c) On the right hand side (RHS) of the equation, place all ionic species which are formed when protons are released.

(d) Each ionic species in the PBE must be multiplied by the number of protons gained or lost when it is formed.

(e) Add $[H_3O^+]$ to the LHS of the equation and $[OH^-]$ to the RHS of the equation.

This is Proton Balance Equation.

Example: 1. For phosphoric acid (H_3PO_4)

$$[H_3O^+] = [OH^-] + [H_2PO_4^-] + 2[HPO_4^-] + 3[PO_4^-]$$

Graphical Solution to pH Problems

Plot of pH vs log[salt]/[acid] results in a straight line. The y-intercept of the graph denotes pKa or the half neutralization point.

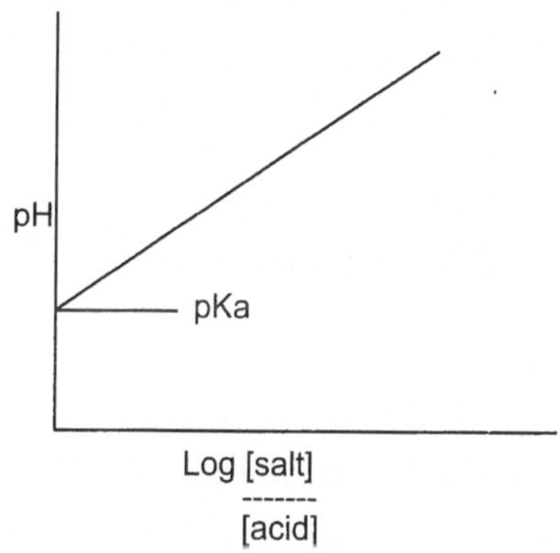

Calculation of pH for Solutions Containing Strong Acids and Bases

When dissolved in water strong acids and bases ionize 100%. When HCl is dissolved in water we get a PBE:

$$[H_3O^+] = [OH^-] + [Cl^-] = \frac{K_w}{[H_3O^+]} + Ca$$

From this we obtain the equation:

$$[H_3O^+] = \frac{C_a + (C_a^2 + 4Kw)^{1/2}}{2}$$

$$[OH^-] = \frac{C_b + (C_b^2 + 4K_w)^{1/2}}{2}$$

For solutions containing conjugate acid and base pairs:

$$[H_3O^+] = K_a \frac{(C_a - (H_3O^+) + [OH^-])}{(C_b - (H_3O^+) - [OH^-])}$$

For solutions containing only a weak acid:

In this case $C_b = 0$ and $[H_3O^+] >>> [OH^-]$

Substituting the above in

$$[H_3O^+] = Ka \frac{(C_a - (H_3O^+) + [OH^-])}{(C_b - (H_3O^+) - [OH^-])}$$

We obtain

$$[H_3O^+] = \frac{-K_a + (K_a^2 + 4K_aC_a)^{1/2}}{2}$$

And when $C_a >> [H_3O^+]$ we obtain

$$[H_3O^+] = (K_aC_a)^{1/2}$$

For solutions containing only a weak base:

In this case $C_a = 0$ and $[OH^-] >>> [H_3O^+]$

We obtain

$$[H_3O^+] = \frac{K_w + (K_w^2 + 4K_aC_b\,K_w)^{1/2}}{2C_b}$$

And when $K_a >> [H_3O^+]$ we obtain

$$[H_3O^+] = (K_aK_w/C_b)^{1/2}$$

$$[OH^-] = \frac{-K_b + (K_b^2 + 4K_bC_b)^{1/2}}{2}$$

And when $C_b >> [OH^-]$ we obtain

$$[OH^-] = (K_b C_b)^{1/2}$$

For solutions containing only a diprotic acid:

This equation describes any solution of any monoprotic acid. For calculation of pH we need to have C_a and K_a:

$$[H_3O^+]^3 + K_1[H_3O^+]^2 - (C_a K_1 - K_1 K_2)[H_3O^+] - 2K_1 K_2 C_a = 0$$

Assuming, $C_a >> K_2$ and $H_3O^+ >> 2K_2$

$$[H_3O^+]^2 + K_1[H_3O^+] - KC_a = 0$$

For solutions containing only a diacidic base:

$$[OH^-] = (K_{b1} C_b)^{1/2}$$

For Solutions Containing Polyprotic Acids

In contrast to a simple monoprotic acid, a polyprotic acid contains more than one acidic hydrogen atoms. A polyprotic acid containing n acidic hydrogens will form n+1 species in solution at equilibrium. A common example is phosphoric acid where, n = 3 (a triprotic acid) when dissolved in solution, equilibrium exists between four species H_3PO_4 (phosphoric acid itself), $H_2PO_4^{-1}$ (dihydrogen phosphate anion), HPO_4^{-2} (hydrogen phosphate anion), and PO_4^{-3} (phosphate anion):

$$H_3PO_a + H_2O \rightleftharpoons H_2PO_a^- + H_3O^+$$

$$K_{a_1} = \frac{[H_2PO_4^-][H_3O^+]}{[H_3PO_4]} = 7.5 \times 10^{-3}$$

$$H_2PO_4^- + H_2O \rightleftharpoons HPO_4^{-2} + H_3O^+$$

$$K_{a_2} = \frac{[HPO_4^{2-}][H_3O^+]}{[H_2PO_4^-]} = 6.23 \times 10^{-8}$$

$$HPO_4^{-2} + H_2O \rightleftharpoons PO_4^{-3} + H_3O^+$$

$$K_{a_3} = \frac{[PO_4^{3-}][H_3O^+]}{[HPO_4^{2-}]} = 2.2 \times 10^{-13}$$

$$[H_nA] = \frac{[H_3O^+]^n C_a}{D}$$

$$[H_{n-1}A^{-1}] = \frac{K_1 [H_3O^+]^{n-1} C_a}{D}$$

$$[H_{n-j}A^{-j}] = \frac{K_1 \ldots\ldots K_1 [H_3O^+]^{n-j} C_a}{D}$$

$$[A^{-n}] = \frac{K_1 K_2 K_3 \ldots\ldots K_n C_a}{D}$$

Calculation of pH for Buffer Solutions

Buffer solution is a mixture of a weak acid and its conjugate base or a weak base and its conjugate acid. Buffer solutions have the capacity to resist changes in pH of the solution upon addition of small amount of acid or base. Buffer solutions are used as a means of keeping pH at a nearly constant value in a wide variety of chemical applications. This pH is resistant to change. This means that the addition of an acid or a base does not affect the hydronium ion concentration. Human blood is an example of a buffer solution. A buffer is usually prepared from roughly equal quantities of a conjugate acid-base pair.

- a weak acid and its conjugate base
- a weak base and its conjugate acid

The pH of a buffer solution can be calculated using the Henderson-Hasselbalch equation.

$$pH = pK_a + \log \frac{[\text{conjugate base}]}{[\text{acid}]}$$

This equation will be useful during a titration when trying to find the pH.

Acid Ionization Constants at 25⁰C

Chemical Substance	Chemical Formula	K_a value
Acetic acid	$HC_2H_3O_2$	1.8×10^{-5}
Aluminum 3+ ion	$Al^{3+}(aq)$	1.4×10^{-5}
Ammonium ion	NH_4^+	5.6×10^{-10}
Arsenic acid	H_3AsO_4	6.0×10^{-3}
	$H_2AsO_4^-$	1.0×10^{-7}
	$HAsO_4^{2-}$	3.2×10^{-12}
Ascorbic acid	$H_2C_6H_6O_6$	6.8×10^{-5}
	$HC_6H_6O_6^-$	2.8×10^{-12}
Benzoic acid	$HC_7H_5O_2$	6.3×10^{-5}
Boric acid	H_3BO_3	5.9×10^{-10}
Butyric acid	$HC_4H_7O_2$	1.5×10^{-5}
Carbonic acid	H_2CO_3	4.4×10^{-7}
	HCO_3^-	4.7×10^{-11}
Chloroacetic acid	$HC_2H_2ClO_2$	1.4×10^{-3}
Chromic acid	H_2CrO_4	1.5×10^{-1}
	$HCrO_4^-$	3.2×10^{-7}
Chromium 3+ ion	$Cr^{3+}(aq)$	6.6×10^{-4}
Citric acid	$H_3C_6H_5O_7$	7.4×10^{-4}
	$H_2C_6H_5O_7^-$	1.7×10^{-5}
	$HC_6H_5O_7^{2-}$	4.0×10^{-7}
Codeine ammonium ion	$HC_{18}H_{21}O_3N^+$	1.1×10^{-8}
Cyanic acid	$HOCN$	3.5×10^{-4}
Dichloroacetic acid	$HC_2HCl_2O_2$	5.5×10^{-2}

Diethylammonium ion	$(C_2H_5)_2\ NH_2^+$	1.4×10^{-11}
Ethylammonium ion	$C_2H_5NH_3^+$	2.3×10^{-11}
Ethylenediammonium ion	$NH_2CH_2CH_2\ NH_3^+$	1.9×10^{-11}
Fluoroacetic acid	$HC_2H_2FO_2$	2.6×10^{-3}
Formic acid	$HCHO_2$	1.8×10^{-4}
Hydrazinium ion	$N_2H_5^+$	1.2×10^{-8}
Hydrocyanic acid	HCN	6.2×10^{-10}
Hydrofluoric acid	HF	6.6×10^{-4}
Hydrogen peroxide	H_2O_2	2.2×10^{-12}
Hydrogen sulfate ion	HSO_4^-	1.1×10^{-2}
	HSe^-	1×10^{-11}
Hydrosulfuric acid	H_2S	1.0×10^{-7}
	HS^-	1×10^{-19}
Hydroxylammonium ion	$HONH_3^+$	1.1×10^{-6}
Hypobromous acid	HOBr	2.5×10^{-9}
Hypochlorous acid	HClO	2.9×10^{-8}
Hypoiodous acid	HOI	2.3×10^{-11}
Hyponitrous acid	$H_2N_2O_2$ (HON=NOH)	8.9×10^{-8}
	$HN_2O_2^-$ ($HON=NO^-$)	4×10^{-12}
Iodic acid	HIO_3	1.6×10^{-1}
Iron 2+ ion	$Fe^{2+}(aq)$	3.2×10^{-10}
Iron 3+ ion	$Fe^{3+}(aq)$	6.3×10^{-3}
Lactic acid	$HC_3H_5O_3$	1.3×10^{-4}
Malonic acid	$H_2C_3H_2\ O_4$	1.5×10^{-3}

Nitrous acid	HNO_2	7.2×10^{-4}
Oxalic acid	$H_2C_2O_4$	5.4×10^{-2}
	$HC_2O_4^-$	5.3×10^{-5}
Phenol	C_6H_5OH	1.0×10^{-10}
Phenylacetic acid	$HC_8H_7O_2$	4.9×10^{-5}
Phosphoric acid	H_3PO_4	7.1×10^{-3}
	$H_2PO_4^-$	6.3×10^{-8}
	HPO_4^{2-}	4.2×10^{-13}
Phosphorous acid	H_3PO_3	3.7×10^{-2}
	$H_2PO_3^-$	2.1×10^{-7}
Propionic acid	$HC_3H_5O_2$	1.3×10^{-5}
Pyridinium ion	$C_5H_5NH^+$	6.7×10^{-6}
Pyrophosphoric acid	$H_4P_2O_7$	3.0×10^{-2}
	$H_3P_2O_7^-$	4.4×10^{-3}
	$H_2P_2O_7^{2-}$	2.5×10^{-7}
	$HP_2O_7^{3-}$	5.6×10^{-10}
Pyruvic acid	$HC_3H_3O_3$	1.4×10^{-4}
Selenous acid	H_2SeO_3	2.3×10^{-3}
	$HSeO_3^-$	5.4×10^{-9}
Succinic acid	$H_2C_4H_4O_4$	6.2×10^{-5}
	$HC_4H_4O_4^-$	2.3×10^{-6}
Sulfurous acid	H_2SO_3	1.3×10^{-2}

Trichloroacetic acid	$HC_2Cl_3O_2$	3.0×10^{-1}
Triethanolammonium ion	$HC_6H_{15}O_3N^+$	1.7×10^{-8}
Triethylammonium ion	$(C_2H_5)_3NH^+$	1.9×10^{-11}
Trimethylammonium ion	$(CH_3)_3NH^+$	1.5×10^{-10}
Zinc 2+ ion	$Zn^{2+}(aq)$	2.5×10^{-10}

Problems

1. The pH of a solution is equal to:

   (a) the hydrogen ion concentration, $[H^+]$
   (b) $\log [H_3O^+]$
   (c) $-\log [H_3O^+]$
   (d) $\ln [OH^-]$
   (e) $-\ln [OH^-]$

   Answer: $pH = -\log [H_3O^+]$

2 Physiological pH is 7.4. What is the hydrogen ion concentration of a solution at physiological pH?

   (a) 6.4 M
   (b) 1.5M
   (c) 2.6×10^{-9} M
   (d) 2×10^{-6} M
   (e) 3.98×10^{-8}

   Answer:

   pH is the negative log of the hydrogen concentration, i.e.

   if $pH = -\log [H^+]$,

   then $[H^+] = \text{antilog}(-pH) = 10^{-7.4}$ M

   Thus, the hydrogen ion concentration of a solution at physiological pH (7.4) is $10^{-7.4}$, which is equal to 3.98×10^{-8} M.

3. What is the pH of a 10^{-10} M solution of HCl?

   (a) 7.0
   (b) 5.8

(c) 6.2

(d) 7.2

(e) 6.3

Answer: The negative log of 10^{-10} gives a pH of 10. This does not make sense because the pH a dilute acid cannot be above 7. In case of pH of very dilute acid solutions, water makes a greater contribution to $[H^+]$ than the dilute acid. So we consider the ionization of water 10^{-7} M $[H^+]$ and hence the effective pH = 7.

4. If the concentration of H^+ in a solution is 10^{-4} M, what will the concentration of OH^- be in the same solution at 25° C?

   (a) 10^{-10} M

   (b) 10^{-11} M

   (c) 3×10^{11} M

   (d) 1×10^{-9} M

   (e) 10^{-12} M

   Answer: In aqueous solutions at 25° C, the product of the H^+ and OH^- concentrations is always 10^{-14}, as expressed in this equation: $[H^+][OH^-] = 10^{-14}$ This allows calculation of the OH^- concentration if the H^+ concentration is known. $[OH^-] = 0^{-14}/[H^+]$ $[OH^-] = 10^{-14} / 10^{-4} = 10^{-10}$ This calculation is used when the solution in question is not pure water, but contains some mixture of acids and bases.

5. Identify the conjugate acids of the following Bronsted-Lowry weak bases

   (a) F^- (b) ClO_3^- (c) SO_4^{2-} (d) NH_3 (e) CH_3NH_2

   For these substances to be acting as bases, they must accept a proton

   Answer:

   (a) HF (b) $HClO_3$ (c) HSO_4^- (d) NH_4^+ (e) $CH_3NH_2^+$

   Calculate the pH of a solution NH4OH if the [OH–] = 2.2 × 10–5 M

CHAPTER 18

Complexation

Complexation ***is the*** *binding or chelation of bi- or multi-dentate ligand.* Chelating agents form multiple bonds with a single metal ion or molecule. Complexes can be broadly classified into two classes: a) molecular complexes, b) coordination complexes.

(a) Coordination complexes: Ion containing a central metal cation bonded to one or more ions or molecules forming coordinate bonds. These complexes play crucial role in many biochemical processes. This interaction is similar to Lewis acid-base reaction in which a metal cation combines with a Lewis base (ligand) by accepting a pair of electrons from the ligand to form a coordinate covalent bond. For example: when HCl is added to a cobalt (II) chloride solution the solution turns blue due to the formation of the complex ion ($COCl_1^{2-}$).

$$CO^{2+}\,(aq) + 4\ Cl^-\,(aq) \rightleftharpoons COCl_4^{2-}\ (aq)$$

Aluminum, tin, and lead, for example, form complexes such as the AlF_6^{3-}, $SnCl_4^{2-}$ and PbI_4^{2-} ions.

Ligands: These are ions or molecules with a pair of nonbonding electrons. Based on the number of linking sites ligands can be classified as monodentate ligands such as halogens (attach to the metal at only one place), bidentate ligand such as ethylenediamine (attach to the metal at only one place), tridentate ligand such as diethylenetriamine (attach to the metal at only one place).

Coordination number: *It is the* integer number of its nearest neighbors or number of nearest neighbors of an atom or an ion in a lattice.

Some examples

Metal Ion		*Ligand*		*Complex*	*Coordination Number*
Ag^+	+	$2\ NH_3$	$\rightleftharpoons$	$Ag(NH_3)_2^+$	2
Ag^+	+	$2\ S_2O_3^{2-}$	$\rightleftharpoons$	$AgCl_2^-$	2

B. Molecular complexes: These are formed by non-covalent interactions between the substrate and the ligand. Non-covalent interactions arise from electrostatic forces which give rise to hydrogen bonding, hydrophobic effects and charge transfer. These complexes occur between small molecules or a small molecule and a macromolecule.

Complexes between small molecules

Complexation of a drug with another drug will result in alteration of "pharmaceutical properties" of a dosage form to a smaller or larger extent.

Pharmaceutical properties affected by complexation

Property	Example
Chemical stability	Caffeine-benzocaine
Permeability	Dialkylamides-prednisone
Dissolution rate	Hexanoic acid-griseofulvin
Solubility	Gentisic acid-caffeine
Absorption rate	Caffeine-salicylamide
Partition coefficient	Caffeine-benzoic acid

Knowledge of complexation between various drug molecules or drug molecules and excipients prevent incompatibilities which may in turn affect patients' therapy.

Complexes between small molecules and macromolecules: Human blood contains various proteins that help in the transport of endogenous and exogenous compounds, neutralization and clearance of microorganisms etc. For example albumin which is abundant in the blood binds to various drugs increasing the circulation for longer periods of time making them unable to enter interstitial fluids and reach cellular targets. This significantly alters the distribution, excretion and pharmacological activity of drugs.

E.g. Warfarin extensively binds to plasma proteins. Co-administration of drugs that has higher affinity for plasma proteins (NSAIDs) displace warfarin from its binding sites. This results in serious hemorrhage to the patient.

Metal Complexes

Metals acts as Lewis acids due to the presence of positive charge. They react with water to form hydrated compounds such as $Na(H_2O)_6^+$. These are also called as coordination compounds. Neutral molecules such as H_2O or NH_3 and anions such as CN^-, CH_3COO^- act as ligands. For example ammonia forms complex with metals such as Ag^+ resulting in formation of silver ammonia complex which is colorless.

$$AgCl\ (s) + 2\ NH_3 = Ag(NH_3)_2^+ + 2\ Cl^-$$

Method of analysis

The strength of any interactions between molecules that form a complex is indicated by stability constant which is also known as equilibrium constant for complex formation. This helps in the estimation of concentration of a particular complex in solution.

Methods of continuous variation

Additive properties such as spectrophotometric extinction coefficient can be used for measurement of complexation.

For a reaction:

$$M + nA = MA_n$$

The stability constant $K = [MA_n] / [M][A]^n$

Here [M] is the concentration of uncomplexed metal, [A] is the concentration of uncomplexed ligand and n is the number of moles of ligand combined with 1 mole of metal ion.

Distribution Method

The distribution of solute between two immiscible solvents will be utilized calculating the stability constant. Complexation of iodine in presence of potassium iodide is an example

$$I_2 + I^- = I_3^-$$

When iodine is distributed between water and carbon disulfide

$$K = \frac{[\text{complex}]}{[I_2]_{free}\,[KI]_{free}}$$

Solubility Method

Excess quantities of drug along with the varying concentrations of complexing agent are placed in well stoppered containers that are kept under constant agitation. At regular time intervals samples are removed from the supernatant and analyzed for drug concentration.

E.g. complexation of p-aminobenzioc acid in presence of caffeine

Absorbance

The absorption curve of a non complexed species significantly shifts from the complexed species within the UV-visible range (200-800 nm). For example iodine in presence of carbon tetrachloride (non-complexing solution) produces a λ_{max} of 520 nm. However, in presence of benzene (complexing solution) λ_{max} was found to be 475 nm.

For a reaction:

Forward reaction: D + A → DA (equilibrium constant k_1)

Backward reaction: DA → D + A (equilibrium constant k_2)

Overall equilibrium constant $K = k_1/k_2$

$$A_o/A = 1/\square + 1/K\square D_o$$

A_o = Initial acceptor concentration (moles/liter)

D_o = Initial donor concentration (moles/liter)

□ = Absorptivity

A plot of A_o/A (vs) $1/D_o$ results in a straight line with slope ($1/K\square$) and intercept ($1/\square$)

Applications of stability constants

- Use of chelation therapy in treatment of various metal-related illnesses, such as iron overload in â-thalassemia
- Use of DTPA as a complexing agent for gadolinium in MRI contrast enhancement. As Gd^{3+} is highly toxic in nature it is complexed with DTPA which is a very strong complexing agent. This ensures very low concentration of free Gd^{3+} (almost negligible) inside the body. The water molecules present in this compound exchanges rapidly with the surrounding fluid and makes this compound into a contrast reagent.
- Disodium EDTA forms strong complexes with divalent cations and hence used in washing powder to act as a water softener by sequestering calcium and magnesium ions.
- Wilson's disease which is characterized by excess copper it treated using triethylene tetramine (TETA) or penicillamine.
- In the similar manner DTPA is used for plutonium poisoning.
- Chelex 100 (ion-exchange resin) contains chelating ligands bound to a polymer. It is widely used as a water softener and in chromatographic separation techniques.
- In all the above mentioned examples ligands are chosen on the basis of stability constants of the complexes formed.

Mathematical analysis of Protein binding

The interaction between a protein (P) and a drug molecule (D) can be written

$$P + D \rightleftharpoons PD$$

$$K = \frac{[PD]}{[P][D]} \quad .....(i)$$

$$\Rightarrow \quad K\,[P]\,[D] = [PD] \quad .....(ii)$$

[D] = unbound drug

[P] = unbound protein

[PD] = concentration of protein-drug complex

K = association constant

Considering the total protein concentration [Ptotal], then

$$[P_{total}] = [P] + [PD] \Rightarrow [P] = [P_{total}] - [PD]$$

Substitute [P] in equation *(II)*

$$K\,[P_{total}]\,[D] - K\,[PD]\,[D] = [PD]$$

$$K\,[P_{total}]\,[D] = [PD]\,\{K\,[D] + 1\}$$

$$\Rightarrow \quad \frac{[PD]}{[P_t]} = \frac{k\,[D]}{K\,[D]+1} \qquad \text{.....(iii)}$$

Let $R = [PD] / [P_{total}]$, the number of moles of drug bound per mole of total protein, then

$$R = \frac{k\,[D]}{K\,[D]+1} \qquad \text{.....(iv)}$$

Inverting the equation *(III)* results in

$$\frac{1}{R} = \frac{1}{K\,[D]} + 1 \qquad \text{.....(v)}$$

For "ν" number of independent available binding sites the expressions for "R" becomes

$$R = \nu\,\frac{K\,[D]}{K\,[D]+1} \qquad \text{.....(vi)}$$

The above equation can be written as

$$R + R\,K\,[D] = \nu\,K\,[D]$$

(or)

$$\frac{R}{[D]} = -RK + \nu\,K \qquad \text{.....(vii)}$$

Transforming data in equation (vii) creates a Scatchard plot

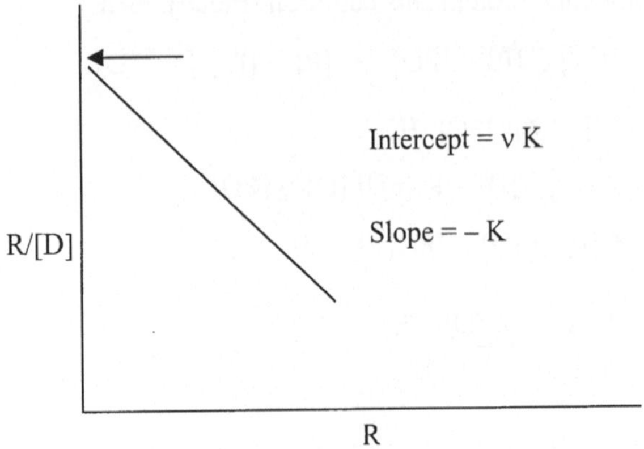

Problems

1. Calculate the concentration of free P-aminobenzoic acid (PABA) solution, if the stability constant of PABA-caffeine (1:1) complex is 59, the concentration of PABA/caffeine is 0.0073 M and the concentration of total caffeine in solution is 0.01 M.

   Answer: 0.0458

2. For the following graph

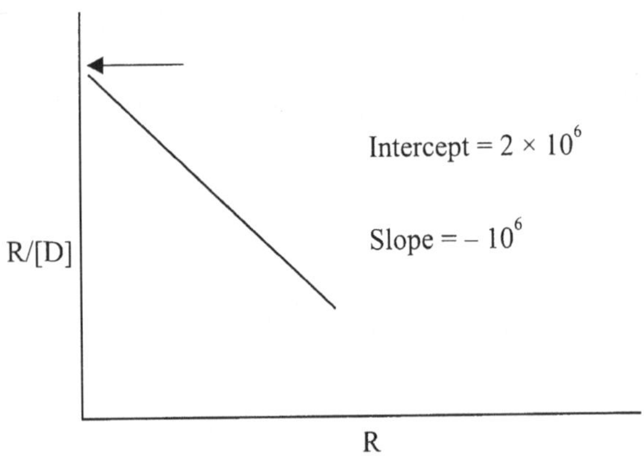

   Calculate (1) the number of binding sites and (2) the dissociation constant for drug-protein complex.

   Answer: (1) 2

   (2) 10^{-6}

CHAPTER 19

Coarse Dispersions

Dispersion is a mixture in which the dispersed phase is uniformly distributed throughout the continuous phase or dispersion medium. They are classified into 3 types:

(a) **Molecular Dispersions**: These are true solutions which consist of a solute phase (dispersed phase) homogeneously dispersed in a solvent phase (dispersion medium). The molecule size of solute phase > 1 nm. E.g.: air (a molecular mixture of nitrogen, oxygen, hydrogen etc), electrolytes (aqueous solutions of salts), alloys (solid solutions of metals).

(b) **Colloids:** These are micro-heterogeneous dispersed systems, in which the size of the dispersed phase particles is within the range 1 - 1000 nm. Colloids phases cannot be separated under gravity and requires centrifugal forces. E.g.: milk (emulsion of fat and some other substances in water), opal (colloidal silica) and fog (aerosol of water micro-droplets in air).

(c) **Coarse Dis persions:** These are heterogeneous dispersed systems in which dispersed phase particles are greater than 1000 nm. These are characterized by relatively fast sedimentation of the dispersed phase by gravity or other forces. E.g.: suspensions, emulsions, foams, some aerosols. These are thermodynamically unstable systems and hence require stabilizers to ensure good stability.

Suspensions: These are heterogeneous fluids containing solid particles that are sufficiently large for sedimentation. Usually the size of suspended particles is greater than 1 μm. Dispersed phase is evenly distributed by mechanical means. Pharmaceutical suspensions are coarse dispersions in which internal or dispersed phase is uniformly distributed throughout the external or continuous phase. Suspensions are classified in several ways:

(a) Based on proportion of solid particles (dilute suspension: 2-10% w/v solid, concentrated suspension: 50%w/v solid)

(b) Based on delivery route (oral suspension, externally applied suspension, parenteral suspension).

Suspension type	Solid contents (%w/v)	Particle size (μm)
Oral	2.5-5.0	~ 1
Topical	≥ 20	~ 1
Parenteral	0.5-5.0	~ 0.5-1

(c) Based on electrokinetic nature of solid particles (flocculated suspension, deflocculated suspension)

(d) Based on size of solid particles (colloidal suspension < 1 μm, coarse suspension >1 μm, nano suspension < 10 nm)

Theory of Suspensions: Suspensions as mentioned above contain dispersed particles which tend to flocculate under gravitational force. This is also known as sedimentation process and is well explained by Stoke's equation. The process of sedimentation (V) depends on several factors such as particle size diameter ($V \alpha d^2$), difference in density of dispersed phase and dispersion media ($V \alpha [\rho_s - \rho_o]$) and viscosity of dispersion medium ($V \alpha 1/\eta_o$).

$$V_{sed} = d^2(\rho_s - \rho_o)g/18\eta_o$$
$$= 2r^2(\rho_s - \rho_o)g/9\eta_o$$

Where, V_{sed} = sedimentation velocity in cm / sec

d = particle diameter

r = particle radius

ρ_s = density of dispersed phase

ρ_o = density of dispersion medium

g = acceleration due to gravity

η_o = viscosity of disperse medium (poise)

From the above equation it is clearly evident that lowering the viscosity of medium increases the sedimentation velocity and increasing the viscosity of medium gives rise to problems in pourability, syringeability and redispersibility.

Limitation of Stoke's Equation

Stoke's equation applicable to spherical particles in a very dilute suspension (0.5 to 2% w/v). However, most of the pharmaceutical suspensions contain more than 5% w/v dispersed particles which hinder the particle settling.

Suspensions are known to:

- improve chemical stability of certain drugs like procaine penicillin G
- increase bioavailability as compared to other dosage forms (solution > suspension > capsule > compressed tablet > coated tablet)
- control the duration and onset of action like protamine zinc-insulin suspension
- mask the taste of unpleasant/ bitter drugs like chloramphenicol

Some disadvantages associated with suspensions include: difficulties in formulation, handling and transport, less physical stability, and less uniformity while dosing.

Characteristics of an Ideal Suspension

- Dispersed particles should not settle rapidly to produce sediment
- Easy to resuspended upon moderate amount of shaking
- Good syringeability
- Should be physically and chemically stable
- Should be sterilizable (parenteral and ophthalmic suspensions)
- Should have pleasing odor, color and palatability (oral suspensions)

Pharmaceutical suspensions are classified into two types flocculated and deflocculated suspensions. Flocculated suspensions refer to the formation of a loose aggregation of discrete particles held together in a network like structure by physical adsorption or van der Waals forces.

Theories Involved in Disperse Phase

Interfacial Phenomenon

Smaller solid particles are employed in the preparation of suspensions. However smaller particles are associated with large surface area and surface free energy making them thermodynamically unstable. Thus the particles possess high energy which leads to grouping together to reduce surface free energy thus leading to formation of floccules. These floccules are held together by weak van der waals forces. However, when particles are adhered by stronger forces they form aggregates resulting in a hard cake. Use of surfactants reduces the surface free energy and increases the thermodynamic stability of the suspension.

Electrical Double Layer and Zeta Potential

Most surfaces acquire a surface electric charge upon contact with aqueous surface. A solid charged surface upon contact with an aqueous medium possesses positive and negative ions. This results in the formation of an electrical double layer consisting of charged particles. Electrical double layer is made up of the charged surface and neutralizing counter-ions (in excess) distributed in a diffused manner in aqueous medium resulting in the development of electric potentials.

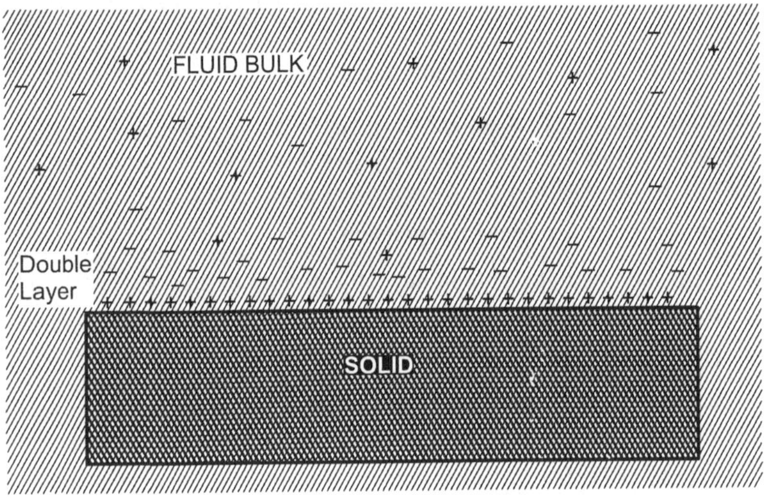

Schematic of double layer in a liquid at contact with a solid

Double layer is separated by a plan also known as stern plane and this occurs at a hydrated ion radius from the particle surface. Zeta potential (denoted by Greek letter zeta, hence *æ-potential*) refers to electrostatic charges present on the particles which propels them to move in electric field towards opposite charge.Its magnitude is measured by microelectrophoresis or any other electrokinetic phenomena. From a theoretical viewpoint, zeta potential l is the potential difference between the dispersion medium and the stationary layer of fluid attached to the dispersed particle. It is used for quantification of electrical charge at the double layer.

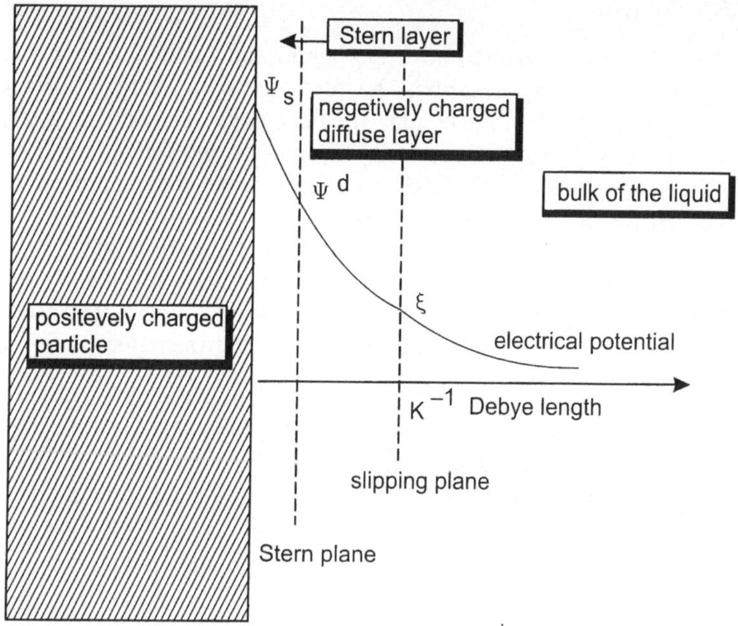

Detailed illustration of interfacial double layer

Colloids with higher zeta potential (negative or positive) are electrically stabilized, while colloids with low zeta potentials tend to coagulate or flocculate as outlined in the table below.

Zeta Potential [mV]	Stability behavior of the colloid
0 to ±5	Rapid coagulation or flocculation
±10 to ±30	Incipient instability
±30 to ±40	Moderate stability
±40 to ±60	Good stability
more than ±61	Excellent stability

Sedimentation Concept

Dispersed particles undergo collision between themselves as a result of Brownian movement. Depending on the forces of interactions-electrical forces such as repulsion, attraction and forces arising due to solvation result in particle collation. Further these collisions result in permanent contact of particles leading to coagulation and formation of larger aggregates. These particles sediment according to stokes' law as mentioned above.

DLVO Theory

The DLVO theory is named after Derjaguin and Landau, Verwey and Overbeek. This theory describes the force between charged surfaces interacting through a liquid medium. The net energy of a colloidal system is determined by the sum of double layer repulsion and the van der Waals attractive forces that the particles experience when they approach one another. However, when the particles collide with sufficient energy to overcome the barrier, then attractive force will pull them resulting in strong adherence which is irreversible. If the particles have sufficiently high repulsion, dispersions will resist flocculation and the colloidal system remain stable. If the repulsion mechanism does not exist then flocculation or coagulation will eventually take place.

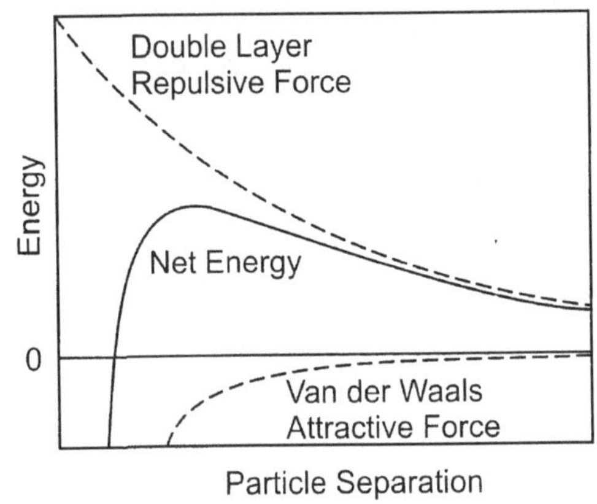

Variation of free energy with particle separation according to DLVO theory

Flocculated Suspensions: These suspensions form loose aggregates and sediment more rapidly when compared to deflocculated suspensions. Sedimentation of flocculated suspensions depend on the size and porosity of flocs. In flocculated suspensions the loose structure of the rapidly sedimenting flocs is due to the amount of entrapped liquid. Hence the volume of final sediment is relatively large and is easily redispersed upon agitation. Flocculating agents decreases zeta potential of suspended charged particle and thus cause aggregation of the particles. Examples of flocculating agents are: neutral electrolytes (KCl, NaCl), calcium salts, alum, sulfate, citrates and phosphates salts. Neutral electrolytes also decrease interfacial tension of the surfactant solution. For highly charged particles such as insoluble polymers and poly-electrolytes species, di or trivalent flocculating agents are used.

Deflocculated Suspensions

In deflocculated suspensions the rate of sedimentation of individual particles is very low. This in turn prevents the entrapment of dispersion medium between the floccules making it difficult to re-disperse upon simple agitation. This phenomenon is known as cracking. The rate of particle sedimientation is directly proportional to their size.

State	Rate of settling	Sediment volume	Nature
Flocculated	Fast	High	Porous, easy to redisperse
Deflocculated	Slow	Low	Compact difficult to redisperse

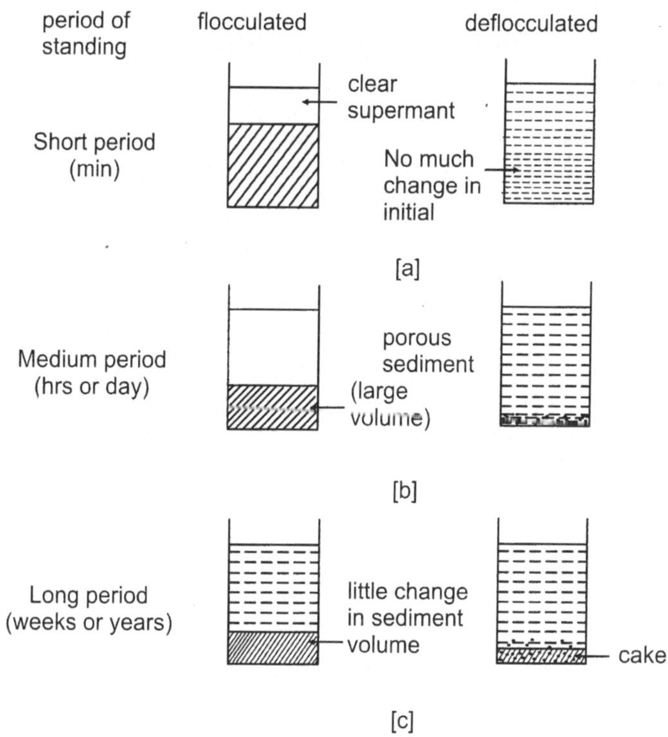

Sedimentation behaviour of flocculated and deflocculated suspensions

Sedimentation volume (F) or height (H) for flocculated suspensions

Sedimentation volume is a ratio of the final or ultimate volume of sediment (V_u) to the original volume of sediment (V_O) before settling.

$$F = V_u / V_O$$

where, V_u = final or ultimate volume of sediment, V_O = original volume of suspension before settling. The value of sedimentation volume can be less or greater than 1. Generally the value of F is less than 1. At flocculation equilibrium the values of F equals to 1 and the suspension does not show any clear supernatant upon long standing. When the network of flocs formed in the suspension are loose and fluffy they possess F values > 1.

Similarly for a deflocculated system the ultimate sedimentation volume is relatively small and can be written as $F_\infty = V_\infty / V_O$

Similarly when a measuring cylinder is used to measure the volume

$$F = H_u / H_O$$

Where, H_u = final height of sediment, H_O = original height of suspension before settling.

Degree of flocculation (β): It is the ratio of F_∞ / F

Also written as $\beta = V_\infty / V_u$

This is a more fundamental parameter as it relates F for a flocculated and a deflocculated suspension.

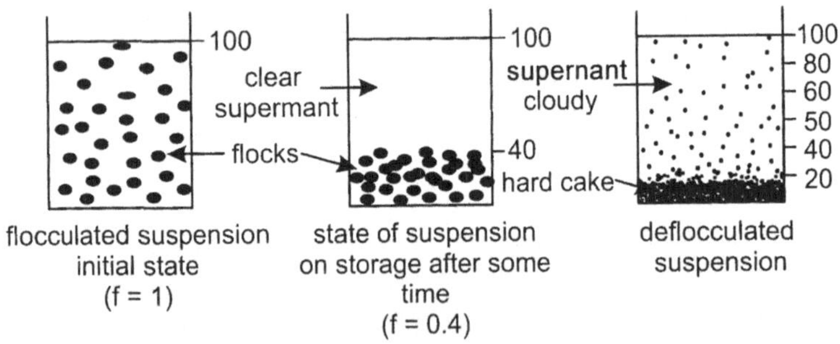

Suspensions quantified by sedimentation volume (F)

Brownian Movement: This is named after the Scottish botanist Robert Brown. It is the random movement of particles suspended in a liquid or gas. Particle theory is used for describing the random movement of particles. This movement depends on: density of dispersed phase and viscosity and density of dispersion medium. According to Brownian movement the kinetic bombardment of particles (size < critical radius) by the molecules of the suspending medium will keep the particles suspending. Brownian motion of the smallest particles can be eliminated by employing high viscosity mediums such as 50%w/v glycerin solution (viscosity ~ 5 cps). The displacement (D_i) due to Brownian motion is given by equation:

$$D_i^2 = RTt/N\pi\eta r$$

Where, R = gas constant

T = temperature in Kelvin

t = time

N = Avogadro's number

η = viscosity of medium

r = radius of the particle

At sedimentation diameter, no sedimentation occurs in the suspensions systems.

Formulation of Suspensions

Suspensions containing diffusible solids: This consists of solids that are insoluble in water but easily wettable. On shaking with water, solid particles diffuse readily throughout the liquid and remain suspended for a long time. Suspensions containing diffusible solids are prepared by following steps:

- triturating the solids in a mortar with sufficient quantity of vehicle to form a smooth cream.
- addition of nonvolatile substance by dissolving it in a small quantity of vehicle.
- addition of more vehicles and filtration through muslin cloth to remove foreign particles.
- addition of volatile components followed by final volume makeup with the vehicle.

Suspensions Containing Indiffusible Solids: This consists of substances which do not remain distributed for long time in the dispersion medium. To ensure the uniformity of dose it is required to shake the emulsion before use. They are prepared by addition of suitable thickening agents to the vehicle. This delays the separation or sedimentation of indiffusible particles by increasing the viscosity.

Suspensions Containing Poorly Wettable Solids: This consists of substances which are poorly soluble and poorly wettable in nature, resulting in formation of clumps making them difficult to disperse. They are prepared by addition of suitable thickening agents to the vehicle. These agents are adsorbed at the solid/liquid interface and promote wetting of the solid particles by the dispersion medium.

Suspensions of Precipitate Forming Liquids: This consists of liquid tinctures which are alcoholic or hydroalcoholic extracts of vegetable drugs. These extracts are resinous in nature. When tinctures are added to water they precipitate into indiffusible and stick substances. They are prepared by addition of suitable thickening agents prior to the addition of the precipitate forming liquid.

Suspensions Produced by Chemical Reactions: These are prepared by mixing two dilute solutions of reactants resulting in the formation of a fine precipitate. These precipitates are diffusible in nature and do not require suspending agents. If precipitate is indiffusible a suitable thickening or suspending agent may be added. They are prepared by dissolving the reactants separately in approximately half volumes of the vehicle and the two portions are then mixed together. Formulation Components: Various components are utilized in the formulation of suspensions. These include:

Components	Function
API	Active drug substances
Wetting agents	Disperse solids in continuous liquid phase.
Flocculating agents	Floc the drug particles
Osmotic agents	Osmotic pressure comparable to biological fluid
Buffers	Stabilize the suspension to a desired pH range.
Thickeners	Increase the viscosity of suspensions.
Coloring agents	For desired color to suspension
Preservatives	Prevent microbial growth.
External liquid vehicle	Construct structure of the final suspension.

Formulation of Flocculated Suspension System: Two important steps are involved in the formulation of flocculated suspensions: a) wetting of particles, b) controlled flocculation. In the primary step adequate wetting of particles is ensured by addition of suitable amount of wetting agents. While in controlled flocculation the product is achieved by addition of optimum concentration of electrolytes, surface-active agents or polymers.

Different Methods are used in the Formation of Floccules

Electrolytes: Addition of electrolyte decreases the electrical barrier between the particles and bring them together to form floccules. These electrolytes reduce the electrical barrier between the particles and resulting in a zeta potential close to zero. This helps in the formation of a bridge between the adjacent particles lining them together into loosely arranged structures. For example bismuth subnitrate when dispersed in water containing increasing concentration of monobasic potassium phosphate, a co-relation between apparent zeta potential and sedimentation volume, caking, and flocculation can be observed as shown below.

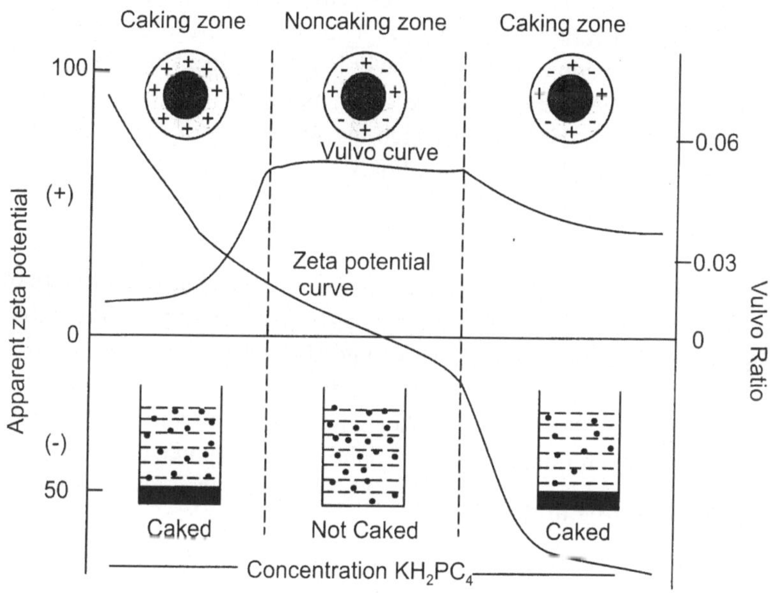

Caking diagram, showing the flocculation of a bismuth subnitrate suspension by means of the flocculating agent (Courtesy: A.Martin and J.Swarbrick, in sprowls, American Pharmacy, 6 th Edition, Lippincott, Philadelphia, 1966, p.205)

Addition of monobasic potassium phosphate to suspension of bismuth subnitrate particles causes a decrease in the positive zeta potential. This may be attributed to the adsorption of negatively charged phosphate anion. However, continued addition of the electrolyte results in zeta potential value near to zero and then increases the value in negative direction.

Surfactants: Both ionic and non-ionic surfactants can be used to bring about flocculation of suspended particles. Surfactants also act as wetting agents and help in reducing surface free energy by reducing the surface tension between liquid medium and solid particles.

Polymers: Polymers possess long chain in their structures. A part of the long chain is adsorbed on the surface of the particles while the remaining part is projected out into the dispersion medium.

Rheology of Suspensions

This helps in determination of the setting behavior and arrangement of vehicle and particle structural features. The rheology of suspensions is measured using Brookfield viscometer mounted on a helipath stand. The T-bar spindle is made to descend slowly into the suspension. Resistance met by the spindle is shown on the dial reading of the viscometer. This technique indicates the level at which the suspension of the structure is greater owing to particle agglomeration.

Emulsion

An emulsion is a colloidal drug delivery system consisting of a mixture of two or more immiscible liquids i.e. the dispersed phase and the continuous phase. Colloids and emulsions are used interchangeably; however emulsion tends to imply that both the dispersed and the continuous phase. Emulsions have gained lot of importance as they contain both oil and water phases which help in the formulation of hydrophilic and lipophilic drugs.

Classification of Emulsions

(a) Based on dispersed phase

- Oil in Water (O/W): Oil droplets dispersed in water or oil is dispersed phase and water is continuous phase. E.g. milk and vanishing cream
- Water in Oil (W/O): Water droplets dispersed in oil or water is dispersed phase and oil is continuous phase. E.g. butter, cold cream and cod liver oil.
- Oil-in-water-in-oil (o/w/o) emulsion
- Water-in-oil-in-water (w/o/w) emulsion

(b) Based on size of liquid or emulsion droplets

Macroemulsions: Size ranges between 0.2 – 50 mm. They are kinetically stable.

Microemulsions: Size ranges between 0.01 – 0.2 mm. They are thermodynamically stable.

Examples of Emulsions Encountered in Daily Life: ice creams and cold creams

General Types of Pharmaceutical Emulsions:

- Lotions
- Liniments
- Creams
- Ointments
- Vitamin drops

Pharmaceutical Application of Emulsions

- O/W emulsions are used for oral delivery
- Used for masking unpleasant taste of drugs
- Used for increasing oral absorption
- Topical application as creams

Preparation of Emulsions

Emulsification: This is a process of making emulsions. Emulsions are made by mixing the dispersed phase and dispersion medium vigorously followed by addition of stabilizing agent. Addition of stabilizer prevents the drops of the emulsion from combining together and separating out as a separate layer.

Demulsification: It is the separation of emulsion into its consistent liquids. Demulsification occurs by freezing or boiling or centrifugation or electrostatic precipitation or chemical methods.

Theories of Emulsification:

According to Bancroft, the size of emulsion droplets should be small enough to remain suspended in the dispersed phase with a sufficiently viscous film around each drop. This prevents the coalescing of emulsion droplets. Many theories have been proposed to explain the mechanism by which the emulsion is stabilized by the emulsifier. Depending on the emulsion type various theories have been postulated.

Electrical Double Layer: The oil globules in a pure oil and pure water emulsion carry a negative charge. The water ionizes to give both H^+ and OH^- ions. Negative charge on the oil comes from adsorption of the OH^- ions around the oil globules. A second layer of oppositely charged H^+ ions forms a layer in the liquid outside the layer of OH^- ions. These two oppositely charged layers are known as Helmholtz double layer. This is a boundary phenomenon and plays an important role in stabilizing emulsions.

Phase-Volume Theory: If spheres of same diameter are closely packed (one sphere is surrounded by 12 others), then the volume the spheres occupy approximately 74% of the total volume. However, when the dispersed phase is increased to more than 74% of the total volume, a reversal of the emulsion will occur. But dispersed phase does not remain rigid in shape and drops flatten out where they come in contact with each other and moreover dispersed particles are not of the same size.

Hydration Theory: Fischer and Hooker stated that hydrated colloids are the best emulsifiers. An emulsifier by which a permanent emulsion is obtained, invariably "proves to be a hydrophilic colloid when water and oil emulsions are concerned.

Oriented-Wedge Theory: It is based on the concept that molecules of an emulsifier align themselves at the interface of the dispersed and continuous phases, forming a wedge. This determines the curvature and the size of the dispersed phase.

Interfacial Film Theory: A film of emulsifying agent prevents the contact and coalescing of the dispersed phase. This is the most universally accepted theory for the formation of emulsions. The process of emulsification is influenced by (1) the mass of the emulsifying agent present, (2) the ease with which this agent is adsorbed at the interfacial separating surface, and (3) the nature of the ions adsorbed by the resultant film. The emulsifier has more affinity to one phase (oil or water phase) and thus lowers the interfacial tension of one liquid to a greater extent. Depending the on this lowering the droplets of smaller size are formed. The type of emulsion formed depends on the nature of the emulsifier. If the emulsifying agent has more affinity to water than the oil, then water becomes the continuous phase. When the tension on each side of the film or the emulsifying agent is the same no emulsion is formed.

Emulsifying Agents: These agents stabilize an emulsion. Pharmaceutically acceptable emulsifiers must

- be stable
- be compatible with other ingredients
- be non – toxic
- possess little odor , taste or color
- not interfere with the stability or efficacy of the active agent

Types of Emulsifying Agents:

(a) Carbohydrate Materials: Acacia, Tragacanth, Agar, Pectin.

(b) Protein Substances: Gelatin, Egg yolk, Caesin.

(c) High Molecular Weight Alcohols: Stearyl Alcohol, Cetyl Alcohol, Glyceryl Mono stearate o/w emulsion, cholesterol.

(d) Wetting agents or surfactants: This can be classified into anionic, cationic and nonionic surfactant molecules. Anionic – sodium stearate, potassium laurate, sodium dodecyl sulfate, sodium sulfosuccinate; Cationic – quaternary ammonium salts, amine hydrochlorides Nonionic – polyglycol, fatty acid esters, lecithin.

(e) Solids: Finely divided solids with amphiphilic properties such as soot, silica and clay, may also act as emulsifying agents

Hydrophilic-lipophilic Balance (HLB)

It is the measure of the degree of hydrophilicity or lipophilicity for surfactants. It is determined by calculating values for different regions of the surfactant molecule, as described by Griffin method. This method is utilized for non-ionic surfactants as follows:

$$HLB = 20 * M_h / M$$

Where, M_h is the molecular mass of the hydrophilic portion of the surfactant molecule and M is the molecular mass of the whole molecule. Generally HLB values of surfactants range from 0 to 20 scale. HLB value of 0 corresponds to a highly hydrophobic molecule and a value of 20 corresponds to a highly hydrophilic surfactant molecule.

The HLB value can be used to predict the surfactant properties of a molecule:

- 0 to 3 indicates an antifoaming agent
- 4 to 6 indicates a W/O emulsifier

- 7 to 9 indicates a wetting agent
- 8 to 18 indicates an O/W emulsifier
- 13 to 15 is typical of detergents
- 10 to 18 indicates a solubilizer or hydrotrope.

In 1957, Davies suggested another method for calculating the HLB values. Unlike the method suggested by Griffin this method takes into account the effect of strong and weak hydrophilic groups for calculating the HLB value. The method works as follows:

$$HLB = 7 + m * H_h - n * H_l$$

Where, H_h - value of the hydrophilic groups; H_l - Value of the lipophilic groups; n - number of lipophilic groups in the molecule and m - number of hydrophilic groups in the molecule.

Emulsion Stability

In general, emulsions are **thermodynamically** unstable. The addition of protective agents induces only **kinetic** stability. However it is possible to choose special surfactant combinations, to generate emulsions with (almost) zero surface tension also known as microemulsions, which have the size of the droplets in nanometers.

If two components are completely compatible or miscible the free energy of mixing is negative and they do not form an interface. E.g. mixture of gases and mixture of miscible liquids. However, incase of two incompatible or immiscible components free energy of formation is positive. The preparation of emulsions hence requires energy to disperse the organic phase in water. The change in the Gibbs free energy of the system (ΔG) is provided by the particular dispersing procedure at constant composition and pressure can be expressed by:

$$\Delta G = \Delta H - T \Delta S$$

Entropy (ΔS) is a measure of the extent of disorder in the system and hence measures the extent of size reduction of the organic phase (or increase in droplet number). The increasing disorder during the formation of an emulsion means a positive ΔS contributing to stability. ΔH is the enthalpy of the system and can be considered as the binding energy of the organic bulk material or the energy input needed to achieve a certain average droplet size. If the volume change during the emulsification is neglected the enthalpy corresponds to the internal energy which is the sum of the work required to expand the interfacial area (ΔW) and an amount of heat which results from wasting a part of the energy input. The increase in the energy of an emulsion compared to the non-emulsified components is equal to ΔW. This amount of energy can be considered as a measure of the thermodynamic instability of an emulsion.

$$\Delta W = \sigma \times \Delta A$$

ΔW is the free energy of the interface and corresponds to the reversible work brought permanently into the system during the emulsification process. This makes an emulsion very prone to coalescence processes which lead to a decrease in ΔA and subsequently in ΔW. The conclusion is straightforward that ultimate stability against coalescence processes is only achieved if σ approaches zero.

Physical Stability of Emulsion: Mechanical strength of the interfacial film prevents the coalescence of dispersed particles.

- *Creaming:* It is the upward movement of dispersed droplets of emulsion relative to the continuous phase due to the difference in density between the two phases
- *Stoke's law:* $dx/dt = d^2 (\rho_i - \rho_e)g/18h$

  Where,

  dx/dt = rate of settling

  D = diameter of particles

  r = density of particles and medium

  g = gravitational constant

  h = viscosity of medium

  Breaking: It occurs when the film surrounding the particles is destroyed. This is an irreversible process. To prevent the breaking of emulsions they should be protected against microbial contamination, extreme cold and heat.

  Coalescence: It is the process by which emulsified particles merge with each to form large particles.

  Aggregation: It occurs when dispersed particles come together and do not fuse.

Ostwald Ripening: The phenomenon was first described by Wilhelm Ostwald in 1896.this phenomenon is observed in emulsions which describe the formation of non-homogenous structure over time. It is a direct consequence of polydispersity of the droplet size distribution. When a phase precipitates out of solid, energetic factors will cause large precipitates to grow, drawing material from the smaller precipitates, which shrink. This is a thermodynamically driven spontaneous process as larger particles are more energetically favored than smaller particles. This stems from the fact that molecules on the surface of a particle are energetically less stable than the ones already well ordered and packed in the interior. As the system tries to lower its overall energy, molecules on the surface of a small (energetically unfavorable) particle will tend to detach and diffuse through solution and then attach to the surface of larger particle. Therefore, the number of smaller particles continues to shrink, while larger particles continue to grow. This can lead to the destabilization of emulsions (for example, by creaming and sedimentation).

Preservation of Emulsions: Addition of preservatives helps in preventing the growth of microorganisms. Preservatives should be in unionized state to penetrate the bacteria and should not bind to other components of the emulsion.

Tests for Emulsion Type (W/O or O/W Emulsions)

1. Dilution test: o/w emulsion can be diluted with water while w/o emulsion can be diluted with oil.
2. Conductivity test: The conductivity of emulsion with continuous water phase is greater than continuous oil phase.
3. Dye-Solubility test: Water soluble dye will dissolve in the aqueous phase and oil soluble dye will dissolve in the oil phase. The emulsion type can be under microscope.
4. Refractive index measurement
5. Filter paper test

Kinetic Stability of Emulsions: The rate of coalescence is used as a measure for emulsion stability. It depends on various factors such as:

(a) ***Physical nature of the interfacial surfactant film:*** The mechanical stability of surfactant films are characterized by strong lateral intermolecular forces and high elasticity. Mixed surfactant system preferred over single surfactant. E.g. A combination of lauryl alcohol and sodium lauryl sulfate are used for hydrophobic interactions.

(b) ***Electrical or steric barrier:*** This is significant only in O/W emulsions. In case of non-ionic emulsifying agents, charge may arise due to the adsorption of ions from the aqueous phase or contact charging (phase with higher dielectric constant is charged positively). However, no correlation exists between droplet charge and emulsion stability in W/O emulsions.

(c) ***Viscosity of the continuous phase:*** Higher viscosity in emulsion s reduces the diffusion coefficient. This results in reduced frequency of collision and therefore lower coalescence. This depends on Stoke-Einstein's equation as shown below:

Stoke-Einstein's equation:

$$D = \frac{KT}{6\pi\eta a}$$

Viscosity may be increased by adding natural or synthetic thickening agents. Moreover, viscosity also increases with increase in number of droplets. So emulsions are more stable in concentrated form than in diluted form.

(d) ***Size distribution of droplets:*** Emulsion with a fairly uniform size distribution is more stable.

(e) ***Phase volume ratio:*** As volume of dispersed phase increases its stability decreases and eventually phase inversion can occurs.

(f) ***Temperature:*** As the temperature increases the emulsion stability decreases. Temperature affects various parameters such as interfacial tension (D), solubility of surfactant, viscosity of liquid, phases of interfacial film.

Inversion of Emulsions (Phase Inversion)

As the temperature increases, the water solubility of some surfactants such as ethoxylated nonionic emulsifiers decreases (the HLB decreases). Phase inversion temperature is the temperature at which hydrophilic and lipophilic characteristics of the emulsifier are equal (relative to the required HLB of the oil phase). At this temperature the emulsion will exhibit a phase inversion. The temperature should be generally 20 °C higher than the storage temperature.

Emulsifiers can be selected by means of the HLB value or by the phase-inversion temperature.

For a typical o/w based emulsion containing ethoxylated emulsifiers when each phase is heated to 75 °C and oil phase is added to water phase the hydrogen bond formation does not occur. Ethoxyiated emulsifiers that normally have HLB of 12 at room temperature, have an HLB of 5 at 75°C. Such low HLB values results in formation of w/o emulsion. As the emulsion cools the hydrogen bond formation occurs and HLB value of emulsifier increases. At phase inversion temperature the emulsion inverts from w/o to o/w form. At this temperature the particle size decreases and the distribution of particles narrows down. Both the conditions help in formation of a good emulsion. Above the phase inversion temperature the emulsion is thin and watery while below that the emulsion becomes white, opaque, glossy and thickened. Alteration in phase volume ratio also results in phase inversion. For example increase in oil/water ratio results in formation of W/O emulsion and vice versa. Phase inversion can also be achieved by addition of electrolytes and other additives. Addition of strong electrolytes to O/W emulsion (stabilized by ionic surfactants) may result in inversion to W/O. E.g. Inversion of O/W emulsion (stabilized by sodium cetyl sulfate and cholesterol) to a W/O type upon addition of polyvalent Ca.

Rheology of Emulsions

Rheological characteristics of an emulsion system depend upon globule size, emulsifier and its concentration and phase volume ratio. The **rheology** emulsions provide critical information for product and process performance in many industrial applications. In order for emulsions to have proper product performance or process efficiently, they must be stable. But these are often complex formulations of solvents (or fluids), suspended particles of varying size and shape, and various additives used to affect stability. Measuring the rheology of a formulation gives an indication of the colloidal state and interactions that are occurring. Rheology based measurements can help predict which formulations might exhibit flocculation, coagulation or coalescence, resulting in undesired effects such as settling, creaming and separation. Moreover it very important as emulsions are marketed in tubes or containers. Most of these products exhibit non-newtonian nature. Some common rheology measurements and parameters include:

- Flow behavior of non-Newtonian materials: This helps in indicating the degree of dispersion and/or flocculation as well as shear thinning or thickening which often helps determine processing behavior.
- Storage modulus and Loss modulus: This determines the degree of stability of a formulation under rest conditions or during transport.
- Creep/recovery tests are used for measuring zero shear viscosity or the maximum viscosity of the fluid phase which must be required to prevent sedimentation

Microemulsion: These are thermodynamically stable, transparent (or slightly translucent) and monophasic dispersions of oil and water. They have gained a lot of attention due to high clarity, stability, ability to incorporate wide number of hydrophilic as well as hydrophobic drugs, ease in preparation, involves less amount of energy, high drug loading capacities, increased bioavailability, and ease of administration. Hoar and Schulman were the pioneers who coined the word "microemulsions". They defined microemulsions as clear and transparent solutions which are obtained by mixing a normal coarse emulsion with medium-chain alcohols. The size of microemulsions range from 10-1000 A^0 and these require relatively large amount of surfactants for stabilizing the interfacial area created by the nanodroplets. Three types of microemulsions exist based on the nature of internal and external phases a) O/W, b) W/O and c) bi-continuous microemulsions. Appropriate fluidity or viscosity can be achieved by addition of small amount of alcohol and the choice of the surfactant system is very important in controlling the surfactant concentration. The formulation of either O/W (hydrophobic) or W/O (hydrophilic) microemulsions depends on the nature of drug molecules. Microemulsions are easy to handle as they have less viscosity. They are characterized by conductivity, transmission electron microscopy, nuclear magnetic resonance spectroscopy, small-angle neutron scattering, small-angle x-ray scattering and dynamic light scattering. The psuedoternary phase diagram depicts the possible regions of microemulsions formation with varying concentrations of oil, water and surfactant.

Problems

1. According to Stokes' law, which of the following changes to a formulation of an o/w emulsion would be expected to decrease the rate of creaming of the emulsion?
   (a) decrease in the size of the oil droplets
   (b) increase in the viscosity of the continuous phase
   (c) increase in the difference in density between the oil and water phases
2. Consider an o/w emulsion with specific gravity of oil and aqueous phase 0.95 and 1.10 respectively. If the diameter of the particles is 6 μm, the external phase has viscosity of 0.6 poise. What is the velocity of creaming in cm per second?

$$V = (6 \times 10^{-4})^2 \times (0.95 - 1.10) \times 981/18 \times 0.6$$

$$= -4.9 \times 10^{-6} \text{ cm/sec}$$

3. Which of the following are attractive interactions between two particles?
   (a) electrostatic forces
   (b) van der Waals forces
   (c) steric forces
   (d) solvation forces
4. Which of the following statements are true?
   (a) The double-layer thickness around the particles is increased.
   (b) Repulsion between particles is decreased.
   (c) van der Waals forces between particles are decreased.
   (d) The height of the primary maximum is decreased.

Chapter 20

Electromotive Force and Oxidation-Reduction Systems

Definitions

(a) Electromotive force is the external work spent per unit of charge for producing an electric potential difference across two open-circuited terminals.

(b) For an electric charge (Q) that passes through a device or electrochemical cell, and gains energy (W), the net EMF is the energy gained per unit charge, or W/Q.

Electromotive force or EMF is denoted by E. The SI unit of EMF is volts or joules/coulomb.

An **electrochemical cell** is a device which is used for generating the electromotive force. The most common example of an electrochemical cell is a standard 1.5-volt battery. There are two types of electrochemical cells.

1. A primary cell is a type of electrochemical cell in which the reaction cannot be reversed and the anode and cathode identities are therefore fixed. The anode is always the negative electrode and cathode is positively charged. The cell can be discharged but cannot be recharged. Most commonly alkaline batteries also carbon-zinc cells with a carbon post as cathode (+) and a zinc shell as anode (-) are used.

2. A Secondary cell or rechargeable cell is the one in which the reaction is reversible. During the process of charging, the anode becomes the positive (+) electrode and the cathode the negative (–). The chemical change, which is responsible for the conversion of chemical energy into electrical energy, is reversible. E.g. Lithium-ion Battery and Nickel Cadmium Battery.

   A galvanic cell consists of two electrodes which are dipped into the same or two different electrolytes. No reaction takes place until a conducting wire joins the two electrodes. Electron transfer takes place when a chemical reaction occurs and all electron-transfer reactions which occur at the surface of the electrode are called electrode reactions. Flow of electrons causes oxidation at anode and reduction at cathode of the electrochemical cell. Thus, half of the overall redox reaction takes place at each of the two electrodes. Therefore, the reaction at each electrode is called half-cell reaction while the combination of an electrode and the solution in which it is dipped is called a half-cell. Galvanic cell is a combination of two half-cells (anodic half-cell and cathodic half-cell). Oxidation occurs at anode and reduction occurs at cathode.

Classification of Electrode Types

Conventional electrodes as half cells for electro-analytical techniques involve redox reactions (electrodes of zeroth, 1st, 2nd and 3rd kinds) as follows:

Class 0: Inert metals are used as electrodes. Ideal inert materials have the capability to exchange electrons reversibly with the electrolyte components and are resistant to oxidation or corrosion.

Class 1: Reversible metal/metal ion electrodes are used. Generally ion exchanging metals are dipped in electrolytes containing their own ions. E.g. Ag/Ag^+.

Class 2: Reversible metal/metal ion with saturated salt of the metal ion and excess anion X^- are used. E.g. $Ag/AgX/X^-$

Class 3: Reversible metal/metal salt or soluble complex/second metal salt or complex and excess second cation are used as electrodes. E.g. Pb/Pb.oxalate/Ca.oxalate/Ca^{2+} or Hg/$HgEDTA^{2-}$/$CaEDTA^{2-}$/Ca^{2+}

An **Ion-selective electrode** is a transducer which converts the activity of a specific ion dissolved in a solution into an electrical potential. This activity can be measured by a voltmeter or pH meter. In theory, this voltage is dependent on the logarithm of the ionic activity. This electrode has a sensing part which is usually made as ion-specific membrane, along with a reference electrode. There are four main types of ion-selective membrane used in ion-selective electrodes: glass, solid state, liquid based, and compound electrode.

Using glass membranes electrodes, the known pH of a reference solution are determined by using two electrodes, a glass electrode and a reference electrode. The voltage (difference in potential) generated between the two electrodes is measured. The difference in pH between solutions inside and outside the thin glass membrane creates electromotive force which is proportional to the difference in pH. This thin membrane is called the electrode membrane. The liquid inside the glass electrode usually has a pH of 7. Thus, if one measures the EMF generated at the electrode membranc, the pH of the test solution can be found by calculation. Generally, silver chloride is used as the material for the internal electrode. Potassium chloride solution maintained at pH 7 is usually used as the internal solution.

Hydrogen Electrode

This is obtained by bubbling hydrogen gas on a platinum (Pt) foil dipped into a solution containing H^+ ions. The H_2 (g) remains in equilibrium with the H^+ ions in the solution. Inert metal like platinum provides electrical contact of this electrode. The Pt foil used is further coated with Pt black and this acts as a catalyst to increase the speed of the attainment of equilibrium between $H_{2(g)}$ and H_3O^+ ions in the solution. The surface of the foil acts as a site for reaction.

Advantages of using platinum for hydrogen electrode:

- inertness of platinum
- capability of platinum to catalyze the reaction of proton reduction
- excellent reproducibility of the potential

When used as an anode, the electrode is denoted by (Pt) $H_{2(g)}$ $H^+_{(aq)}$ and, when used as a cathode, it is denoted by $H^+_{(aq)}$ $H_{2(s)}$ (Pt)

The electrode reactions are:

$$H + (aq) + e^- \underset{\text{oxidation}}{\overset{\text{reduction}}{\rightleftarrows}} 1/2\ H_2(s)$$

Calomel Electrode

It consists of mercury which is in contact with calomel (Hg_2Cl_2) dipped in a solution containing chloride ions (e.g., a solution of KCl). The half-cells in calomel electrode are written as,

As an anode: $Hg_{(l)}$ $Hg_2Cl_{2(s)}$ $Cl^-_{(aq)}$ oxidation

As a cathode: $Cl^-_{(aq)}$ $Hg_2Cl_{2(s)}$ $Hg_{(l)}$ reduction

Electrode reactions for the calomel electrode are

$$2Hg_2Cl_2(s) + e^- \underset{\text{oxidation}}{\overset{\text{reduction}}{\rightleftarrows}} Hg(1) + Cl^-(aq)$$

Generally, 0.1 M or 1 M or a saturated solution of KCl is used in a calomel electrode and this is used as secondary reference electrode. When saturated solution of KCl is used in calomel electrode then it is called as saturated calomel electrode (SCE).

Microelectrodes

These are very small electrodes (size of hypodermic needle or micropipette) which are used for studying electrical characteristics of living cells and tissues. They have metal or glass tips with diameter of 1 μm or less. They can sterilized and implants in animals for pharmacological studies.

Nernst Equation

Nernst equation is named after the German physical chemist Walther Nernst. In an electrochemical cell the Nernst equation is used to determine the equilibrium reduction potential of a half-cell or total voltage for a full electrochemical cell.

EMF of a half-cell:

$$E_{red} = E^0_{red} - \frac{RT}{zF} \ln \frac{a_{Red}}{a_{Ox}}$$

EMF of a total-cell:

$$E_{Cell} = E_{Anode} - E_{Cathode}$$

$$E_{cell} = E^0_{cell} - \frac{RT}{zF} \ln Q$$

where,

E_{red} is the half-cell reduction potential

E°_{red} is the *standard* half-cell reduction potential

R is the universal gas constant: $R = 8.314$ □ 472 J □K^{-1} □ mol^{-1}

T is the absolute temperature

a is the chemical activity for the relevant species

z is the number of electrons transferred in the cell reaction or half-reaction

Q is the reaction quotient.

F is the Faraday constant, the number of coulombs per mole of electrons (or) $F = 9.64 \times 10^4$ C□mol^{-1}

E_{cell} is the cell potential (electromotive force)

E°_{cell} is the *standard* cell potential

The above equation can be further simplified. At room temperature of 25 °C, *RT/F* can be written as a constant 25.693 mV for cells. Nernst equation can be expressed in terms of base 10 logarithms:

$$E = E^0 - \frac{0.05916}{z} \log_{10} \frac{a_{Red}}{a_{Ox}}$$

Standard electrode potential and the equilibrium constant of a redox reaction can be related in the following manner.

At equilibrium, $E = 0$ and $Q = K$. Therefore,

$$0 = E^0 - \frac{RT}{nF} \ln K$$

$$\ln K = \frac{nFE^0}{RT}$$

At standard temperature,

$$\log 10\ K = \frac{nE^0}{59.2\,mV} \text{ at } T = 298\ K.$$

Some Important Applications of Nernst Equation

Nernst Equation – Equation Potential as Function of pH

$$E = E_0 + 0.0591 \log \left(\frac{[H^+_{inside}]}{[H^+_{outside}]} \right)$$

(or)

$$E = E_0 + 0.0591 \, (pH_{outside} - pH_{inside})$$

If pH_{inside} of the electrode has constant value the above equation can be reduced to:

$$E = E'_0 + 0.0591 \, pH_{outside}$$

Electric potential of a cell membrane with respect to one type of ion can be found using Nernst equation.

$$E = \frac{RT}{zF} \ln \frac{[\text{ion outside cell}]}{[\text{ion inside cell}]}$$

When the cell membrane is in thermodynamic equilibrium the membrane potential equals to Nernst potential. However, in physiology the active ion pumps present on the inside and outside of a cell are not in equilibrium.

Reduction Potential

It is the intrinsic property of a chemical species to reduce upon acquisition of electrons. The more positive the potential, the greater is the affinity of species' to gain electrons and be reduced.

For aqueous solutions, the reduction potential is the tendency of the solution to either gain or lose electrons when a new species is added. A solution with a higher positive reduction potential than the new species will have a tendency to gain electrons from the new species and a solution with a lower negative reduction potential will have a tendency to lose electrons to the new species. It is measured in volts (V) or Eh (1 Eh = 1 mV). Reduction potentials are defined relative to the standard hydrogen electrode (SHE) which is arbitrarily given a potential of 0.00 volts. Standard reduction potential (E^0), is measured at a temperature of 25°C, and concentration of 1 M for each ion participating in the reaction.

E_h and pH of a solution are related.

For a reaction: $aA + bB = cC + dD$

Half cell standard potential (E_0) is given by:

$$E_0 \text{ (volts)} = -\frac{\Delta G}{nF}$$

where

ΔG = Gibbs free energy change

n = is the number of electrons involved

F = Faraday's constant.

The Nernst equation relates pH and E_h:

$$E_h = E_0 + \frac{0.05916}{n}\log\left(\frac{[A]^a\,[B]^b}{[C]^c\,[D]^d}\right) - \frac{0.05916h}{n}\text{pH}$$

Problems

If the voltage of a cell is 0.389V in a 0.500 M solution of Fe^{+2}, 1 atm pressure of H_2 at 25°C, what is the hydrogen concentration in the solution?

$$Fe|Fe^{+2}||H^+|H_2$$

- $Fe(s) \rightarrow Fe^{+2}(aq) + 2e^-$ $E^0 = +0.409$ V
- $2H^+(aq) + 2e^- \rightarrow H_2(g)$ $E^0 = +0.000$ V

Solution:

The standard cell voltage is: 0.409 + 0 = 0.409 V.

Two electrons are transferred during the reaction. Hence the balanced equation is

$$Fe(s) + 2H^+(aq) \rightarrow Fe^{+2}(aq) + H_2(g)$$

The Nernst equation is

$$E = E^0 - (RT/nF)\ln(Q)$$

Reaction quotient $(Q) = P_{H2}{*}[Fe^{+2}]/[H^+]^2$

$$Q = 1{*}0.500/[H^+]^2$$

Now plug everything into the Nernst equation and find out hydrogen ion concentration.

At 25°C, the term RT/F= 0.0257 V

$$E = E^0 - (RT/nF)\ln(Q)$$

$$0.389 = 0.409 - (0.0257/2)*\ln(0.5/[H^+]^2)$$

$$4.74 = 0.5/[H^+]^2$$

$$[H^+] = 0.325 \text{ M}$$

Chapter 21

Some Basic Formulae Useful for Calculations

Scientific calculations are frequently handled by expressing quantities in scientific notation. Such operations require simple manipulation of exponents, usually exponents of 10. When the same base is used (e.g., 10), the following rules apply :

1. When the operation involves multiplication, add the exponents algebrically.
   - example : $103 \times 10^4 = 10^{(3+4)} = 10^7$
   - example : $10^5 \times 10^2 \times 10^{-3} = 10^{(5+2+(-3))} = 10^4$
2. When the operation involves division, subtract the divisor exponent from the numerator exponent.
   - example : $10^5/10^3 = 10^{(5-3)} = 10^2$
   - example : $10^7/10^{12} = 10^{(7-12)} = 10^{-5}$
   - example : $10^8/10^{-3} = 10^{(8-(-3))} = 10^{11}$
   - example : $(10^6 \times 10^4)/(10^3 \times 10^2) = 10^{(6+4-(3+2))} = 10^5$
3. When the operation involves powers or roots, multiply the exponent by the power number or divide the exponent by the power number, respectively.
   - example : $(10^5)^3 = 10^{(5\times3)} = 10^{15}$
   - example : $(10^{-7})^4 = 10^{-(7\times4)} = 10^{-28}$

Quite often we come across the use of logarithms in physics and chemistry apart from mathematics. Two kinds of logarithms are used in chemistry :

Briggian or common logarithms : The power to which a base of 10 nmust be raised to obtain a number is called the common **logarithm** (log) of the number.

Napierian or natural logarithms : The power to which the base e (e = 2.718281828 ....) must be raised to obtain a number is called the **natural logarithm** (ln) of the number.

Using log10 ("log to the base 1") :

$\log_{10} 100 = 2$ is equivalent to $10^2 = 100$

where 10 is the base, 2 is the logarithm (i.e., the exponent or power) and 100 is the number.

1. Using natural logs (loge or ln) :

   Carrying all numbers to 5 significant figures,

   ln 30 = 3.4012 is equivalent to $e^{3.4012} = 30$

2. Many equations used in chemistry were derived using calculus, and these often involved natural logarithms. The relationship between ln x and log x is :

   $$\ln x = 2.303 \log x$$

   why 2.303? Let's use x = 10 and find out for ourselves.

   Rearranging, we have (ln 10)/(log10) = number.

   We can easily calculate that ln 10 = 2.302585093 ... or 2.303 and log 10 = 1.

   So, the number has to be 2.303.

   The rest of this mini-presentation will concentrate on logarithms to the base 10 (or logs). One use of logs in chemistry involves pH, where pH = –log10 of the hydrogen ion concentration.

   Here are some simple examples of logs.

Number	Exponential Expression	Logarithm
1000	10^3	3
100	10^2	2
10	10^1	1
1	10^0	0
1/10 = 0.1	10^{-1}	–1
1/100 = 0.01	10^{-2}	–2
1/1000 = 0.001	10^{-3}	–3

For any log, the number to the left of the decimal point is called the **characteristic**, and the number to the right of the decimal point is called the **mantissa**. The characteristic only locates the decimal point of the number, so it is usually not included when determining the number of significant figures. The mantissa has as many significant figures as the number whose log was found. So in the above examples :

Example 1: log $5.43 \times 10^{10} = 10.735$

The number has 3 significant figures, but its log ends up with 5 significant figures, since the mantissa has 3 and the characteristic has 2.

Example 2: log $2.7 \times 1^{-8} = -7.57$

The number has 2 significant figures, but its log ends up with 3 significant figures.

Natural logarithms work in the same way :

Example 3: ln $3.95 \times 10^{6} = 15.18922614 \ldots = 15.189$

Application to pH Problems

pH = –log (hydrogen ion concentration) = –log [H+]

Example 4: What is the pH of an aqueous solution when the concentration of hydrogen ion is 5.0×10^{-4} M?

$$pH = -\log [H^{+}] = -\log (5.0 \times 10^{-4}) = -\ (-3.30) = 3.30$$

( )

1. Sometimes we know the mogarithm (or ln) of a number and must work backwards to find the number itself. This is called finding the antilogarithm or inverse logarithm of the number.

Example 5: log x = 4.230; so, x = inverse log of 4.203 = 15958,79147.... (too many significant figures)

There are three significant figures in the matissa of the log, so the number has 3 significant figures. The answer to the correct number of significant figures is 1.60×10^{4}.

Example 6 : log x = – 15.3;

so, x = inv log (–15.3) = 5.011872336... x $10^{-16} = 5 \times 10^{-16}$ (1 significant Fig.)

Natural logarithms work in the same way

Example 7: ln x = 2.56; so, x = inv ln (2.56) = 12.93581732 ... = 13 (2 sing. Fig.)

pH = – log (hydrogen ion concentration) = – log $[H^+]$

Example 8 : What is the concentration of the hydrigen ion concentration in an aqueous solution with pH = 13.22?

$$pH = -\log [H^+] = 13.22 \log [H^+] = -13.22$$

$$[H^+] = \text{inv} \log (-13.22)$$

$$[H^+] = 6.0 \times 10^{-14} \text{ M (2 sig. Fig.)}$$

Because logarithms are exponents, mathematical operations involving them follow the same rules as those for exponents.

Common Logarithm	Natural Logarithm
log xy = log x + log y	ln xy = ln x + ln y
Log x/y = log x – log y	ln x/y = ln X – ln y
$\log x^y$ = y log x	ln x^y = y ln x
$\log^y$ = 10g $x^{1/y}$ = (1/y) log x	ln = ln $x^{1/y}$ = (1/y) ln

Example 9 : log 5.0 × 10^6 = log 5.0 + log 10^6 = 0.70 + 6. = 6.70

Hint : This is an easy way to estimate the log of a number in scientific notation!

Example 10 : log (154/25) = log 154 – log 25 = 2.188 – 1.40 = 0.788 = 0.79 (2 sig. Fig.)

Example 11 : log (5.46 × 10^{-3})6 = 6 log 5.46 × 10^{-3} = 6 × (–2.263) = – 13.58

Example 12 : log (4.35)1/4 = 1/4 log 4.35 = 0.160

If you memorize

$$\ln(2) = 0.693... \text{ (0.7 is often good enough)}$$

$$\ln(10) = 2.302... \text{ (2.3 is often good enough)}$$

then you can readily compute the natuiral logrithm of any number to a good approximation using the laws of logarithms and the Taylor series expansion. It is sometimes helpful, but not really necessary, to know

$$e = 2.718281828...$$

where e is defined by ln (e) = 1.

Another approximation worth remembering is ln (20) = ln (2*10) = ln (2) + ln (10) = 2.995... = 3.00.

From the Taylor series

$$\ln (1 + x) = x - x^2/2 + x^3/3 - x^4/4 + \dots,$$

which is easy to remember-recall the derivation where we passed from $1/(1 + t)$ to $1 - t + t^2 + \dots$ to $t - t^2/2 + t^3/3 - \dots$ by integration–we get the useful two-decimal place approximations

$$\ln (1 + x) = x \text{ for } |x| < 0.1$$

(this is an overestimate when $x > 0$, because the next term would be negative)

$$\ln (1 + x) = x - x^2/2 \text{ for } |x| < 0.23$$

(this is an underestimate when $x > 0$, because the next term would be positive).

Here are some examples.

ln(3) = ln (2*5/4 *6/5) = ln(2) + ln(1 + 0.25) + ln (1 + 0.20) = (underestimate) $0.693 + 0.25 - 0.25^2/2 + \dots + 0.20 - 0.20^2/2 + \dots = 0.69 + 0.25 - 0.031 + 0.20 - 0.02 = 1.092$ (the correct answer is 1.0986...). This example also illustrates why, if you want your answer to two decimal places, you really should compute intermediate results to three decimal places.

Here are some more examples of computing logs to two decimal places.

ln(4) = 2*ln(2) = 1.39.

ln(5) = ln (10/2) = ln (10) – ln(2) = 2.302 – 0.693 = 1.61.

ln(1/2) = – ln(2) = –0.69.

ln (100) = ln (10^2) = 2*ln(10) = 2*2.302 = 4.60.

ln (1000) = ln (10^3) = 3*ln (10) = 6.91.

ln (1,000,000) = 6*ln(10) = 13.82.

ln (0.8) = ln(2^3/10) = 3*ln(2) – ln(10) = 3*0.693 – 2.302 = – 0.22 (rounded).

It's very easy to compute the logrithms of nastier numbers, too; just look for the closet number for which you can reliably estimate the log from values you already know, then use the Taylor series approximation :

ln(0.79) = ln(0.8*(1–1/80)) = –0.22 – 1/80 = – 0.23.

ln (4.4) = ln (4*1.1) = ln(4) + ln(1 + 0.10) = 1.386 + 0.10 – 0.01/ 2 + ... = 1.48.

ln (17) = ln (16* (1 + 1/16)) = 4*ln(2) + 1/16 –... (because 1/ 16 is much less than 0.1, we need only one term in the series) = 2.772 + 0.0613 = 2.83.

ln(Pi) = ln (3 + 1/7, approximately) = ln(3*(1 + 21)) = 1.10 + 1/ 21 – ... = 1.15 (a slight overestimate; the correct value is 1.14 to two decimal places).

If you're not being finicky and just want to know the logarithm roughly, life is easy:

ln(93) = ln (100 * 0.93) = 2* ln(10) + ln(1 – 0.07) = 4.6 – 0.07 = 4.5, roughly

ln (560 000) = ln (5.6 * 105) = ln)5 * 1.12 * 105) = ln(106/2 *1.12) = 6* 2.3 – 0.7 + 0.12 = 13.2 (it's actually 13.236...).

You should begin to see why you need only four simple things for rough computationof logs :

1. The laws of logarithms
2. ln(2) = 0.7
3. ln(10) = 2.3
4. The Taylor series approximation ln (1 + x) = x (or sometimes $x - x^2/2$, just to be more accurate)

The computation is so straightforward you can readily accomplish it with mental arithmetic if you just want the log to one decimal place, which is often good enough. An earlier version of this material, which

Simple derivaties of some simple functions follow.

$$\frac{d}{dx}\ln x = \frac{1}{x}$$

$$\frac{d}{dx}\sin x = \cos x$$

$$\frac{d}{dx}\cos x = -\sin x$$

$$\frac{d}{dx}\tan x = -\sec^2 x$$

$$\frac{d}{dx}\csc x = -\csc x \cot x$$

$$\frac{d}{dx}\sec x = -\sec x \tan x$$

$$\frac{d}{dx}\cot x = -\csc^2 x$$

$$\frac{d}{dx}e^x = e^x$$

$$\frac{d}{dx}a^x = (\text{In } a)\, a^x$$

$$\frac{d}{dx}\sin^{-1} x \frac{\sqrt{1}}{1-x^2}$$

$$\frac{d}{dx}\cosh x = \sinh x$$

$$\frac{d}{dx}\tanh x = \text{sech}^2 x$$

$$\frac{d}{dx}\coth x = -\text{csch}^2 x$$

$$\frac{d}{dx}\text{csch } x = -\text{csch } x \coth x$$

$$\frac{d}{dx}\text{sn } x = \text{cn } x \text{ dn } x$$

$$\frac{d}{dx}\text{cn } x = -\text{sn } x \text{ dn } x$$

$$\frac{d}{dx}\text{dn } x = -k^2 \text{ sn } x \text{ cn } x$$

Integration formulae

$$\int cf(x)\,dx = c\int f(x)\,dx$$

$$\int f(x) + g(x)\,dx = \int f(x)\,dx + \int f(x)\,dx$$

$$\int x^n\,dx = \frac{x^{n+1}}{n+1} + C$$

$$\int x^{-1}\,dx = \ln|x| + C$$

$$\int \sin(x)\,dx = -\cos(x) + C$$

$$\int \cos(x)\,dx = \sin(x) + C$$

$$\int \sec^2(x)\,dx = \tan(x) + C$$

$$\int \csc^2(x)\,dx = -\cot(x) + C$$

$$\int \sec(x)\tan(x)\,dx = \sec(x) + C$$

$$\int \csc(x)\cot(x)\,dx = \csc(x) + C$$

$$\int e^x\,dx = e^x + C$$

$$\frac{1}{\sqrt{\int 1 - x^2}}\,dx = \arcsin(x) + C$$

$$\frac{1}{\sqrt{\int 1 + x^2}}\,dx = \arcsin(x) + C$$

Exponentials

Exponents are abbreviated notations used for denoting the multiplication of the same number by itself. For example, the shorthand for multiplying five copies of the number "4" is shown on the right-hand side (RHS) of the "equals" sign in $4 * 4 * 4 * 4 * 4 = 4^5$. The "exponent" in this example is "5" and the number that's being multiplied "4", is called the "base". In many pharmaceutical calculations exponent (base 10) of decimal numbers are commonly used and are denoted as E *n* which is equal to 10^n.

Conversion scale in power of 10's

10^n	E *n*	Symbol	Prefix	Scale
10^{24}	E 24	Y	Yotta	Septillion
10^{21}	E 21	Z	Zetta	Sextillion
10^{18}	E 18	E	Exa	Quintillion
10^{15}	E 15	P	Peta	Quadrillion
10^{12}	E 12	T	Tera	Trillion
10^9	E 9	G	Giga	Billion
10^6	E 6	M	Mega	Million
10^3	E 3	k	Kilo	Thousand
10^2	E 2	h	Hector	Hundred
10^1	E 1	da	Deca	Ten
10^{-1}	E -1	d	Deci	Tenth
10^{-2}	E -2	c	Centi	Hundredth
10^{-3}	E -3	m	Milli	Thousandth
10^{-6}	E -6	µ	Micro	Millionth
10^{-9}	E -9	n	Nano	Billionth
10^{-12}	E -12	p	Pico	Trillionth
10^{-15}	E -15	f	Femto	Quadrillionth
10^{-18}	E -18	a	Atto	Quintillionth
10^{-21}	E -21	z	Zepto	Sextillionth
10^{-24}	E -24	y	Yocto	Septillionth

Proportions

These are equations that contain two ratios of equal value. The proportion uses an equal sign or double colon to demonstrate that the ratios on both sides of the equal sign (double colon) are equal.

We can use apply desire, have, vehicle, and give to proportions as follows:

Example: 8 : 16 :: 2 : 4,

(or)

$$\frac{8}{16} = \frac{2}{4}$$

The fractions can be reduced to their lowest terms resulting in:

$$\frac{8}{16} = \frac{1}{2} \qquad \frac{2}{4} = \frac{1}{2}$$

In proportions the product of extremes should be equal to the product of means.

Example: 8 : 16 :: 2 : 4

The product of the means is always equal to the product of the extremes in true proportions.

Example: 8 × 4 (extremes) = 16 × 2 (means)

Example:

A physician must administer 25 mg of a medication intravenously. The drug is available as 50 mg/2 mL. How much will the physician administer?

50 mg : 2 mL :: 25 mg : X

(50) (X) = (25) (2)

50X = 50

Therefore: X = 1 mL

Laplace Transformations

The Laplace transformations are useful in solving certain types of differential equations when certain initial conditions are mentioned. Generally, the initial values will considered as zero in Laplace transformations. The Laplace transform is named in honor of a famous mathematician and astronomer Pierre-Simon Laplace.

For a function $f(t)$ when $t > 0$ the Laplace transform is defined by the following integral defined over 0 to ∞:

$$\mathcal{L}_{\{f(t)\}} = \int_0^\infty e^{St} f(t)\, dt$$

The resulting expression is obtained as a function of s, which can be written as $F(s)$.

$$\mathcal{L}_{\{f(t)\}} = F(s)$$

Similarly, the Laplace transform of a function *h*(*t*) would be written:

$$\mathcal{L}_{\{h(t)\}} = H(s)$$

The following table of Laplace Transforms is very useful for solving problems in pharmacy.

Function	Laplace Transform	
1	$\frac{1}{S}$	s > 0
A	$\frac{A}{S}$	s > 0
t	$\frac{1}{S^2}$	s > 0
t^n (*n*, a positive integer)	$\frac{n!}{S^{n+1}}$	s > 0
t^{e-t}	$\frac{1}{(S+1)^2}$	s > –1
e^{at}	$\frac{1}{S-a}$	s > a
$1 - e^{-t/T}$	$\frac{1}{s(1+T_s)}$	s > –1/T
$\frac{1}{(\alpha-\beta)}[\alpha \exp(-\alpha t) - \beta \exp(-\beta t)]$	$\frac{s}{(s+\alpha)(s+\beta)}$,	$\beta \neq \alpha$
$\frac{1}{(\beta-\alpha)}[\exp(-\alpha t) - \exp(-\beta t)]$	$\frac{1}{(s+\alpha)(s+\beta)}$,	$\beta \neq \alpha$
$\frac{1}{\alpha\beta} + \frac{\exp(-\alpha t)}{\alpha(\alpha-\beta)} + \frac{\exp(-\beta t)}{\beta(\beta-\alpha)}$	$\frac{1}{s(s+\alpha)(s+\beta)}$,	$\beta \neq \alpha$

Appendix

Table A.1 Concentration of acids.

Acid	Specificgravity	Percent by weight	Approximate normality
HCl (conc.)	1.19	37.89	11 N
HCl (dil.)	—	—	5 N
H_2SO_4 (conc.)	1.84	96.01	36 N
H_2SO_4 (dil.)	—	—	5 N
HNO_3 (conc.)	1.41	69.80	16 N
HNO_3 (dil.)	—	—	5 N
CH_3COOH (conc.)	1.06	99.51	17 N
CH_3COOH (dil.)	—	—	5 N

Table A.2 Physical constants of liquids at 20° C.

Liquid	Molecular weight	Index of refraction for D-Sodium Line	Density (gm/ml)
Acetic acid	60.05	1.3721	1.049
Aniline	93.12	1.5863	1.622
Acetone	58.08	1.3588	0.792
Benzene	78.11	1.5011	0.879
Chloroform	119.39	1.4464	1.4984

Table A.2 Contd...

Liquid	Molecular weight	Index of refraction for D-Sodium Line	Density (gm/ml)
Ethyl alcohol	46.07	1.3611	0.785
η - Heptane	100.20	1.3876	0.6837
η - Hexane	86.19	1.3749	0.6603
Methyl alcohol	32.04	1.3288	0.7917
Toluene	92.13	1.4969	0.8669

Table A.3 Transition temperatures of hydrates.

Substance			Temperature (^{0}C)
$Na_2CO_3 \cdot 10H_2O$	⇆	$Na_2CO_3 7H_2O$	32.10
$Na_2SO_4 \cdot 10H_2O$	⇆	Na_2SO_4	32.40
$Na_2CrO_4 \cdot 10H_2O$	⇆	$Na_2CrO_4 \cdot 6H_2O$	19.73
$Na_2CrO_4 \cdot 10H_2O$	⇆	$Na_2CrO_4 \cdot 7H_2O$	19.52
$MnCl_2 \cdot 4H_2O$	⇆	$MnCl_2 \cdot 2H_2O$	58.35
$NaBr \cdot 2H_2O$	⇆	$NaBr$	50.69
$SrCl_2 \cdot 6H_2O$	⇆	$SrCl_2 \cdot 2H_2O$	61.37

Table A.4 Specific conductivity of KCl solution.

Temperature (°C)	N Solution	N/Solution 10	N/Solution 100
20	0.10207	0.01167	0.001278
21	0.10400	0.01191	0.001305
22	0.10594	0.01215	0.001332
23	0.10789	0.01239	0.001359
24	0.10984	0.01264	0.001386
25	0.11180	0.01288	0.001413
26	0.11377	0.01313	0.002819
27	0.11574	0.01337	0.002873
28	....	0.01362	0.002927
29	....	0.01387	0.002981
30	....	0.01412	0.003036
35	....	0.01539	

Table A.5 Surface tension of liquids.

Substance	°C	Surface tension
Acetic acid	20	27.6
Acetone	20	23.7
Benzene	20	28.88
Carbon terachloride	20	26.8
Chlorobenzene	20	33.2
Chloroform	20	27.1
Cyclohexane	20	25.3
Ethyl acohol	20	22.9
Ethyl alcohol	20	22.3
Formic acid	20	18.4
n-Hexzne	20	22.6
Methyl alcohol	20	28.4
Toluene	20	37.6
Water	20	72.75

Table A.6 Interfacial tension at 20° C.

Liquid	γ	Liquid	γ
Benzene - Mercury	357	Water-n-Hexane	51.1
Ether- Mercury	379	Water-Mercury	375
Water-Benzene	35	Water-n-Octane	50.8
Water - Carbon Tetrachloride	45	Water-Ether	10.7

Table A.7 Viscosity of liquids.

Liquid	Viscosity (centi poise)	Liqid	Viscosity (centi poise)
Acetaldehyde	0.255 (10°) 0.22 (20°)	Chlorobenzene	0.799 (20°) 0.631 (40°)
Acetic acid	1.31 (15°) 1.155 (25°) 1.04 (30°)	Chloroform	0.58 (20°) 0.542 (25°) 0.514 (30°)
Acetone	0.337 (15°) 0.316 (25°) 0.295 (30°)	Cyclohexane Ethyl acetate	1.02 (17°) 0.455 (20°) 0.441 (25°)

Table A.7 Contd...

Liquid	Viscosity (centi poise)	Liqid	Viscosity (centi poise)
Aniline	3.71 (25^0) 3.16 (30^0)		0.400 (30^0)
		Ethyl alcohol	1.200 (20^0)
Benzene	0.652 (20^0) 0.564 (30^0) 0.503 (40^0)		1.003 (30^0) 0.834 (40^0)
		Ethylene glycol	19.9 (20^0)
Carbon tetra-Chloride	0.969 (20^0) 0.843 (30^0) 0.739 (40^0)	Glycerine	1490 (20^0) 954 (25^0) 629 (30^0)
		Toluene	0.590 (20^0) 0.526 (30^0)
iso-Butyl alcohol	4.703 (15^0)		0.471 (40^0)
iso-propyl alcohol	2.86 (15^0) 1.77 (30^0)	Turpentine	1.487 (20^0) 1.272 (30^0) 1.070 (40^0)
Methyl alcohol	0.597 (20^0) 0.547 (25^0)		

Table A.8 Critical solution temperature. (CST).

System	Temp. (^{0}C)	Composition	System	Temp. (^{0}C)	Composition
Water-Phenol	65.9	66%	Gylcerol - m-Toluidine	6.7 120	.....
CH_3OH-Cyclohexane	49.2	29%			......
Methyl ethyl ketone-Water	–6 +33	....	Nicotine-water	60.8 208	....

Table A.9 Parachors and refractivities.

Element	Parachor	Refractivity	Group or linkage	Parachor	Refractivity
Carbon	4.8	2.591	Double bond		23.2 1.575
Hydrogen	17.1	1.028	Triple bond		46.6 1.977
Oxygen	20.0	1.764	3-membered ring	17.0	...
			5-membered ring	8.5	-0.10
Sulphur	48.5	...	6-membered ring	6.1	-0.15
Chlorine	54.3	5.844	Semi polar bond	-1.6	...
Bromine	68.0	8.7141			
Iodine	91.0	13.954			

Bibliography

1. Alfred Martin, 1996, Physical Pharmacy, 4th Ed ; B.I. Waverly Pvt Ltd, New Delhi.
2. Leon Lchman, H.A. Lieborman, J.L.Kanig ; 1991, The Theory and Practice of Industrial Pharmacy, 4th Ed ; Varghese Publishing House, Indian Reprint, Bombay.
3. E. A. Rawlins (Ed), 2004, Bentley's Textbook of Pharmaceutics, 8th Ed; Bailliere Tindall, London.
4. H. J. Arnikar, S.S. Kadam, K.N. Gujar, 1992, Essentials of Physical Chemistry and Pharmacy, 1st Ed ; Orient Longman Limited, Bombay.
5. U. B. Hadkar, 2001, A Textbook of Physical Pharmacy, 2nd Ed, Nirali Prakashan, Pune.
6. D. W.A. Bourne, L.W. Dittert, 1990, Modern Pharmaceutics, 2nd ed, [Bankar, G.S. and Rhodes C.T., Eds.], Marcel Dekker Inc, New York.
7. S. K. Dogra and S. Dogra, 2004, Physical Chemistry Through Problems, 1st Ed ; New Age International Publisheres, Delhi.
8. A. R. Gennaro ; 2000, Remington: The Science and Practice of Pharmacy, 20th Ed ; Mack Publishing House, Eston, Pennsylvenia.

9. P. D. Sethi, 1997, Quantitative Analysis of Drugs in Pharmaceutical Formulations, New Delhi.
10. M. E. Aulton, 2003, Pharmaceutics, 2nd Ed; Churchill Livingstone, Spain.
11. S. H. Maron and C. F. Prutton, 1972, Principles of Physical Chemistry, 4th Ed, Oxford IBH publishing Co. Pvt. Ltd; New Delhi.
12. B. S. Bahl; G.D. Tuli, Arul Bahl; 2002, Essentials of physical chemistry, 24th Ed; S. Chand and company Ltd; New Delhi.
13. P. L. Soni and O. P. Dharmarha, 1990, Textbook of Physical Chemistry; 17th Ed, Sultan Chand and Sons, New Delhi.
14. S.Gasstone, 1998, Textbook of Physical Chemistry, 2nd Ed; MacMillan India Limited, New Delhi.
15. M. L. Schrooff, 1970; Professional Pharmacy; part IV; Five Star Enterprises.
16. H. A. Lieberman, M.M. Rieger ; G. S. Banker, 1996 ; Pharmaceutical Dosage Forms, Dispense Systems ; Volume - II ; 2nd Ed, Marcel Dekker, Inc, New York.
17. J. C. Edmundson, 1967, Advances in Pharmaceutical Sciences, volume - II, (Eds) H. S. Bean, et.al., Academic press, London.
18. Indian Pharmaceopoeia; 1985, 3rd Ed; The Controller of publications, Delhi.
19. Water Lund (Ed); 1994; The Pharmaceutical Codex, Principles and Practice of Pharmaceutics, 12th Ed; The Pharmaceutical Press, London.
20. J. T. Carstensen ; 1997 ; Pharmaceutics of solids and solid Dosage Forms; John Wiley and Sons, New York.
21. G. S. Banker and C. T. Rhodes, 1996; Modern Pharmaceutics; 3rd Ed; Volume 72 ; Marcel Dekker Inc; New York.
22. L. V. Allen, M. G. Popvich, H. C. Ansel; 2005 ; Ansel's Pharmaceutical Dosage Forms and Drug Delivery Systems; 8th Ed; Indian Edition; Lippincott Williams and Wilkins; Philadelphia; PA.
23. C.V.S. Subrahmanyam 2000; Textbook of Physical Pharmaceutics; 2nd Ed; Vallabh Prakashan, Delhi.

Index

T

U

V

W

Y

Z